YOUR BEST INVESTMENT

SECRETS TO A HEALTHY BODY AND MIND

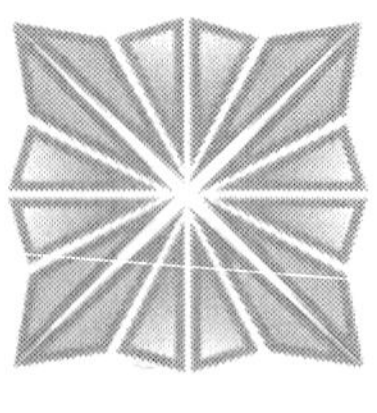

IHB Publishing, LLC

Your Best Investment

Secrets to a Healthy Body and Mind

Edwin Lee M.D., F.A.C.E.
Author of *Feel Good Look Younger: Reversing Tiredness Through Hormonal Balance*

with Alison Gordon B.S.
and Laura Gavin M.S.

DrEdwinLee.com

This publication contains the opinions and ideas of the author. It is intended to provide helpful and informative material on the subjects addressed in the publication. It is sold with the understanding that the author and publisher are not engaged in rendering medical, health, psychological or any other kind of personal professional services in the book. At the time of publication, all links to Internet references were valid; however, over time, those links may become invalid. If the reader requires personal medical, health, other assistance or advice, a competent professional should be consulted. The author and publisher specifically disclaim all responsibility for any liability, loss or risk, personal or otherwise, that is incurred as a consequence, directly or indirectly, of the use and application of the contents of this book.

Published in the United States of America by
IHB Publishing, LLC, Florida, USA

Library of Congress Cataloging-in-Publication Data
Your Best Investment: Secrets to a Healthy Body and Mind
Edwin N. Lee
Library of Congress Control Number: 2011944799

ISBN: 978-0-9829193-2-3

Printed in the United States of America
First Edition, Revised

"DON'T THINK OF THIS AS JUST ANOTHER DIET BOOK. RATHER, WHAT DR. LEE HAS CREATED IS THE ULTIMATE MAP OF DIFFERENT PATHS FOR YOU TO TAKE ON YOUR WAY TO A HEALTHIER YOU."

— RAUL SANTOS M.D.
BOARD CERTIFIED IN
NEPHROLOGY AND ANTI-AGING

"Dr. Lee will forever change your perception of how simple applications of optimal nutrition can transform your life. This is THE diet book that you definitely need to embrace and fully understand."

— Mark Houston M.D., M.S., FACP, FAHA
Associate Clinical Professor of Medicine
Vanderbilt University Medical School

Dedicated to my amazing wife, Su-Eun.
Thank you for supporting my many ambitions.
Without you, Su-Eun, none of my greatest
accomplishments would have been possible.

To my sons, Connor and Nathan.
I pray that you will always be healthy,
always be happy,
and always be blessed with many friends.

And to my parents, Stewart and Young-Ja.
Thank you for helping guide my journey in life.

Acknowledgements

I would like to thank Jim Huth for helping me on this, my second book. The idea for this book has been in my head for some time, and without his help I could have never brought it to print. I am so blessed that he is gifted in writing, and that he knows how to take what I've written and shape it into a cohesive and engaging story. Just be careful on that bike Jim!

In addition, I would like to thank Dr. Mark Gordon for introducing me to Alison Gordon, who helped with the nutritional plan. She has incredible passion for her work, and her recipes are always innovative. I wish her the best of luck with medical school and her future endeavors. I would like to thank Laura Gavin, as well, for writing part of the nutritional plan, and for always helping me out when I first started my new practice. I am so glad that you followed your dreams and went back to school and obtained your Master of Science in Human Nutrition. Congratulations Laura.

Two other amazing friends that I met recently on my path of life are John Strelecky and David Dobson.

John is an international best-selling author whose books include *The Why Cafe* and *Life Safari*. He is also an international speaker on personal development, and he was recently honored along with Oprah Winfrey, Lance Armstrong, Deepak Chopra and Tom Peters as one of the 100 Most Influential Thought Leaders in the field of leadership and personal development. Whenever I call John for advice on writing, his insightful answers are always on target—and no matter what we talk about, I always come away feeling enlightened and inspired!

David is a professional photographer whose famous subjects have ranged from Mother Teresa, to B.B. King, to Moby. During a recent photo session with David (for this book's back cover), I was pleasantly surprised to learn that I do have a great smile after all.

Thanks are due as well to Dr. Angeli Maun Akey and Jean Henne for their valuable help in proofreading and fact checking.

Olympic athletes are all-time heroes, and it has been an honor for Gold Medalist Glenn "Ed" Moses to endorse my book. What a great privilege to receive an endorsement from an American Olympic Gold Medalist. I wish Ed the very best for the 2012 Olympic Games.

I would also like to thank my family for their moral support, and to thank my parents for helping out with my children's homework while I was working on this book. And of course, to thank my beautiful wife, Su-Eun, for her unconditional love and support, which is always and forever appreciated.

Last but definitely not least, I would like to thank my wonderful staff. Without them, I could not have such a successful practice—as evidenced in many of the patient testimonials featured throughout this book. My assistant, Jason Holland, consistently goes above and beyond to exceed expectations—at work and in everything he does. I am so glad that he is now a faster runner than I am—but watch out Jason, you've given me a new goal to achieve! Melanie Shaginaw really is the boss in the office, and she is blessed with amazing communication skills for relating to my patients. Susan Hyatt has her amazing laboratory skills, and she has this magic touch when it comes to the needle. As always, I am indebted to Jennifer Sidman for her flexibility in the laboratory and in the office.

Of course, my wonderful patients have my most genuine gratitude as well. I sincerely thank my patients for allowing me to participate in their health care.

THANK YOU FOR INVESTING THE TIME TO READ THIS BOOK.
MANY COLLEAGUES AND FRIENDS HAVE CONTRIBUTED TO
THE SUCCESS OF MY APPROACH TO NUTRITIONAL HEALTH,
AND NOW I HOPE THAT YOU WILL ALSO BENEFIT
FROM WHAT WE HAVE LEARNED.

Table of Contents

FOREWORD

by Dr. Mark Gordon

Living in California and close to the Hollywood scene, you are exposed to famous people trying to mimic each other in their homes, cars, manner of dress... and the units of Botox® they use. However, the most challenging goal they all have in common is the goal to attain a younger and healthier appearance, with very little attention to the quality and manner in which they achieve that appearance.

Starvation diets, such the HCG Diet, encourage you to eat no more than 500 calories a day while skipping breakfast and injecting yourself with a product that originates from the urine of pregnant women (at least it's better than the hormones that come from pregnant horse urine). The other extreme option is having your guts cut out, or a rubber band tied around your stomach, diminishing its size and ability to expand, thereby forcing you to eat less; that is, eat less of the same unhealthy foods you were eating before the surgery.

Why do we do this? In our fast-paced lives where there is little desire (and little time) to learn how to eat correctly by choosing more healthy quantities of good foods, we would rather put our bodies into yo-yoing cycles of feeding and fasting, which causes our hormones to alter, thereby creating subtle yet significant damage to our internal parts. Many diabetics die of what is known as a silent MI (myocardial infarction, or heart attack). Why is it called silent? Because they never heard it coming.

In practicing endocrinology, I have seen patients attempting to alter their bodily shapes via diets that have come and gone in the blink of an eye. Many of them were picked up and promoted by the "famous of the famous" here in Beverly Hills and Hollywood—becoming known, for example, as the Beverly Hills Diet or the Hollywood Diet. Having such names has lured many innocent people into thinking these diet programs would imbue them with the qualities of the regions for which they are named.

Over the years, the only reality that I have come to believe is that the control of insulin is mandatory in order for one to manage their weight and distribution of body fat. Insulin has, in my lifetime, always been referred to as the "hormone of storage." So why have we spent over 60 years trying to convince the past few generations that fats are the culprit of weight gain? The simple answer: "I don't know!"

Nonetheless, what we know about insulin is that if you have too little, the sugar that enters your body does not get into the cells and therefore accumulates in the blood. This is the more common form of diabetes—type 2 diabetes, which requires improving your body's production of insulin with either medication or the replacement of insulin by daily injections.

Neither of those options are what we would embrace openly if there was a way to improve it naturally or more healthily with exercise or better eating habits. Right?

The other form of diabetes (which may soon be more prevalent than even type 2 diabetes) is metabolic syndrome. In this condition, your body progressively produces more and more insulin because your body increasingly fails to recognize and use insulin. As this condition progresses, blood sugar rises, as do fats, causing damage to blood vessels throughout the body, brain, eyes, heart and kidneys, along with the possibility of inflammation to the pancreas. In the past, healthcare providers failed to fully assess this condition with an insulin blood test and often missed the diagnosis.

As I stated above, insulin is known as the "hormone of storage" and therefore, as the levels rise, much of the sugar that is consumed is forced into the cells as fat—leading to the characteristic "bursting belly," which is characterized by an enlargement of the waist that's overshadowed by a bulging gut. We've all seen this, and some of us reading this now are now gazing down at what we may have been carrying for years.

In the year 2000, the Massachusetts Male Aging Study (1987-2004) published a preliminary article to address their findings relative to metabolic syndrome. What they found was a relationship between three things: males over 50 years of age, the development of metabolic syndrome, and low levels of free testosterone. Two years later, the same was found for women with low testosterone.

In dealing with any form or stage of diabetes, the recognition of diet and exercise—along with the correction of underlying hormonal deficiencies and insufficiencies—allows us to better manage and possibly correct, if not reverse, the condition.

All of this and more is eloquently explained by Dr. Edwin Lee in the pages that follow as he steers you toward synergistically achieving a healthy body internally, and an attractive body externally. It is a definite win/win. Plus, the recipes are delicious and nutritional! I know this as a fact since my daughter, Alison Gordon, worked with fellow nutritionist Laura Gavin to create the recipes for Dr. Lee.

Eat well, and look great while doing so!

Mark L. Gordon M.D., FAAFP
Medical Director, Millennium Health Centers, Inc.
Medical Director, CBS Studios
Clinical Professor, USC Keck School of Medicine
Author of *The Clinical Application of Interventional Endocrinology*

Preface

While writing my first book, *Feel Good Look Younger: Reversing Tiredness Through Hormonal Balance*, I made a conscious effort to abbreviate the section on insulin resistance and type 2 diabetes because I knew this subject alone was going to require another book—a book that began as a way to help people lose their belly fat, but has now evolved into so much more.

In my previous medical practice, where I would sometimes see 30 patients with diabetes a day, medical insurance plans only allowed me about ten minutes per patient. During those precious ten minutes, I would have to evaluate their blood sugar control (usually their blood sugars would be elevated or all over the place), blood pressure, erectile dysfunction in male patients, lipids (cholesterol) and kidney or eye damage. Also, while trying to write down their instructions—since most people will forget about half of their doctor's instructions before making it to the parking lot—I would try to answer their many questions. The one question I most often got was, "How can I lose my belly fat?" If I had even two minutes to spare, I would have asked what they normally ate and drank.

The answers I usually heard were indicative of a very serious pattern. Most of my patients would not eat breakfast, but instead drank one or two cups of coffee with Splenda® or sugar. Or, if they did eat breakfast, it was a bagel, cereal or oatmeal. Lunch then consisted of a sandwich, or a burger with fries, and a soda. Dinner was some type of meat with potato or rice and some wine or alcohol. Also, there was some type of dessert with either cake or ice cream, or both cake and ice cream. Such eating habits are typical of the appropriately abbreviated Standard American Diet (SAD), and exactly why the current SAD is the main reason for three interrelated conditions: type 2 diabetes, insulin resistance and belly fat.

In my previous busy practice of seeing many patients in my office and in the hospital, I did not have a dietician in my office to work with me. I would have to educate my patients to eat healthier (usually in less than two minutes). I remember giving advise to one of my patients to eat more vegetables. He was single and didn't know how to cook, so I recommended that he steam some vegetables. He asked me how do you steam vegetables? I looked at him and smiled and said that he reminded me of myself before going to college. Fortunately, he had a daughter in town that was able to help her dad in teaching him how to steam his vegetables.

Also, in my previous practice of helping patients with their diabetes I would see some challenging patients that were traveling all the time. Most of those patients were truck drivers that would see me for their diabetes. They would have a huge challenge in finding fresh vegetables at the truck stops. My recommendation was to carry a cooler with them so that they could carry them their vegetables. If you can't find it then you have to bring it with you. For most of my patients, when they changed their diet to a plant based diet with more fiber and less refined sugars then their blood sugars would significantly improve and I could either take them off one or two of their diabetes medication or even reduce their insulin. Some of my patients—with proper diet and change of their medications—I could even get them off their insulin. Although patients with type 1 diabetes will always need to take their insulin.

In addition to improving their blood sugars, most of my patients would also lose weight and their blood pressure would improve with their lipids. The best part would be that they would have more energy and would also be proud that they would lose their belly fat.

One of the most important things you can do for your body is to feed it well with plant based foods that are high in fiber and low in sugar content. In this book I will cover the topic of why high sugar (although tasty) is really not healthy for you. High-refined sugars will increase insulin levels. High insulin levels are associated with chronic inflammation that is a gateway to chronic disease. In other words, a high insulin level is really the devil in your body.

It turns out that everyone in my family is a good cook—except for me! In my family I am not even allowed to carve the turkey on Thanksgiving. This year, my brother-in-law, who is a turkey junky, carved the turkey since my brother couldn't make it. I won't even try to fillet a fish when I catch one in the ocean so that I can have sashimi. I let my friend fillet it since he is a surgeon and a fishing enthusiast.

In this book I have simple recipes that do not take a long time to prepare and feature ingredients that are easy to obtain. I have looked at many diet books and I turn my eyes upwards whenevr I see that there are 15 or more ingredients and half of them are very difficult to obtain. I also get turned off when the meal preparation time is very long. My cooking skill set leans toward quick and easy. I am so glad that my wife is an excellent cook!

In my current practice in age management endocrinology, I recommend to my patients that they need four weeks to eliminate their "white sins," such as pasta, bread, rice and potatoes, as well as oranges, grapes, sugar and desserts. After four weeks, the patient can reintroduce whole grains into their diet. The book has Phase One and Phase Two diets, and there is information on juicing and on super foods.

As the father of western medicine Hippocrates once said, "Let food be your medicine." However, you also need to choose wisely—and you need to know what food sensitivities you have. (More on that topic in chapter 6.)

If we all knew how to eat healthy and all had active lifestyles then we would not have an epidemic of obesity, diabetes and chronic disease. Unfortunately the U.S. is ranked 37th in the world for healthcare and the current medical system is broken. One has to be more proactive in one's health.

I was recently at an Anti-Aging conference and I met someone who went to Europe for stem cell treatment. He mentioned that he had a bad heart and that he now has a second chance in life with his "new heart." I was happy for him but in the back of mind I was thinking if he does not change his lifestyle and lose weight, then his heart disease will come back again and he may not have a third chance in life. As I always say to my patients, if you want anything in life, then you need to work at it and you need to sacrifice to obtain your goals.

Introduction

Your genes are like a loaded gun,
and your lifestyle is the trigger.

Imagine a world where you can live a life that is longer and healthier than anyone has ever lived before—where the technology and the understanding for a healthier body and mind are at your disposal.

It's not science fiction, or even the future... it is now—but only if you know where to invest your time and your resources. While society continues on its epidemic path of obesity, the people who understand and follow the principles and secrets in this book are the type of people who will achieve optimal health.

While obesity charges on, the overweight and unhealthy are beginning to increasingly outnumber the fit and healthy. Fifty years ago, you just didn't see as much obesity. Today, it's everywhere—despite that we now know more, and have more tools at our disposal, to keep us healthier and more youthful for much longer than ever before.

While rampant marketing drives us toward consumeristic lifestyles, those lifestyles are geared toward making money, not making you healthier.

Yet, there are growing numbers of people becoming aware that there are better options—better investments—for them to make. It does take work, and it will sometimes require you to go against the tide, but the results are amazing. I know. I see those results in my office every day. I read about them in medical publications. I discuss it with other doctors around the world. There is a growing rift between those who let society tell them what to eat and how to live, and those who decide for themselves on what they should be doing for nutrition and health.

With this book, you'll gain insight and essential information to understand why, as a society, we are losing the obesity battle—and what it will take for you to win that battle.

The most important job that I do in my current practice is educate my patients on obtaining optimal health. That is what I do for many different patients from around the world—including attorneys, physicians, world-class athletes, successful business owners, builders, scientists, college students, firefighters, ambassadors, teachers, professors, investors, advisors and many homemakers.

For my patients who change their lifestyles and invest in their health, their "return on investment" is enjoying a new sense of vitality, energy and youth. For those that do not change their habits and invest in their health, then they struggle with life.

I always tell my patients that I will give you the direction and set you on a path to optimal health; however, it's up to you if you want to walk down that path.

"OUR FOOD SUPPLY HAS BECOME SO CONTAMINATED WITH ARTIFICIAL CONCOCTIONS THAT ARE PASSED OFF AS FOOD THAT WE DON'T KNOW HOW TO FEED OURSELVES ANYMORE. THERE IS SO MUCH MISINFORMATION OUT THERE ABOUT WHAT TO EAT THAT WE'RE BOUND TO EAT THE WRONG THING. WE NEED TO START TEACHING NUTRITION IN SCHOOLS AND EDUCATING CHILDREN FROM A YOUNG AGE ABOUT WHAT IT MEANS TO EAT THE RIGHT WAY. UNDERSTANDING THE FOOD WE EAT IS OF THE UTMOST IMPORTANCE TO OUR PHYSICAL AND MENTAL HEALTH."

— LINDSEY SHAW
ACTRESS AND NUTRITION ADVOCATE

1

America's Secret Recipe for Obesity

"Companies spend billions to make sure that you know their product.
In 2001, on direct media advertising, McDonald's spent 1.4 billion dollars.
Pepsi spent more than a billion dollars.
To advertise candy, Hershey spent a mere 200 million dollars.
In its peak year, the Five-a-Day Vegetable Campaign's
total advertising budget was a lowly 2 million dollars—
100 times less than the direct media budget of one candy company."
— Morgan Spurlock in the 2004 documentary, Super Size Me

Your best investment is in obtaining optimal health, period. There is no shortcut, no pill for obtaining optimal health. All the money in the world can't buy optimal health, and you can't depend on your active past for a healthy future. It takes work, along with an appropriate and ongoing active lifestyle, but you can achieve optimal health.

In my current practice I see many successful patients who have achieved financial freedom; however, with their current lifestyle (lack of exercise, overeating, smoking, excessive drinking, etc.) they are only indenturing themselves to an accelerated aging process. Thankfully, one of the most remarkable features of your body is that it can recover... unless it is just too late.

So don't let another day slip by! If you really want to understand the secrets to a healthy body and mind, then you need to learn and embrace the principles in this book. To begin, this chapter will provide some necessary history and revealing insight on why our food industry and government are the main cause behind today's obesity epidemic, which has led to the downfall of our nation's state of health.

To better understand how we as a nation have gotten fat, you need to first understand why too much insulin (or having a high insulin level) will make you fat—while also increasing your risk of memory loss, high blood pressure, autoimmune disease, stroke, heart disease, diabetes and an earlier death.

It All Comes Down to Insulin

It's very simple. When you consume too much refined sugar—like bread, pasta, potatoes, grapes, rice, oranges, cereals, cakes, oatmeal, cookies, candy, ice cream, pancakes, waffles or soda—your body's insulin level will rise. Higher insulin levels are very dangerous in that they accelerate your aging process and, as you will soon learn, that comes with consequences more dire than looking old before your time.

What is amazing, though, is that people who are over 100 years old and still mentally "with it," they all have one thing in common, and that is a very low insulin level. High insulin levels "tell" your body to develop belly fat, or obesity. High insulin levels also reflect a condition called insulin resistance. More about the dangers of insulin resistance will be covered in the next chapter.

One of the most important secrets for achieving optimal health is to have low insulin levels, and you achieve low insulin levels by restricting or limiting your consumption of refined sugars.

"I would never have suspected pre-diabetes."

Despite being a physician, I always thought that pain was a part of exercising. After a day of golf, my body would ache so much that I was having difficulty walking up or down the stairs. Regular exercise was not fun—knowing that my body would ache so much at the end of the day. My previous three endocrinologists had diagnosed me with low testosterone levels for the past 15 years; however, not one ever recommended hormone replacement therapy.

Reading Dr. Edwin Lee's first book, "Feel Good Look Younger," *was an eye opener for me. Here is someone who has mastered the knowledge of conventional medicine, and has combined it with functional medicine. A few days after I read his book, I flew to Florida to see him. It turned out to be the most important trip I have ever taken for myself.*

He started me on testosterone replacement and a medical regimen to help me lose weight and treat my newfound, pre-diabetic condition. Until Dr. Edwin Lee skillfully discovered and diagnosed my pre-diabetes, I would never have suspected pre-diabetes in myself.

I have also improved upon my lifestyle and changed my diet—primarily by increasing my vegetable intake, reducing my refined sugars (such as bread, pasta, rice, potatoes and sweets) and by adding some nutraceuticals (to help lower my insulin levels).

So far I have lost 23 pounds, and four inches have vanished from my waist. I'm exercising regularly—without pain—and best of all, I've gained 30 yards off the tee. Plus, it just keeps getting better, like when I played six consecutive days of golf on a recent trip to Phoenix—with absolutely no pain!

I feel great, thanks to Dr. Edwin Lee!!

— James Lee M.D. (no relation, really!)

Don't Fight Nature, Because You Will Lose

Another important secret for achieving optimal health is to never forget that when you go against nature, you will lose. If you build a city where earthquakes are known to happen regularly, then someday a major earthquake will damage that city. If you eat processed foods that are filled with chemicals and preservatives, then medical problems will not be far away.

Our ancestors did not have the "diet" that we have today, nor did they have today's chronic diseases (such as epidemic obesity) because they ate much healthier than we currently do, and they were not exposed to the thousands of chemicals and preservatives in their foods as we are. Our bodies are not designed or built for today's passive lifestyle and its chemical-laden convenience foods.

It's crucial to not eat processed foods that are low in nutrition and high in calories and in chemicals. Your body and mind need the nutrients that nature has provided for us. Yet we feed ourselves and our children thousands of man-made chemicals and toxins that are clearly poisoning our bodies.

The Food and Drug Administration maintains a list appropriately entitled, *Everything Added to Food in the United States*. As of this writing, there are more than 3,000 synthetic food additives and chemicals on this comprehensive list. To see every additive and chemical, simply go to: www.fda.gov/food/foodingredientspackaging/ucm115326.htm.

While most of the additives and chemicals listed there are benign, many are proven to have harmful effects. However, because there are strong food lobbyists supporting the use of those chemicals, they are in our foods—poisoning us, and our children.

"It's Not Nice to Fool Mother Nature!"

In the 70s there were some popular television commercials with Mother Nature getting fooled by a margarine that tastes like butter, and then proclaiming, "It's not nice to fool Mother Nature," as thunder boomed and different forest animals became afraid. Looking back on those commercials with today's understanding of how harmful such products are—with their chemicals, preservatives and petroleum byproducts—it's quite ironic that they chose to say, "It's not nice to fool Mother Nature."

Flash forward to today, and those Mother Nature commercials are a faded memory; however, the products remain. Yet, although we now know about the ingredients, we still buy them. Even a popular standup comedian, Jim Gaffigan, has a routine about such foods, which includes a joke about the time he didn't put his groceries into the refrigerator soon enough, and his margarine melted into diesel fuel.

In the 70s we just didn't know, so we bought those products. Today, even though we should know, we still buy those products, while we laugh about the dangers.

Chief among those newer dangers are aspartame, olestra, partially hydrogenated vegetable oil, butylated hydroxytoluene (BHT) and butylated hydroxyanisole (BHA)—just to name a few.

(1) Aspartame

Aspartame is found in diet sodas and in many other food products as an artificial sweetener. I used to drink many diet sodas, then switched to diet ice tea, and later to diet lemonade. However, when my father became ill, I started reading about nutrition—something which most doctors have very little education in—and quickly learned about the dangers of aspartame.

Aspartame has been linked to brain tumors, seizures, depression, headaches and neurotoxicity. Aspartame is composed of ten percent methanol, and methanol breaks down into deadly chemicals that the body has a hard time getting rid of—the most damaging of which are formaldehyde, formic acid and diketopiperazine (a known carcinogen).

In addition, diet sodas are very acidic, so when you drink it your body wants to neutralize the acid by releasing calcium from your bones. Sodas with caffeine act as a diuretic, which causes you to lose your calcium through your urine, and this can lead to osteoporosis or bone loss.[1]

Since diet sodas with aspartame are very sweet (approximately 200 times sweeter than sugar) then you will need to eat increasingly more refined sugars to satisfy your "addiction," your "need," for food and drink that is 200 times sweeter than normal. Consequently, as more refined sugars are eaten, your insulin levels will increase, which will then cause many more problems.

I have many patients that are addicted to diet sodas, or to regular sodas, but once they stop their soda habit they all feel like their brain fog has disappeared, and many of them also lose weight.

"I was addicted to sugar, soda and caffeine."

My weight loss journey began at the age of 37. At 5'2" I weighed 151 pounds, and was having a difficult time losing weight after the birth of my third child. Two years later, I still hadn't lost much weight and I was becoming discouraged.

Dr. Lee explained that weight loss was possible for me—if I completely changed my eating habits. I was addicted to sugar, soda and caffeine. To feel like I was making a good choice, I would often use a sugar substitute like Splenda®. I agreed to follow Dr. Lee's plan of NO Splenda®, which also included most sugar substitutes because of the aspartame. And, I eliminated all sugar and simple carbohydrates from my diet.

Over the next several months my extra weight disappeared. I noticed that my clothes were becoming too big. Even my pre-pregnancy size-eight clothes were loose. Today, I still adhere to a healthy diet of veggies and lean proteins. I find that when I do give in to the temptation and eat sugar, I just feel awful afterwards—I'm cranky and tired. So I've decided that cheating is just not worth it.

I've lost a total of 30 pounds! I feel great and haven't been this size since my teens. I love the new me!

— Terri Smith

(2) Olestra

Olestra is a fat substitute not found in nature, but it is found as Olean®, the Procter & Gamble brand of olestra. Olean® is used in certain foods, and as a no-fat cooking oil, shortening and butter substitute. Since 1996, according to the Procter & Gamble website, more than five billion servings of foods containing Olean® have been sold.

Unfortunately, a recent study has concluded that rats, when given foods made with olestra—over time—gained weight because olestra slowed down their metabolisms; hence, their long-term weight gain.[2]

Olestra does have zero calories; however, your stomach's digestive enzymes can't break down olestra's large, synthetic molecules. Therefore, your body's vital ability to absorb nutrients is impaired by olestra, which is also why it can give you diarrhea.

By the way, Procter & Gamble recently found another use for olestra. Sefose®—their olestra-based "cousin" of Olean®—is now being used for paints and lubricants.

(3) Partially Hydrogenated Vegetable Oil

With more than 70,000 heart attacks a year to its credit, partially hydrogenated vegetable oil has been banned in New York City. Thankfully, many restaurants across the country have followed suit and also switched to healthier frying oils. However, since this product is relatively cheap to produce and buy, it is still found in many restaurants, and in many products on grocery shelves.

We don't need to use partially hydrogenated vegetable oil! Nature provides plenty of healthy fats that keep your cell membranes strong, help your brain to work better and are important in your body's production of hormones. Some of these healthy fats from nature are olive oil, avocados, flax seeds, nuts and fish.

Although vegetables are important for obtaining optimal health, partially hydrogenated vegetable oil is not found anywhere in nature. So, why do we need to be exposed to an artificial fat that has been linked to heart disease?[3]

"I was placed on Pravachol®, Zocor®, Lipitor®, Crestor® and Zetia®—nothing worked."

In August 2007, my primary care physician began prescribing medication to lower my cholesterol. On the first blood test, my total cholesterol was 238. Over the next several years, I was placed on Pravachol®, Zocor®, Lipitor®, Crestor® and Zetia®—nothing worked. We tried each medication at several different dosage levels before moving on to the next drug.

During this time, my lowest total cholesterol was 206. On January 3, 2011, my primary care physician's test results revealed that my cholesterol had climbed to 291. She wanted me to continue taking Crestor® 40 mg and Zetia® 10 mg daily.

When I first met with Dr. Lee, my primary focus was simply to lose weight. Dr. Lee suggested focusing on eating 50 to 75 percent of each meal as vegetables. He also suggested that I give up diet colas, all artificial sweeteners, bread, rice, potatoes and pasta.

I began his diet regimen on January 31, 2011, and increased my daily walking activities. On March 3, 2011, my primary care physician and I were both astounded by my routine blood tests for cholesterol.

After only one month of following Dr. Lee's nutritional plan, my total cholesterol had dropped from 291 to 151. My primary care physician reduced my cholesterol medication, and wants to follow up on my progress in two months.

— Jean Summers Stinson

(4) BHT and BHA

Two other, equally scary additives that our food industry is using are butylated hydroxytoluene (BHT) and butylated hydroxyanisole (BHA). These are petroleum derived antioxidants and preservatives that, according to the Department of Health and Human Services, BHA is "reasonably anticipated to be a human carcinogen." Yet, the FDA allows BHA to be used in food products. In addition, BHT has been linked to cancer in animals.[4] Common foods in which you will find these chemicals are certain gums, crackers and cereals.

The good news is that foods found in nature will not have these chemicals or poisons. If you want optimal health, then stay away from foods that come from a box or that are packaged. Instead, eat real foods that come from the land and sea—while they are in season, not preserved beyond their normal shelf life, and not laden with pesticide residue—like those in the Dirty Dozen™.

Dirty Dozen™ and Clean 15™

Are you ready to start eating fewer pesticides? Then it's time to learn about the Dirty Dozen™.

While eating only organic means you won't be eating pesticide residue, it will cost more to do so. As a more affordable alternative—because certain foods have less pesticide residue (like those listed on the Clean 15™)—your food budget will go further whenever you focus your organic purchases on the Dirty Dozen™ (foods with the most pesticide residue), while buying the Clean 15™ as non-organic.

Thanks to the Environmental Working Group's annual lists of the Dirty Dozen™ and the Clean 15™ [5] (see Appendix B), it is estimated that you will reduce your exposure to pesticide residue by a whopping 80 percent if you switch to organic when buying the twelve foods on their Dirty Dozen™ list.

(1) Dirty Dozen™

These foods contain the highest levels of pesticides. Whenever possible, buy these foods as organic.

Apples
Celery
Strawberries
Peaches
Spinach
Nectarines
Grapes

Sweet bell peppers

Potatoes

Blueberries

Lettuce

Kale / collard greens

(2) Clean 15™

These foods have been found to have low levels of pesticides. To help stretch you grocery dollar, the non-organic versions of these foods are nearly as safe as their organic versions.

Onions

Corn

Pineapples

Avocado

Asparagus

Sweet peas

Mangoes

Eggplant

Cantaloupe

Kiwi

Cabbage

Watermelon

Sweet potatoes

Grapefruit

Mushrooms

The China Study

An amazing study has recently proven that profoundly beneficial health results are associated with: eating foods from nature, reducing refined sugars, lowering insulin levels and reducing the amount of animal protein.

T. Colin Campbell, Professor Emeritus of Nutritional Biochemistry at Cornell University, recently published the findings of his study on the relationship of the consumption of animal protein with cancer, diabetes, bowel disease, heart disease, autoimmune disease and other conditions. His findings quickly became famously known simply as, The China Study.

According to the New York Times, this was the "Grand Prix of epidemiology studies" as it was conducted over 20 years and included 880 million people. Campbell chose to conduct his study in China because the nation has a genetically similar population that tends to live in the same place and eat the same foods for their entire lives. Also, China has a genetically similar population with significant regional differences in disease rates, dietary habits and environmental exposures. These characteristics of China's population-at-large provided Campbell with a somewhat controlled setting, almost like a laboratory.

The conclusion of his study was that animal proteins increased the risk of the diseases they were studying, but plant based foods lowered the risk. As for diabetes, there was a diabetes diet study which looked at 50 diabetics. All the diabetics were taking insulin and they were on the American Diabetes Diet. Campbell then switched them to a high fiber diet ("lots" of vegetables, which lowers insulin resistance) and the amazing results were that they required much less insulin—or some even got off their insulin all together.[6]

The main principle of The China Study of food and health that I found most significant was this: ***The same nutrition that prevents disease in its early stages can also halt or reverse it in its later stages.***

The mechanism of "cause and effect"—why the consumption of animal protein is bad for your health—is as follows: animal protein is very acidic; your body has to neutralize the acidity by releasing calcium from your bones; this inhibits the production of the active vitamin D that helps regulate your immune system. Whereas, plant-based foods are not acidic, and they contain higher amounts of antioxidants to help protect your body (especially your DNA) from any damage due to free radicals.

Another important piece of information that The China Study presents—with which I totally agree—is that if all Americans switched to a plant-based diet, then a lot of wealthy industries would stand to lose a lot of revenue.

Although I am not a vegan, I have dramatically reduced my animal protein intake for some time. For those that are vegans, then it is crucial to supplement your diet with vitamin B12 (preferably injections).

Cheap Corn

Another reason we have an epidemic of obesity, diabetes and chronic disease is that we have cheap foods, as well as cheap sweeteners—all based on corn. An excellent documentary, called King Corn, explains where our food comes from and the importance of corn in our food supply.

The tipping point of our government policy was the U.S. farm policy, as written by President Nixon's Secretary of Agriculture, Earl Butz, who radically rewrote the U.S. farm policy—trying to make the U.S. into the breadbasket of the world by subsidizing farmers to produce corn.

Corn is also used for animal feed and the production of high fructose corn syrup, which is a cheap sweetener. Corn is high in sugar content and thus will spike your insulin levels, and that will definitely lead to obesity.

The next time you're in a fast food restaurant, compare the price of fries, a hamburger and a soda to a grilled chicken salad. The fries are fried in oil from corn, the meat of the hamburger is derived from the cows eating corn to quickly fatten them up, and the sodas are made from high fructose corn syrup. Therefore, that burger, fries and soda are going to cost less than a grilled chicken salad almost every time. Cheap foods that are filled with chemicals, and our own government subsidizes it all.

Try this little science experiment at home. Buy a cheap burger and then watch it stay "alive" for many years. I have one, still in its original paper and never refrigerated, that has not molded or decomposed, thanks to being laden with chemicals. With the incredible marketing and advertising of the fast food industry, it's no wonder why it's also a billion dollar industry.

Two Decades — From Pyramid to Plate

Twenty years ago, the American government developed a guideline to promote better health; but, unfortunately, it had no science behind it and was instead "written" by the big food industry. Our first such guideline was known as the Food Pyramid, and it was created in 1992 by the U.S. Department of Health.

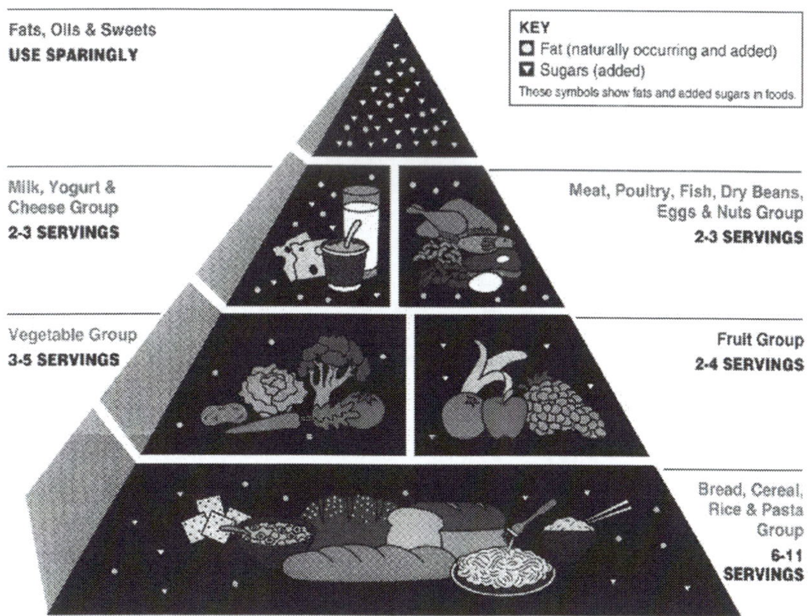

The Food Pyramid, introduced in 1992 by the U.S. Department of Health, heavily emphasized the consumption of grains.

The food pyramid heavily emphasized the consumption of grains such as rice, pasta, bread and cereals (six to eleven servings daily!).

Because of this, and many other misleading recommendations, I believe—and I see the evidence daily in my practice—that the government's food pyramid guidelines have increased your risk for developing insulin resistance and gaining weight.

Since 1992, the food pyramids have appeared in countless books, magazines, hospitals and textbooks; in schools, universities and health clinics; and on websites. Every time, the message was dominated by an emphasis on grains such as rice, pasta, bread and cereals. (More on this later—refined grains will raise your insulin levels, and that will promote belly fat.)

I am sure that before each food pyramid was released, there were many food industry lobbyists wanting their products on the food pyramid. The resulting tragedy of this flawed process led to the recommendation of eating an astounding six to *eleven* servings a day of grains—bread, pasta, rice, white potatoes and so on—all of which increase insulin levels, increase morbid obesity, and increase the risk of heart disease and cancer.

Many experts, such as Dr. Walter Willett, a Harvard nutritionist (see, *What a Food Pyramid Should Be,* later in this chapter), believe that the pyramids did not reflect the current research, even back then. For example, certain dietary items had already been associated with heart disease, such as three cups of whole milk and an eight ounce serving of hamburger daily—which were recommended under the pyramids!

The 1992 food pyramid also drew an imaginary line in the air and limited the amount of all fats. While there are many types of fats, there are healthy fats that are essential for optimal health and they tend to come from fish, olive oil, nuts and avocados, for example.

Long before the first pyramid was developed, nutritionists already knew that some types of fats were essential to health. The theme for the 1992 food pyramid was that carbohydrates are good and all fats are bad. Then, in 2005, the Department of Health released My Pyramid.

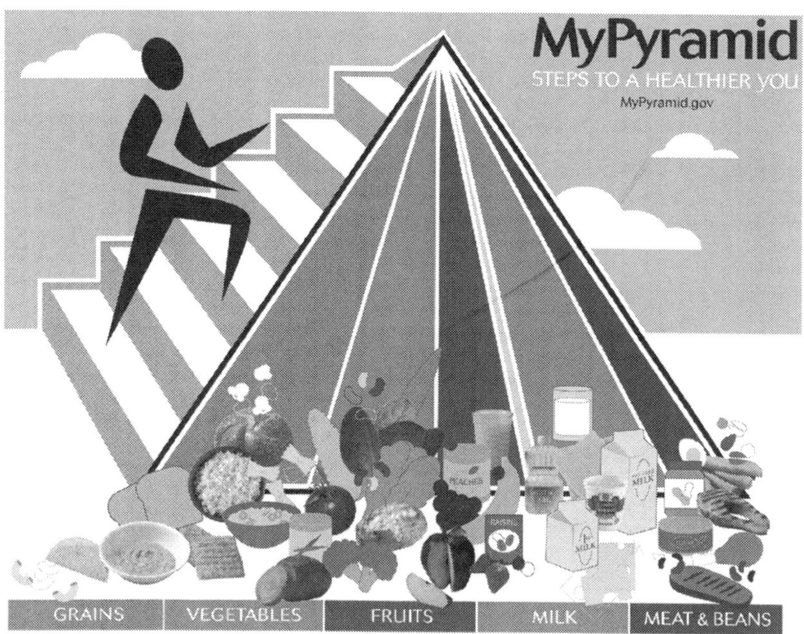

By the time My Pyramid was phased out in 2011, 34 percent of Americans 20 years and older were obese.[9]

The new pyramid was designed to be simple, without much text. On my first look, I had no idea what it was. You have to reference a government website to interpret it—although not every American has Internet access.

For this release of the pyramid, it is still quite obvious how the food industry influenced the recommendations, instead of the scientific evidence.[7] The only thing I liked about My Pyramid were the steps with a stick-figure climbing them—to represent physical activity.

Regarding the grains, My Pyramid indicates that half the grains should be refined carbohydrates—which will only increase your insulin levels and increase your risk of developing many chronic diseases like heart disease or diabetes! What a shame.

As for protein, My Pyramid lumps all protein in one group: red meat, poultry, fish and beans. Then My Pyramid wants you to make choices that are low fat or fat-free—despite the evidence that certain fats are very healthy—like those from fish.

Another issue is that My Pyramid recommends drinking three servings of milk, or eating three servings of dairy products, every day to prevent osteoporosis. Those extra 300 calories from drinking that much milk every day will add up quickly. With the current epidemic of obesity, that would be like putting gasoline on a fire.

Also, millions of Americans have been diagnosed with lactose intolerance—and many more have some degree of undiagnosed lactose intolerance. For most of my patients, when I take them off dairy, it's amazing how much better they feel. In addition, there is a lack of evidence that links the consumption of dairy products with any prevention of osteoporosis.[8]

The two things America's food pyramids did accomplish are that the average American has ballooned in weight (34 percent of Americans 20 years and older are now obese) while our nation has declined significantly in overall health.[9] Yet, even more sadly, our nation's next generation is already being targeted by food industry marketing to continue the legacy.

For the many reasons presented in this chapter, I firmly believe that the government's food pyramids were flawed in many ways, with little scientific data supporting them, and they have long since taken their toll on America.[10]

"I weighed 407 pounds and was struggling with diabetes, high blood pressure, acid reflux, asthma and sleep apnea."

By the time I first came to Dr. Lee, I weighed 407 pounds and was struggling with diabetes, high blood pressure, acid reflux, asthma and sleep apnea. I wore size 50 pants with 4X and 5X shirts, and every day I had to take two sugar pills and eight shots of insulin.

So, when Dr. Lee said, "I am going to save your life," I listened. He wrote out my diet and I started following it immediately. In the first two weeks I lost 33 pounds. Now, five months later, I've lost 100 pounds so far!

Already, my life is much better and I have more self-esteem—just by being able to sit in a booth at a restaurant, being able to walk easier, bend over to tie my shoes, and having plenty of energy to play with my two-year-old. I'm now wearing size 36 pants and 2X shirts, taking only half a sugar pill in the morning and at night, and I no longer need acid reflux pills or a BiPap machine for sleep apnea.

I accomplished it all by following the diet that Dr. Lee created for lowering my insulin levels—and that meant more vegetables, while avoiding bread, oatmeal, cereals, pasta, rice, corn, potatoes, oranges and grapes.

Being on Dr. Lee's diet really did save my life—just like he said on the day I met him. Thank you so very much, Dr. Lee.

— Greg Strickland

Finally realizing their new guidelines for the health of America were yet another misstep, in June 2011 the Department of Health replaced My Pyramid with My Plate.

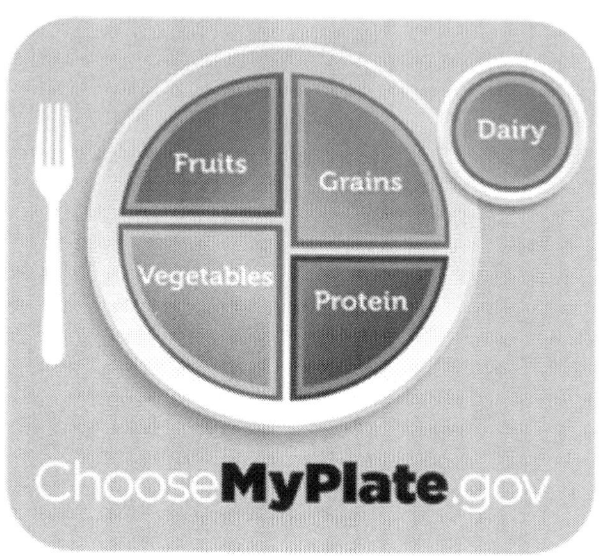

Like its predecessors, My Plate fails to differentiate between grains, while still emphasizing dairy.

Regrettably, the government's My Plate approach falls short of the mark as well. While somewhat better than its predecessors, My Plate is still rife with ambiguity, and still fails to effectively differentiate between grains, while also suffering from an oversimplified "food for dummies" style.

What a Food Pyramid Should Be

Most notable of the many critics of the food pyramids has been the Harvard School of Public Health. In fact, Harvard went so far as to label the government's food pyramids as not being helpful to the public. I really like the food pyramid developed from Harvard, which is featured below. I agree with Harvard that a sound nutritional guideline will place an emphasis on a plant-based diet, with an active lifestyle, and with limits on red meat, refined sugars and dairy.

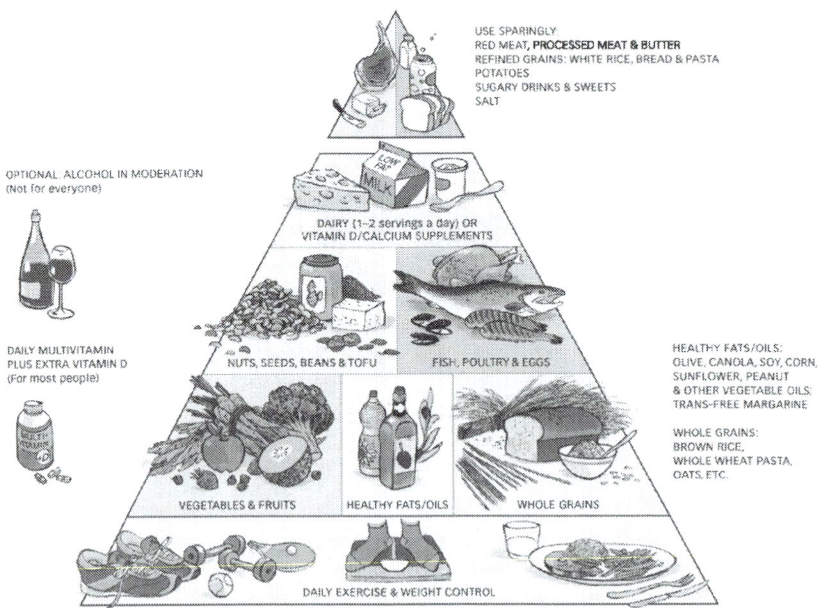

For more information on Harvard's Healthy Eating Pyramid, please visit www.thenutritionsource.org.

Your best investment truly is in obtaining optimal health, and that investment begins with a sound nutritional plan, like the one developed at Harvard—and not by Washington lobbyists looking to line the pockets of their constituents. Just be aware that there are many poor quality foods that are convenient and inexpensive. You have to invest in healthy foods for your body—the most important investment you will ever make.

"Over the years, I had accumulated some extra pounds."

Dr. Edwin Lee was recommended to me by my wife. I was very impressed with the health improvements she had received from his protocol.

After some very thorough analysis, Dr. Lee stated that I was pre-diabetic, my hormones were out of balance, I was obese, and I needed to lose about 40 pounds.

Over the years, I had accumulated some extra pounds, mostly around my midsection. I didn't think at my age, 75, I would ever be able to lose any major weight; however, I couldn't stand that word, "obese."

By following part of Dr. Lees' recommendations I began to feel much better, but I didn't follow all of his advice (only what I chose to follow), so I wasn't losing the weight.

Then, about a year later—after reading Dr. Lees' book, Feel Good Look Younger, *I got more serious about following his instructions (specifically, about staying away from fast food restaurants, increasing my vegetable intake, reducing my refined sugars and increasing my walking).*

Before I knew it, over a four month period, I lost 35 pounds while significantly lowering my insulin levels. I feel like a new man, thanks to a brilliant physician.

— Baylis Carnes

Conclusion

The key to achieving a healthy body and mind is lowering your insulin levels—and you can do it simply by consuming more plant-based foods. I doubt that the food industry has all those Washington lobbyists in place with the intention to lose profits while improving your health. So remember, it's your body, your mind and your health in which you need to invest.

No doubt about it, you need to reduce your refined carbohydrate. For the best results, just follow the recommendations on Harvard's Healthy Eating Pyramid. A big shocker for many people is to limit dairy, which is very acidic. Many people are lactose intolerant, or have a delayed food allergy to dairy, and they will benefit from less dairy.

Also, always remember to not go against nature, because nature will always win. Humans have evolved to be hunters and gatherers, which means that we need to eat real food, provided by nature, and avoid the foods that come in a box filled with chemicals and preservatives (even those that are fortified with vitamins).

Certain non-organic foods have high levels of pesticides, while other non-organic foods have low levels. Use the Dirty Dozen™ and the Clean 15™ as a handy guide when deciding whether you should buy non-organic or organic.

Although it may be more expensive to eat organic and/or fresh vegetables and meats that are cage-free or grass-fed, it is worth the investment. Enjoy the foods that Mother Nature has provided and your body and mind will thank you.

CHAPTER 1 REVIEW

— High levels of insulin will cause belly fat, since insulin is a fat storing hormone.

— Obesity is a growing epidemic around the world due to the higher intake of refined sugars (such as bread, pasta, rice, potatoes, sodas, cakes, grapes, oranges, cookies and candy). These foods will increase your insulin levels.

— The original food pyramid of 1992 promoted eating more refined sugars or grains (thus increasing insulin levels) and mistakenly emphasized that all fats are bad, which has contributed to the current obesity epidemic.

— The Harvard School of Public Health has developed a great food pyramid that is based on science, not food lobbyists.

— The key to reducing belly fat is lowering your insulin levels by reducing your intake of refined sugars and substituting grains (refined sugars) for greens (more vegetables).

— Stretch your grocery dollar when you buy organic versions of the Dirty Dozen™, and non-organic versions of the Clean 15™. For handy charts, see Appendix B.

— Eat real foods from nature, not something mixed with chemicals and preservatives in a box.

2

The Consequences of Insulin Resistance

"Nothing in life is to be feared, it is only to be understood.
Now is the time to understand more, so that we may fear less."
— Marie Curie

Now that you know insulin resistance affects everyone—not just people with diabetes—and that insulin resistance will make you overweight, you need to realize insulin resistance has consequences far more dire than the numbers on your bathroom scale, or the muffin top above your waistband.

To put the far-reaching issues of insulin resistance and its many consequences into perspective, consider Laura McCarthy's story.

"Dr. Lee was the key for unlocking everything."

Today, I am 41, healthier than I have probably ever been, and—after ten years of trying and failing—we just celebrated the birth of our first child, a beautiful baby boy. Regaining my health, and then becoming a mother, has been a very long and difficult journey, to say the least, but it thankfully led to Dr. Lee.

My weight and my health had been an ongoing struggle for about nine years. I had long suspected a thyroid issue, but none of my blood work ever revealed a problem. My initial symptoms were exhaustion, sleep issues, skin problems, foggy thinking and poor memory. I was told by doctors how these were symptoms "in line" with a woman in their 30s, and they tried to prescribe antidepressants. I knew there had to be more to this picture. Soon, my list of symptoms grew longer and longer: intolerance to cold, dry skin, hair loss, decreased libido, periods of depression, and my most intolerable symptom... infertility.

My husband and I had been seeing a reproductive endocrinologist who labeled us as "unexplained infertility." A bitter pill to swallow, but we began with initial treatments to become pregnant. After trying for months, and then moving on to injectable medications and intrauterine insemination, we finally conceived. This unfortunately resulted in miscarriage.

After almost two years we decided to take a break from it all. While doing so, I focused on just being healthy. During this time, out of the blue, I had an episode of bleeding that led me to having laparoscopic surgery, which revealed endometriosis. This diagnosis started to explain some of my symptoms.

At least we had a new outlook, and we decided to continue trying to conceive on our own. All the while, I returned time and time again to have my thyroid checked—but the results always came back in the "normal range." So, I just continued to focus on good health while taking up yoga, seeing an acupuncturist regularly and eating a very clean diet. I also began to read extensively on the subject of women's hormones. I was beginning to suspect I had polycystic ovary syndrome (PCOS, an insulin resistance condition).

After about a year, I was feeling better, but still had many of the symptoms. My acupuncturist encouraged me to see another reproductive endocrinologist. I was apprehensive, but decided to start the process again. While waiting in the exam room for the doctor, there was a divine intervention. I began reading a magazine with an article describing the symptoms of thyroid disease. The article suggested I should ask for a full thyroid work-up—not just the usual test for thyroid-stimulating hormone—and to check for antibodies. After some extreme arm twisting, the doctor agreed.

Then, during our second meeting to go over my test results and create a plan for treatment, the doctor said all the tests came back normal except for one that was high... my thyroid antibodies. I asked what the normal range was and he said normal was around 60, and that mine was a whopping 825! He then insisted this would "not be a problem" for conception. "Not a problem!" I was furious! We decided not to continue with that doctor.

Then one day, my acupuncturist said she thought my thyroid looked swollen. I went to see my family doctor and my long-held suspicions were finally confirmed. I had hypothyroidism that had now turned into Hashimoto's disease. Finally, I had some answers and it felt as though help was on the way—or so I thought.

I was referred to an endocrinologist who treated me with Synthroid® for over a year. I still was not feeling a lot better. I asked if we could try something more natural that I had read about: Armour® Thyroid. The doctor ridiculed me for reading too much on the internet and refused to prescribe it. I was feeling almost broken.

Then, out of nowhere, I received a flyer in the mail for Dr. Lee. I saw this and felt I should give him a try. When I walked into Dr. Lee's office I was cautiously optimistic. I had been let down by the medical profession time and time again, but I decided to take a deep breath and see what he had to say.

Dr. Lee listened to my story very intently, asked me a few questions, and then he said, "I think I already know what is wrong." Then, after I answered a few more questions, he said these words that I will never forget, "I can help you feel better, and I can help you have a baby."

Tears of joy flowed. I could not believe it. Simply put, Dr. Lee is my hero. He did thorough tests and prescribed the right hormones for me. He confirmed that I had PCOS and started me on Byetta®, which helped me lose weight. I also began treatment for my thyroid problems with natural thyroid hormones, and I started to take progesterone. My body responded beautifully, miraculously.

Then, as we began treatment with another reproductive endocrinologist, Dr. Lee was so supportive and helpful. He advised me to stay on progesterone throughout the beginning of the pregnancy, and he monitored my thyroid.

Everything worked! After many doctors, tests and heartbreaks, Dr. Lee was the key for unlocking everything. I am forever grateful for his compassionate approach to medicine. He put an end to my long health crisis, and returned balance to my hormones—and to my life!

— Laura McCarthy

With all Laura was going through, it's important to remember—even though she hit many brick walls—she never stopped trying. Her story is a testament to the many benefits of always being aware of your healthcare options—and an aware lifestyle starts when you're an active participant in your healthcare, not just a patient! (More on this in Chapter 4.)

When someone is not health-aware, there will inevitably be health problems. Many of those problems begin with nutrition—or, the lack thereof—and manifest with insulin resistance. In the beginning, insulin resistance can be interpreted as a warning flag. If corrective action is taken because of that flag, then the problem can usually be avoided. However, when insulin's warning flag is ignored, there will almost inevitably be consequences.

How Insulin Works

Simply stated, insulin resistance is a condition where it takes more insulin than normal to bring fuel (especially glucose) into your cells. As your resistance to insulin builds (typically because of obesity), your body requires ever-increasing amounts of insulin to compensate.

Meanwhile, as long as your pancreas can work overtime to produce more and more insulin, blood glucose levels remain somewhat normal; however, as your overworked pancreas reaches its maximum level of production (or burns itself out), and there's no longer enough insulin to keep overcompensating, your blood glucose levels will rise and diabetes will present itself, along with chronic inflammation. Also—because you are now resistant to insulin—your muscles, fat, brain and liver do not respond properly to insulin, and other conditions begin presenting themselves as well.

Insulin is a hormone made in your belly, in an organ called the pancreas. The pancreas also makes digestive enzymes that help digest your food—as well as other hormones, such as glucagon, somatostatin and pancreatic polypeptide. The pancreas is unique since it is a dual function organ that helps with digestion and with the regulation of blood glucose or sugar. Below is an illustration on the anatomy of the stomach, gallbladder, small intestine and pancreas.

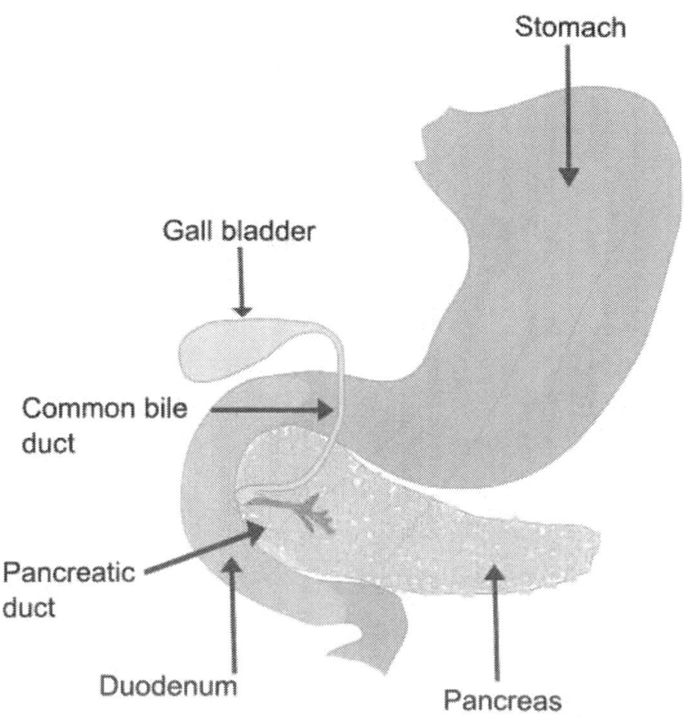

What Insulin Does

To begin with, let's briefly touch on the basics of what insulin does. Insulin is made from the special cells of the pancreas called the islet cells of Langerhans. Insulin is made in the pancreas and stored as a hexamer (a unit of six insulin molecules) and requires the mineral zinc to help it hold the hexamer together. The active part of insulin is when the hexamer dissolves into single monomers (single units of insulin). You have about one to three million islets of Langerhans that make the hormone insulin. When someone loses about 90 percent of their insulin-making cells, then they will require the use of insulin to help control their high glucose, or diabetes.

Insulin is very important in helping regulate carbohydrate (glucose or sugar) and fat metabolism. Insulin helps deliver the glucose into the liver, muscles, brain and fat. Insulin is considered a fat storing hormone—meaning that high levels of insulin prevent the body from using fat as energy. The more insulin you have, then the more belly fat you will have.

Insulin also helps potassium and amino acids enter the cells. In addition, insulin helps store of glucose in the liver, which is then called glycogen. After the liver produces enough glycogen, then it converts the extra glucose into fatty acids. One interesting fact for weight loss is that after you burn all your glycogen storage for energy, then your body can begin burning fat for energy. This is why the top athletes (lean, mean, fat burning machines) are in shape. They are very efficient in using fat as energy.

Another fact is whenever there is too much storage of glycogen and fat in the liver, then you'll have a fatty liver—and that can lead to liver failure or cirrhosis.

Insulin Resistance

Insulin resistance is a condition where the muscles, fat cells, liver, brain and other organs that need insulin now require a higher level of insulin. For example, in a normal patient, if it takes one molecule of insulin to lower glucose by ten points, then in an insulin resistant patient it will take ten molecules of insulin to lower glucose by ten points.

In other words, the body's cells are resistant to insulin action. Thus, the pancreas needs to pump out higher levels of insulin in order to keep the glucose regulated.

The good news is that insulin resistance is a reversible condition. It is associated with two things: chronic inflammation, and what we put in our mouths (foods high in carbohydrates).

When your pancreas burns out in producing insulin, then you will develop diabetes—a condition where the blood glucose is elevated. An interesting fact is that around 1552 B.C., an Egyptian physician named Hesy-Ra described diabetes as frequent urination, with urine that is sweet tasting.

In fact, in ancient times, doctors would test for diabetes by tasting a patient's urine. A sweet taste meant the patient had diabetes. I am so glad urine tasting was not required in my training!

Nowadays, insulin resistance can be attributed to certain medications such as prednisone, certain psychiatric medications (such as Abilify®, Clozaril®, Zyprexa®, Geodon® Seroquel® and Risperdal®), birth control pills, hydrochlorothiazide and beta blockers (such as, propranolol).

Regardless of the cause, any elevated levels of insulin are potentially lethal and are undeniably associated with heart disease, dementia, loss of memory, depression, neurodegenerative brain disease and other conditions such as… belly fat—which brings us to the first on our list of the dangers of insulin resistance.

Insulin Resistance and Fat

As a fat-storing hormone, the most common area where high levels of insulin will cause you to develop fat is around your belly.

Furthermore, insulin inactivates hormone-sensitive lipase, which breaks down fatty acids. So, high levels of insulin will increase your storage of fat. Therefore, if you have high levels of insulin, or if you eat foods that spike your insulin levels, then you will have trouble burning fat.

Other names for insulin resistance are metabolic syndrome, CHAOS (in Australia) cardiometabolic syndrome and syndrome X. But whatever you call it, one quick way to gauge if you likely have it is simply to measure your waist. If you are a male with a waist of more than 40 inches, or a woman with a waist of more than 35 inches, then you most likely have insulin resistance.[1]

For a more thorough assessment, the American Association of Clinical Endocrinologists has established the clinical criteria for insulin resistance[2] as:

- Body mass index 25 or higher
- Triglyceride level of 150 mg/dL or higher
- HDL cholesterol of less than 40 mg/dL in men or less than 50 mg/dL in women
- Blood pressure of 130/85 or higher
- Fasting glucose level of 110 to 125 mg/dL

Insulin resistance is also a condition of chronic inflammation, and chronic inflammation is a notorious gateway to chronic disease. For more information on this aspect of chronic inflammation, please see my first book, *Feel Good Look Younger: Reversing Tiredness Through Hormonal Balance*.

To learn more on diagnosing insulin resistance, please refer to Appendix A of this book. For more information on fat, please see Chapter 3 of this book.

Insulin Resistance and the Brain

Insulin helps bring glucose into your cells, and—as we are just beginning to learn—into your brain. This is noteworthy since it has long been believed insulin was only needed below the brain for metabolism. Now that insulin receptors have been identified in the brain, for the first time, insulin has been shown to cross the blood brain barrier to affect brain metabolism.[3-4]

A high level of insulin is a lethal disease associated with early heart disease or dementia. Within the next ten years, it is predicted there will be an explosion of dementia or severe memory loss due to insulin resistance. Who knows if this will break our current health care system, which is already strained.

One of the most common causes of dementia is Alzheimer's disease. Although I am not an expert in neurology, one of the pillars for obtaining Alzheimer's disease is having insulin resistance. Alzheimer's disease is a heterogeneous disease consisting of genetic defects of the Apolipoprotein E4 gene or the clusterin gene, multiple infarct or multiple small strokes of the brain, and insulin resistance—which is the biggest part.[5-9]

In the Rotterdam Study they found that levels of insulin and insulin resistance were associated with a higher risk of developing Alzheimer's disease. The most amazing finding was that insulin resistance influences the clinical manifestation of Alzheimer's disease within three years![10]

In my first book, *Feel Good Look Younger: Reversing Tiredness Through Hormonal Balance*, the main theme of the book is to achieve optimal health by reducing chronic inflammation. In Alzheimer's disease, the root problem is inflammation of the brain.[11-12] Furthermore, there is high level of insulin or insulin resistance in Alzheimer's disease.[13]

It has been mentioned in medical literature that Alzheimer's disease is a type 3 diabetes or diabetes of the brain. (Type 1 diabetes is where one is deficient on insulin and depends on insulin for survival and type 2 diabetes does not depend on insulin for survival.) With the high levels of inflammation of the brain this eventually leads to the formation and deposition of Amyloid plaques and tangles.[14]

Amyloid is a protein your body normally makes. In the healthy brain, the amyloid plaques are normally broken down and eliminated. By the way, the genetic defect of the clusterin gene has to do with eliminating the amlyoid plaques. If you have the genetic defect of the clusterin gene, then your risk of Alzheimer's disease is much higher than the normal population.

As for the tangles that are formed in the brain cells of Alzeheimer's disease, these are twisted fibers that destroy the microtubule structures, which are involved with transporting nutrients from one part of the nerve cell to another. Thus, without proper nutrients, your brain cells will slowly die off, as illustrated below.[15]

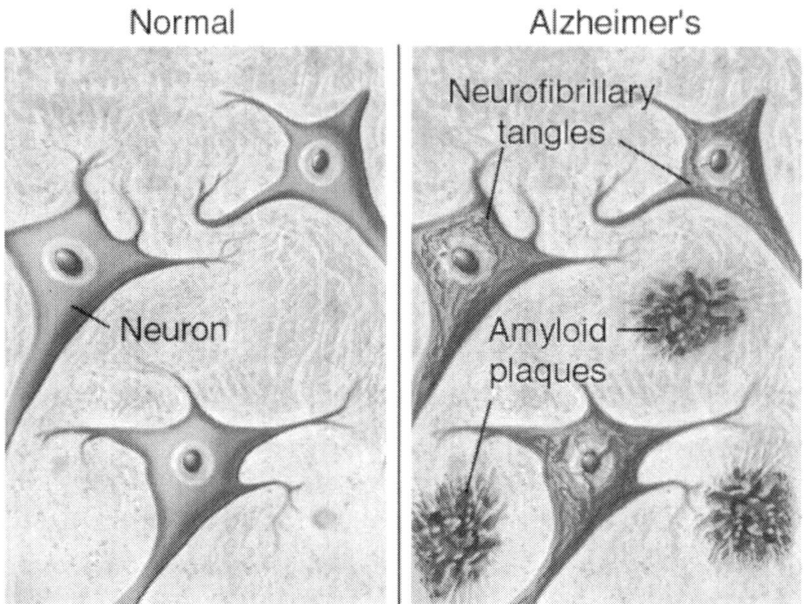

Recently, one of my professional golfer patients wanted to know if he was going to get Alzheimer's disease—since both his parents developed Alzheimer's disease. Some of the tests I did were to screen for insulin resistance—a genetic test called the Apolipoprotein E (ApoE) gene. Studies have shown that if you have two of the copies of the Apo E4 gene, then the risk is between 10 to 30 times of developing Alzheimer's disease by age 75. Apo E comes in different forms like E2, E3 or E4. It is believed Apo E4 does not break down the Amyloid plaque in the brain as well as Apo E2 or E3.[16]

He unfortunately has the double hit of the Apo E4 gene, which increases his risk. I can't change his genes, but the most important thing he can do is to reverse insulin resistance, and the good news is that insulin resistance is reversible.

I should point out that not only is insulin resistance involved with Alzheimer's disease, it is associated with depression, autism, schizophrenia and Parkinson's.[17-20]

Although not everyone with Alzheimer's, Parkinson's, depression, autism or schizophrenia will have insulin resistance, the clear majority of them will. The underlying treatment should focus on the root problem of the disease rather than treating the symptoms. Unfortunately, the concept of functional medicine, or figuring out the root problem, is not yet widely accepted in conventional medicine.

The body truly is the most complex and amazing machine, and the brain is the most remarkable organ in that machine—proven every day by people everywhere. However, the brain is nothing more than a metabolic living organ, which means there are many ways for it to die or become impaired, as with dementia.

I often think of the brain as having a thousand light bulbs. When we are young and active, all those light bulbs are lit up. When you start losing memory, then some of these light bulbs don't light up anymore. Then, by the time conventional medicine has diagnosed you with dementia, you have damage to the wiring of the light bulbs, or your light bulbs have burned out. Unfortunately, if you wait until conventional medicine has diagnosed you with dementia, then it's too late to reverse the damage. However, please know that serious memory loss is not a part of the normal aging process.

Insulin Resistance, Erectile Dysfunction and Heart Disease

So, insulin resistance can cause belly fat, dementia, loss of memory, depression, autoimmune disease, strokes, infertility, neurodegenerative brain disease and—it is directly related to the one thing that will most likely kill you—heart disease. Dr. Gerald Reaven, an Endocrinologist from Stanford University, gave a talk in 1988 at the American Diabetes Association meeting. Reavan discussed how syndrome X (now known as insulin resistance) could be a predictor of heart disease. Later, a landmark study in 1996 showed that insulin resistance is indeed an important predictor of heart disease.[21]

There are many pathways, or mechanisms, through which insulin resistance can cause heart disease. A common theme is that insulin resistance is a pro-inflammatory condition—or, in other words, it is the source of chronic inflammation. As mentioned before, chronic inflammation is the gateway of chronic disease. Insulin resistance activates the pro-inflammatory pathway for increasing the development of atherosclerosis of the heart arteries. Some of the markers of inflammation that have been shown to be elevated are CRP (C-reactive protein), TNF (tumor necrosis factor) and IL-6 (interleukin-6).

In addition, the elevated levels of insulin can stimulate a special, bad fat called visceral fat. Visceral fat produces markers of inflammation—as well as special hormones made in the fat cells (leptin, adiponectin and resistin). This cascade of increased markers of inflammation then produces a condition of endothelial dysfunction and atherosclerosis.[22]

Atherosclerosis is a condition in which an artery wall is filled up with plaque, or a fatty material with cholesterol, and the white blood cells that responded to the chronic inflammation of the artery wall.

Insulin resistance accelerates atherosclerosis. If the plaque ruptures from the artery wall, then a larger clot can form and cause complete blockage of the artery and lead to death of the tissue within five minutes. This is the final step in having a heart attack or stroke caused by loss of blood supply. A reliable test to see if you are going to have a heart attack or stroke—due to a loss of blood supply—is to have a lipoprotein phospholipase A2 (Lp-PLA2) blood test to determine if the plaque is prone to rupture.[23]

While endothelial dysfunction sounds like erectile dysfunction, or ED, they are different yet very similar. As almost everyone knows, erectile dysfunction is male impotence, or a condition characterized by an inability to develop or maintain an erection. Erectile dysfunction is actually a precursor of early heart disease. Medical studies have shown that men with erectile dysfunction have a higher chance of having a heart attack.[24]

Thus, low testosterone and insulin resistance should be identified in patients with erectile dysfunction, and should be corrected to lower the risk of heart disease.

Endothelial dysfunction is an important complication of insulin resistance. It is a condition where the inside of the blood vessels lose their elasticity (their ability to dilate). In certain conditions, you want the blood vessels to dilate and bring more oxygen to an area. Endothelial dysfunction is a precursor of atherosclerosis and is associated with most cardiovascular disease—such as hypertension, coronary artery disease, chronic heart failure, peripheral artery disease, diabetes and chronic renal failure. Endothelial dysfunction is characterized with the reduction of the production of nitric oxide.[25] Erectile dysfunction has been associated with endothelial dysfunction.[26]

Treatment with Viagra® actually increases the production of nitric oxide to help the penis vessels to dilate and cause an erection. Viagra® has helped millions of men with erectile dysfunction; however, it is really not addressing the root problem of their erectile dysfunction, which is endothelial dysfunction from insulin resistance. The key is to treat the insulin resistance and other causes of the chronic inflammation to improve on the endothelial dysfunction.

To recap, insulin resistance can cause brain damage, heart disease, stroke, erectile dysfunction (in men), belly fat and—the next subject I am addressing, cancer.

Insulin Resistance and Cancer

High levels of insulin have been closely related to breast cancer and colon cancer. What's more, it has been noted that prostate cancer is likewise associated with insulin resistance.[27]

High doses of human insulin used in the laboratory have been found to promote cancer. In 2000, the FDA approved a long-acting insulin called glargine (marketed as Lantus® insulin) to help diabetics control their blood sugars. Currently there is a hot and heavy debate whether this particular insulin can cause cancer—thanks to several studies done in Germany, England, Sweden and Scotland that were published in 2009—trying to see if there was a relationship between insulin (Lantus® in particular) and cancer.

The concern is that Lantus® insulin can increase the binding to the insulin-like growth factor-1 (IGF-1) receptor about eight times more than human insulin and stimulate cell growth. In the Sweden study during 2006 and 2007 it showed how women using glargine insulin had an increased risk of breast cancer.[28]

In the German study it was shown how glargine insulin also had a higher incidence of cancer.[29] In the Scottish study there was no association of increased cancer and the use of glargine.[30] In the UK study there was higher risk of colorectal and pancreatic cancer with the use of insulin.[31]

These recent studies have caused much debate in the diabetes world. Currently, the FDA, American Diabetes Association, American Association of Clinical Endocrinologists and the European Association for the Study of Diabetes have all formally stated that patients should continue to use glargine insulin until more information is available. Long-term studies are needed to answer if this particular insulin can cause cancer. However, high levels of insulin—or insulin resistance—have already been linked to cancer.

My personal opinion on insulin resistance increasing the risk of cancer is that insulin resistance is definitely part of the overall problem. The high levels of insulin stimulating the IGF-1 receptor for cell growth, high levels of inflammation, oxidative stress and the generation of free radicals are contributing to the pathway of cancer. Moreover, a weak liver that does not detox well (or eliminate free radicals and toxins) can lead to damage of the most precious material you have in your body—your DNA.

Once you damage your DNA, that damage can then "turn on" cancer growth. Even the 2010 President's cancer panel has said environmental toxins are a greater cause of cancer than previously believed.[32]

Insulin Resistance and PCOS

A classic connection with insulin resistance is polycystic ovary syndrome (PCOS). This is a condition in women that is presented with acne, irregular periods, extra hair on the face, weight gain and patches of dark skin on the back of the neck called acanthosis nigricans. Acanthosis nigricans is a dermatologic disorder of too much insulin (or insulin resistance) that activates the insulin receptors in the skin, forcing it to grow abnormally.

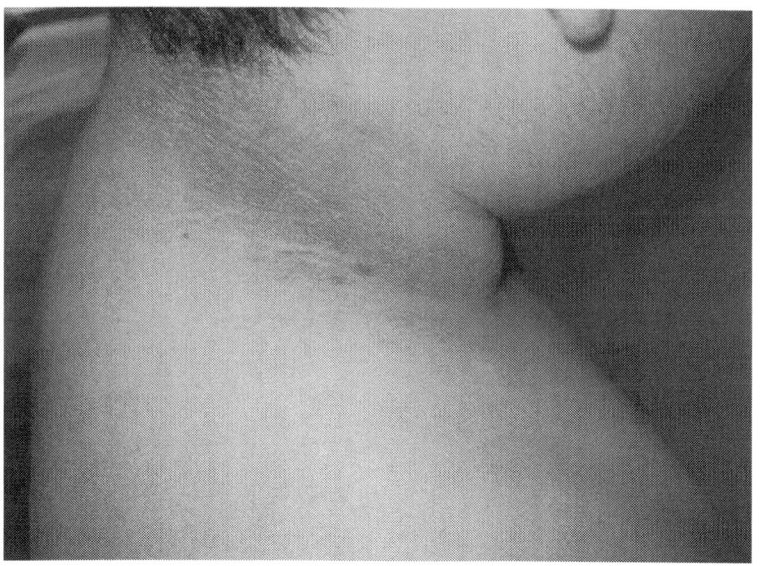

Acanthosis Nigricans (darkening of the skin on the back of the neck) is a sign of insulin resistance.

In addition, PCOS can cause many women to have problems with fertility. It is estimated that five million women of childbearing years have PCOS, and it affects about 10 to 20 percent of women.

The reason women with PCOS have issues with acne and fertility issue is that insulin resistance "turns on" the ovaries to make more testosterone, which causes unwanted hair growth and acne. Additionally, in PCOS there is an elevation of a hormone called LH that controls ovulation, and in PCOS there is no surge of LH so there is no ovulation and the periods are irregular. In my practice I have helped women get pregnant by reducing their insulin resistance, which in turn will improve on their PCOS. Unfortunately, many women with PCOS who are not treated for their insulin resistance will become diabetic over time, or develop early heart disease.

Because chronic inflammation is involved with PCOS, the resulting combination of high insulin and high glucose generates oxidative stress, as well as free radicals. This will turn on the master switch for inflammation—called nuclear factor kappa beta (NFKB). Women with PCOS have markers of inflammation in their blood that are elevated (not a good sign)—like TNF, IL-6 and CRP.[33]

With the high markers of inflammation in PCOS patients, it has been shown there is a higher level of triglycerides (a form of fat), higher insulin levels and higher blood pressures. The high insulin levels again promote belly fat; and, with this condition of high inflammation, these women have a higher risk of developing diabetes, atherosclerosis and heart disease.[34]

Insulin Resistance and Diabetes

Something I need to clarify is that insulin resistance starts before you develop pre-diabetes—and insulin resistance still exists should you become diabetic. There are about 60 million Americans with diabetes and it is still growing—even exploding, in our children. The majority of those 60 million Americans have type 2 diabetes, which results from insulin resistance and is sometimes combined with a deficiency of insulin.

I think every person with insulin resistance should spend some time or volunteer in a diabetic clinic or in a dialysis unit, just so they can see, firsthand, the horrible complications caused by diabetes. Maybe then they will realize how serious insulin resistance is.

Some of the complications of uncontrolled diabetes range from early heart disease, strokes, blindness, amputations of toes and even legs. There are more complications of diabetes, but the reason for the complications of diabetes is that the high blood glucose is like broken glass floating in your blood. This can cause nerve and blood vessel damage and can affect any organ in the body. This in turn will turn on more chronic inflammation in the body, which is not healthy. One of the worst complications is called hypoglycemic unawareness, which is usually in type 1 diabetes but can be in type 2 diabetes. It is a debilitating condition where one does not recognize when their blood sugar is dropping, and so it can lead to passing out or having a seizure.

I remember a very humbling experience with one of my diabetic patients. He was a physician with type 1 diabetes (no insulin production), and he kept passing out at work because he wanted to keep his blood sugars under tight control to prevent the complications of diabetes. Unfortunately, he lost the ability to recognize low blood sugars. Usually, if a person has low blood sugar, there are warning signs of sweating, tremors, headache, pallor, dilated eyes, difficulty speaking, dry mouth or confusion.

The physician was eventually fired from his job since he was scaring the patients when he would pass out, have a seizure and 911 had to be called. He soon moved to Florida to be with his mother who was retired and, despite changing him to the best insulin and technology at the time, he failed the insulin pump and later was found in his house seizing for over twelve hours. His last grand mal seizure fried his brain and he eventually died in the hospital from many complications. Unfortunately, he passed away at a young age of 40 and all he wanted to do was practice medicine to help others.

Another complication of diabetes that sticks out in my memory is the time I had to deny someone a driver's license because they had a low blood sugar and had passed out at the wheel, causing an accident. I really felt bad and sympathized with them because to live without a car is like taking your freedom away, but I had to consider the safety of other motorists and bystanders.

Another complication I will never forget happened when a young grandmother—who could not recognize her low blood glucose levels—was not allowed (because of safety concerns) to babysit her grandchildren. I could probably write an entire book on the complications of diabetes that I have seen, but I just wanted to end with this last case of a chef who had his own restaurant—one of the best in town. He lost one eye from diabetes and soon was losing his other eye from diabetes and had to quit because of his poor vision.

Diabetes is like a sugar cancer, and it will attack you from head to toe. If you currently have insulin resistance (pre-diabetes) then you really have to take this condition seriously because your best chance to reverse it (before it goes from "pre-" into full-blown diabetes) is with lifestyle modification. Also, should you even suspect you may have pre-diabetes, please have yourself checked out.

Insulin Levels and Longevity

At a cellular level, the mechanisms inside our cells are also affected by insulin resistance. At the cellular level, insulin resistance decreases a vital protein for cell survival—the transcription factor protein known as the cyclic-AMP response element binding (CREB) protein. CREB has many functions in many different organs, and has mostly been studied in the brain.[35]

A study—using mice genetically engineered to have no CREB in their brain—was performed to see if the lack of CREB affected their offspring. In this study, the CREB was not present in the developing mouse embryos and the offspring died immediately. CREB has some unique functions, and one of them is cell survival.[36] So, who wants cells that do not survive?

Conversely, in the famous Baltimore Longitudinal Study of Aging (BLSA) it was found that low insulin levels are linked to longevity.[37]

The joke I often tell my patients is, "The people who live the longest have one thing in common, and it doesn't matter if they're from Europe, Asia or South America. The one thing they have in common is they don't speak English." Actually, the thing they do have in common is they have very low insulin levels. Most of these people are not on hormones or any supplements, but they do eat very healthy and consume very few refined sugars.

A book called, *The Blue Zones: Lessons for Living Longer From the People Who've Lived the Longest*, by Dan Buettner, looks at the areas around the world with the longest longevity. Blue Zones are regions where people live beyond the age of 100 and have very active lives. Some of these areas are Okinawa, Japan, Sardinia, Italy, Loma Linda, California, Nicoya Peninsula, Costa Rica and Ikaria, Greece.

The people living in the Blue Zones have several lifestyle characteristics contributing to their health. Those characteristics include: the practice that family comes first; no smoking, plant based diet (thus, low insulin levels); moderate physical activity and social engagement (where people of all ages are socially active and integrated into their communities). We could probably all learn from the secrets of people living in the Blue Zones.

"The proof that Dr. Lee has helped me is in these test results."

I found Dr. Lee in mid-2009 through a friend. My friend and I are both health-aware, and take care of ourselves by eating right and exercising. I'd had surgery six months prior, and although healing fine, I didn't feel quite like my self. I've always had high energy and been optimistic, but now I had trouble sleeping and felt tired and anxious.

Dr. Lee ran several tests and he found I had an imbalance in my estrogen and progesterone levels, as well as low serotonin levels. I'd brought him my recent DEXA scan recording on my bone density, and my recent thyroid scan depicting a troubling nodule. Dr. Lee recommended supplements and hormones to address all my issues. I immediately regained my optimistic outlook and started sleeping again. He adjusted my supplements and hormones as my test results warranted, and he carefully monitored my progress.

In 2010, our family had some devastating news. Cancer had reoccurred in my sister and only sibling. The stress of her illness, and then her death later that year, caused me to experience inflammation in my digestive tract. I lost ten pounds I could ill-afford to lose. Dr. Lee put me on a probiotic (a powdered medical food) as well as intravenous vitamin infusions. I can only imagine how sick I would have been without this intervention. All this was followed and approved by my gastrointestinal doctor.

By the end of 2010, I'd regained my weight. The gastrointestinal doctor gave me a clean bill of health, saying the crisis was over and my intestinal tract was well. The endocrinologist, who'd monitored my thyroid for twelve years had even better news—the nodule was no longer there. Best of all, my December 2010 DEXA scan done at Mayo Clinic showed a six percent increase in the density of my spine—the first increase in bone density in 20 years. I've also stopped having urinary tract infections, which had plagued me for decades—and I now endure much fewer, and less severe, respiratory ailments.

I'd say the proof that Dr. Lee has helped me is in these test results, as well as in the way I feel. I'm better and stronger than I've ever been. Dr. Lee is knowledgeable and caring, and celebrates his patients' successes—the best of concierge medicine. I'm so glad to be his patient!

— *Kyle Miller*

Insulin Resistance and Autoimmune Disease

Your immune system is under constant battle (self-defense mode for fighting enemies such as virus, bacteria, parasites, yeast) round the clock. Sometimes a glitch occurs where the immune system mistakes some part of your body as a foreign substance and starts attacking it. An analogy of this is like "friendly fire," where the immune system starts attacking our own body, and that is why it's called autoimmune disease.

There are many different autoimmune diseases that can affect any part of the body—including the blood system, the brain, the joints, the ear, the digestive track and even the lungs. Some of the autoimmune diseases associated with insulin resistance are rheumatoid arthritis, ulcerative colitis, lupus and ankylosing spondylitis.

Although this is not yet widely accepted, I truly believe the cause for many autoimmune diseases has to do with a leaky gut (intestinal hyperpermeability). Usually, a leaky gut is caused from delayed food intolerance(s)—and there are some foods you can eat that will cause an immune reaction (where your intestinal wall opens up and leaks bacteria, microbes and toxins into your blood system).

My theory on this is that since insulin resistance can cause endothelial injury (blood vessel injury), then insulin resistance can damage the intestinal permeability that can lead to or worsen a leaky gut. With insulin resistance and a leaky gut, this produces the "perfect storm" for the immune system to be altered and thus, an autoimmune disease can develop.[38-40]

Furthermore, a leaky gut can over-stimulate your immune system to start attacking your own body. One such classic disease is celiac disease, where gluten in the diet can cause an autoimmune disease of the small intestine and it has trouble absorbing nutrients. The treatment is the avoidance of gluten (a certain protein found in rye, wheat and barley).[41]

In this way, food intolerance can be the cause of autoimmune disorder. Dr. Loren Cordain, author of *The Paleo Diet*, explains, "All autoimmune diseases develop because of interactions between the genes and one or more environmental factors, such as a viral or bacterial infection or exposure to a certain food."

Surprisingly, we have found that many common gut bacteria fragments are made up of the same molecular building blocks as those found in certain immune system proteins, and in some of the tissues under attack by the immune system. This three-way matchup—of gut bacteria or food protein, immune system protein and body tissue protein—may confuse the immune system, causing it to attack the body's own tissue.

A clear example of this is where gluten can cause celiac disease (autoimmune disease of the intestine) in certain patients who have the genes prone for celiac disease. Not everyone develops celiac disease when one eats gluten, but if you have the gene for it, then you can increase the chance of developing it if you overeat foods high in gluten.

Patients with rheumatoid arthritis have a four times higher risk of dying early with heart disease. Similar to patients with rheumatoid arthritis, patients with lupus also have a higher risk of dying from heart disease, which is even higher (up to eight times higher) in younger patients. For patients with rheumatoid arthritis and lupus, there is higher rate of metabolic syndrome—and, higher levels of inflammation in the blood have been shown to lead to a higher risk of developing a clot that can cause an early heart attack.[42]

Most autoimmune diseases are treated with prednisone to decrease the inflammation, but I am not sure that prednisone is actually getting to the root problem (which may be a leaky gut). A recent article showed how using prednisone in a dose over 7.5 mg a day increased insulin levels, while increasing insulin resistance. The authors believe the use of prednisone may even contribute to the cardiovascular risk.[43]

A study done in South Africa (on patients with rheumatoid arthritis who were also insulin resistant) tested a diet that combined these two things: eating fish four times a week and reducing sugar intake. After three months on this healthy diet, the markers for inflammation improved, insulin resistance improved, cholesterol levels improved and obesity levels were reduced—and, because this diet lowered insulin levels dramatically, it reduced their risk of an early death from heart disease.[44]

Another article has noted how the Mediterranean diet improves insulin resistance, increases longevity, lowers blood pressure and reduces the risk of early death from heart disease or cancer. In addition, it notes there is evidence the Mediterranean diet lowers insulin levels, and that fish intake can help patients with rheumatoid arthritis. Also, the combination of fish and olive oil in a diet has improved joint pain, handgrip strength and other variables among rheumatoid arthritis patients.[45]

Conclusion

The real beauty of treating insulin resistance is how changing your lifestyle habits will change your life. It sounds easy, but you really have to work at it. Like anything in life, if you put in the effort, then the results will come. You can't just buy your health, you have to respect your body and work at it daily. Moreover, the key is in education; so, if you have read this far, then you probably know more than most of your doctors about insulin resistance (the key root problem for early brain loss, heart disease, hypertension, PCOS, endothelial dysfunction, obesity, male impotence, diabetes and early cell death).

The key in your life (and to reducing your belly fat) is to reduce your insulin levels. I personally think that, as a country, we have a food addiction, which makes this matter so much more difficult to address. As I mentioned before, we are failing as a society to be healthy. For the past 40 years we have all gotten heavier—including our children and the elderly. Food addiction should be on our radar like the addiction of alcohol, gambling and tobacco. Just watch the commercials on television and see how many commercials are sponsored by the food industry. Now count how many commercials you see that promote healthy eating with organic foods, or grass-fed cattle, or non-farmed fish, and then you'll clearly see how the food industry wins when it comes to advertising their products.

The secret to successfully reducing insulin resistance—or lowering your insulin levels—lies in what we put in our mouths. Most people tend to have a high intake in refined sugars or white foods. For example, breakfast for most people will include oatmeal, cereals, grits, bagels, toast, pancakes, French toast or a breakfast sandwich with a tall glass of orange juice or a diet soda. There is absolutely nothing nutritious in such a breakfast. Likewise, timing of the meal is crucial. You need to have your largest meal in the morning and the smallest in the evening. How many of us skip breakfast because we're not hungry? The most important meal (like you've heard before) is breakfast. However if you overindulge at nighttime, by morning your body is still trying to digest that food and is telling your brain that you are not hungry in the morning. The advice I tell my patients is to do a modified fast by skipping dinner and drinking water throughout the night. You should wake up more hungry in the morning and then you can reset your eating habits.

My goal is for you to understand that refined carbohydrates will spike your insulin levels and higher insulin levels will promote fat storage. If you want to lose the belly fat, then you need to exchange your grains for greens. I recommend having two to three servings of vegetables (except for corn and carrots, which will spike your insulin levels) with each meal—including breakfast.

When I tell my patients to eliminate their high carbohydrate breakfast and avoid breads, pasta, rice, cereals, oatmeal, and potatoes, they look at me and ask, "Then what will I eat?" The answer is in the back of this book. It's a two-step diet. The first step is a four-week program that is low in refined carbohydrates. The second step is a reintroduction of whole grains—while still trying to avoid the white foods (white sins).

CHAPTER 2 REVIEW

— Insulin resistance is a condition where the muscles, fat cells, liver, brain and other organs that need insulin now require a higher level of insulin. For example, if a healthy person takes one molecule of insulin to lower glucose by ten points, then an insulin resistant person will need ten molecules of insulin to lower their glucose by ten points. In other words, the body's cells are resistant to the insulin's action.

— High levels of insulin are a sign of insulin resistance.

— High insulin levels are in fact a lethal disease that is associated with Alzheimer's disease, impotence, heart disease, infertility, polycystic ovary syndrome, endothelial dysfunction (early blood vessel disease where the blood vessel becomes stiff), stroke, cancer, autoimmune disease, shorter longevity and diabetes.

— I recommend having two to three servings of vegetables (except for corn and carrots, which will spike your insulin levels) with each meal, including breakfast.

— To learn more about how to diagnosis insulin resistance, see Appendix A. An optimal fasting insulin level is less than five microIU/ml.

3

Fighting an Epidemic Battle of the Bulge

"Don't dig your grave with your own knife and fork."

— *English Proverb*

The one question I most often hear—even after adding years to someone's life and improving their health—is, "How can I lose my belly fat?"

Although the most common patient complaint is about always being tired, "How can I lose my belly fat?" is definitely the most asked question. Ironically, as it turns out, tiredness and belly fat are partners in crime.

There are two types of fat in humans: brown fat (brown adipose tissue) and white fat (white adipose tissue). When compared to white fat, brown fat has many more blood vessels and mitochondria (the machinery in our cells that produces energy). Babies, since they cannot shiver, have an abundance of brown fat to keep them warm and help them survive. As the infant grows, its brown fat will diminish.

An interesting fact is that an adult rodent has a considerable amount of brown fat, whereas most adult humans have very little brown fat. The question I have is, why does brown fat tend to disappear as we age? A recent article has addressed the interesting finding that adults with low levels of brown fat have higher levels of obesity, insulin resistance and cardiovascular disease—whereas, adults with higher levels of brown fat maintain lower body weight and exhibit superior health as they age. Currently, two of the best ways to increase your level of brown fats are: restrict your amount of calories while increasing the level of your active lifestyle. As for the future, there is now research in age management that is using stem cell injections to increase levels of brown fat.[1]

Understanding Belly Fat

The belly has two types of fat: subcutaneous (underneath the skin) fat—which makes up about 80 percent of all body fat—and visceral (around the organs) fat.

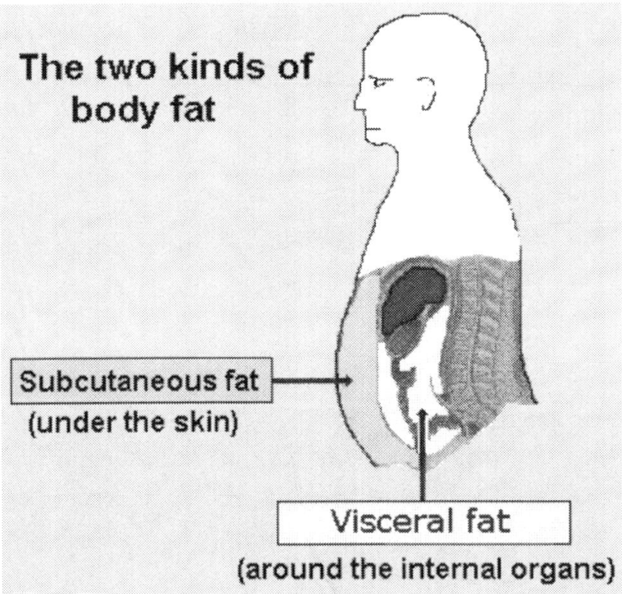

Recent studies have shown that levels of visceral fat are associated with insulin resistance and inflammation.

The best way to see how much visceral fat you have is with a computed tomography (CT) or an MRI scan. While such scans are used in research studies of fat, it would not be cost effective in clinical practice—not to mention the higher risk of radiation. A more practical way is to indirectly look at visceral fat by measuring your blood fasting insulin level, glucose and triglyceride—or by simply measuring your waist size.

Visceral fat (deeper fat in the belly) is very dangerous since it is associated with insulin resistance. The more visceral fat you have, the higher your insulin resistance will be. By the way, subcutaneous fat is not associated with insulin resistance.

In a recent 2011 study, it was shown that only visceral fat—and not subcutaneous fat—is associated with insulin resistance. Also, the more visceral fat that a person has is associated with more inflammation markers—like TNF (Tumor Necrosis Factor), CRP (C-reactive protein) and oxidized LDL (low density lipoprotein, or "bad" cholesterol). Furthermore more visceral fat causes to lower a protective hormone called adiponectin (not a good sign) and a worsening of endothelial dysfunction—with thickening of the carotid artery (stiffness to the main artery to the brain).[2]

Another study examined 40 overweight premenopausal women and showed how only visceral fat—and not subcutaneous fat—is associated with insulin resistance. Interestingly, there was no association noted for insulin resistance and how physically fit they were.[3]

In medical school I learned that fat cells are storage for energy, and that fat cells do not increase in number but only in size. Now, with newer research, it has been shown how obesity increases the size and the number of fat cells. Different, as well, from what I learned in medical school is how visceral fat is now considered an endocrine gland, and that it's involved with insulin resistance.

Recently, it has been shown how visceral fat releases several hormones—like leptin, resistin and adiponectin. A quick note on leptin is that it was the first fat hormone identified, and it is involved with food intake. As for adiponectin, it's involved with insulin sensitivity and helps lower fatty acids in your body. Having low levels of adiponectin correlates with high insulin levels and insulin resistance.

Resistin was discovered in 2001 and termed resistin because of the observed insulin resistance in mice injected with it. High levels of resistin are associated with insulin resistance and with obesity.

Visceral fat also releases chemicals called cytokines, which stimulate the immune system and inflammation. They secrete several chemicals like TNF, plasminogen activator inhibitor type 1 and IL-6 (interleukin-6), which promotes the blood to thicken up (not desirable) and to promote more inflammation (also not desirable).[4]

By the way, if someone undergoes liposuction to help "sculpt" their body, it only removes the subcutaneous fat and has no effect on visceral fat. I know there are people who want to take the easy way out, and perhaps someone is considering surgery to remove their inner fat, but a recent study showed that surgery to remove visceral fat did not improve on insulin resistance. Additionally, the study concluded that removing higher volumes of visceral fat is technically difficult and potentially dangerous.[5]

However, the good news is that you can reduce your visceral fat by improving your nutrition and increasing physical activity, which will be discussed later in this chapter.

"I am now completely off the three major prescriptions."

Dr. Lee gave me back my life, literally. He saved me from the total fatigue and exhaustion that made it difficult to function each day. Plus—as if that wasn't enough—I now have tons of energy, and I look great after losing 22 pounds! I get compliments almost daily from coworkers and friends.

It has been five years since Dr. Lee got me to my healthy weight and lifestyle. Because of that, I am now completely off the three major prescriptions I had been taking for 20 years.

Dr. Lee is incredible for helping me build such a healthy lifestyle!

— Debbie Cook

Causes of Belly Fat

Belly fat, or simply being overweight, has many causes. I consider belly fat a symptom rather than a disease. So, to address it, one has to look for the cause. For example, with some people it is more about what is "eating them," being a bigger issue than what "they are eating." In those cases, the solution lies in figuring out how they can deal with the stress so they don't instead overindulge in wasted calories.

Also, the fast food industry has inexpensive, high-calorie foods that—although convenient—are "supersizing" us. I do admit I have had my share of fast food, but that was before I learned about proper nutrition.

Another cause is lack of physical activity. I often hear, "I was fit in high school and played sports, but now I can't even climb a flight of stairs without getting short of breath." One concept I encourage in all my patients is to develop an active lifestyle. Some people just have a slow metabolism with a sluggish thyroid, but by optimizing their thyroid they can lose weight as well. Others may have poor digestion and are very constipated, but if I can help them to have daily bowel movements that produce a complete evacuation, then they can reduce their belly fat.

There are other causes of weight gain—besides being sedentary and having poor diet. Cushing Syndrome is an endocrine condition where someone has too much production of cortisol, which can cause weight gain and the development of diabetes. Other endocrine conditions are growth hormone deficiency and testosterone deficiency—where both of those hormones (growth hormone and testosterone) are deficient and thus the person is lacking anabolic hormones, which promotes belly fat.

Another cause that has been linked to belly fat is lack of sleep. Sleep is vital for a healthy body and mind, but how many of us really sleep as much, and as well, as we need?

A rare and interesting medical condition is Prader-Willi Syndrome, which is associated with short stature and borderline low intelligence; but, with an extreme and insatiable appetite that often results in morbid obesity. While there are other rare causes of obesity, these are the more common causes.

"I find it easy to maintain my new weight."

Not sure where to start, as the benefits I've received from being treated by Dr. Lee could easily fill the pages of a book.

I first saw Dr. Lee in 2009 for a follow-up on my treatment for a thyroid condition. In conversation, I mentioned that my energy level wasn't all that good. He asked if I would like to do some tests to check my overall health. Saying yes was the best decision I've ever made. I never dreamed of the rewards I was about to reap from that decision.

He found I was lacking a number of things essential to good health—such as no zinc and a very low testosterone level. Dr. Lee treated me for my hormone imbalance, as well as my lack of zinc.

Since then my lifestyle and health have changed dramatically. A typical breakfast used to be fried eggs, bacon or sausage, biscuits and gravy. Now it's a boiled egg, a glass of V8® (low sodium) and some sliced cucumbers. Throughout the day, I eat vegetables, soups, salads and small portions of meat. I have lost 13 pounds since my initial visit and I find it easy to maintain my new weight. I awake each morning feeling rested, with plenty of energy.

The knowledge I've gained from Dr. Lee about diet, my body and my health has been life-changing—like winning the lottery! In seeing Dr. Lee, I not only found a great physician, but I gained a true friend.

I could go on forever, but let me simply say that Dr. Lee has changed my life, my health and my outlook on life. For example, I drag race competitively, and while at a race recently, I noticed how my reaction times were much better, and that I'm as comfortable at speeds of 200-plus miles per hour as I am at 65 miles per hour. I attribute this, and my higher confidence levels, to Dr. Lee.

I'll leave you with this thought, "There should be a law against a 64-year-old man feeling this good." Thank you again Dr. Lee!

— Darlow "Rex" Rexroat

As I said at the beginning of this chapter, the one question I most often hear is, "How can I lose my belly fat?" It does not matter what nationality you are—whether you are Asian, Caucasian, Indian, Middle Eastern—nor does your age matter, because I can help reduce your belly fat and improve your lifestyle.

You just have to be motivated and willing to change your lifestyle, and you'll need to embrace a healthy diet. You will have to sacrifice, but it is worth the effort. Remember, you can't expect to lose your belly fat by eating cake and drinking wine since both of them will increase your insulin levels, which will cause weight gain. The most important thing you can do is educate yourself on the reasons why certain foods will promote weight gain.

In the past 40 years, Americans have gotten fatter and we are failing as a society. The impact of being overweight is estimated to cost 150 billion dollars in unnecessary health expenses. With the recent passage of the new health bill, I think the bigger issue is that we need to overcome obesity—for us, but especially for the younger generation.

About 190 million Americans are overweight, which is about two out of every three. How many of us can run a mile or bike three miles without getting short of breath?

Another depressing fact is that childhood obesity has tripled, and it is now being said that we might outlive our children.

I strongly believe that terrorism will not harm our country nearly as much as having to endure the experience of our next generation—our currently overweight children—dying earlier than us from weight related heart disease or cancer.

Body Mass Index

The terms "overweight" and "obese" are defined by a simple measurement. It's called the body mass index (BMI). The BMI takes your weight in kilograms and divides it by the square of your height in meters. According to the World Health Organization (WHO), "overweight" is defined as having a BMI of equal or greater than 25, and "obesity" is having a BMI of equal or greater than 30.

height	weight in pounds 120	130	140	150	160	170	180	190	200	210	220	230	240	250
4'6"	29	31	34	36	39	41	43	46	48	51	53	56	58	60
4'8"	27	29	31	34	36	38	40	43	45	47	49	52	54	56
4'10"	25	27	29	31	34	36	38	40	42	44	46	48	50	52
5'0"	23	25	27	29	31	33	35	37	39	41	43	45	47	49
5'2"	22	24	26	27	29	31	33	35	37	38	40	42	44	46
5'4"	21	22	24	26	28	29	31	33	34	36	38	40	41	43
5'6"	19	21	23	24	26	27	29	31	32	34	36	37	39	40
5'8"	18	20	21	23	24	26	27	29	30	32	34	35	37	38
5'10"	17	19	20	22	23	24	26	27	29	30	32	33	35	36
6'0"	16	18	19	20	22	23	24	26	27	28	30	31	33	34
6'2"	15	17	18	19	21	22	23	24	26	27	28	30	31	32
6'4"	15	16	17	18	20	21	22	23	24	26	27	28	29	30
6'6"	14	15	16	17	19	20	21	22	23	24	25	27	28	29
6'8"	13	14	15	17	18	19	20	21	21	22	24	25	26	28

The BMI is the world standard for measuring obesity in men and women, age 20 and over. This version is converted to pounds and inches. The top line is weight and the vertical line on the left is height. So, if a person has a weight of 200 pounds and a height of five feet one inch, then their BMI is 38, which is considered obese. If that person were to lose 50 pounds, their BMI would drop to 28, which is considered overweight. To bring their weight into a healthy BMI, that person should weigh 120 to 125 pounds.

According to the WHO, in 2005 there were 1.6 billion overweight people in the world, with at least another 400 million considered obese. Furthermore, at least 20 million children under the age of five are overweight globally in 2005. The future projections of 2015 are even more shocking, with 2.3 billion adults projected to be overweight, with more than 700 million projected to be obese.[6]

For a perspective on those staggering projections, the current U.S. population is about 307 million, with South America at about 385 million—which means that in 2015, the number of obese people in the world will be equal to the current total population of the U.S. and South America combined!

When BMI Fails

BMI is a great tool to screen for obesity, and it's used around the world; however, a high BMI in someone who is physically fit and has low body fat may be falsely determined to be obese.

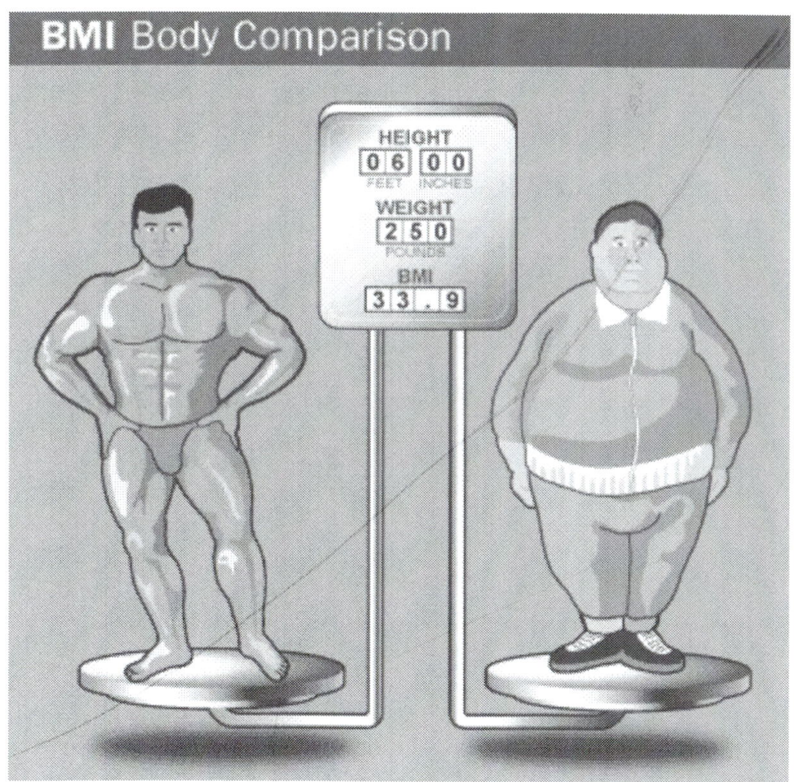

While the BMI is a valuable tool for the general population, people who are exceptionally fit may be improperly rated.

For my patients who like to work out with weights, when I calculate their BMI they are all listed as obese; however, in reality, they are not since they have a measured body fat that is low. The most important number for showing that you have low body fat is your percentage of body fat because, as you lose pounds you want to lose body fat and not muscle.

Many times, I am surprised when I evaluate a young woman who is complaining of body fat when her measurement of body fat is around 35 percent. Ideally a woman should have less than 25 percent of body fat; but, for some of my women patients, I'm happy if they are less than 30 percent. For men, their body fat should be less than 20 percent. However, if someone starts at 45 percent and then achieves a body fat of 25 percent then that is a wonderful achievement. So, body fat is relative to where you start—but the key is to reduce it.

A word of warning, though, about measuring body fat yourself at home with calipers and the bathroom scale. That method is only an estimate of your body fat, and it is usually way off. One should be directly measured with a DXA (Dual Energy X-Ray Absorptiometry) machine, which is the gold standard for measuring body fat. In fact, the television show "Biggest Loser" measures body fat with a DXA machine.

Other Considerations

While there are 190 million Americans who are overweight, the rest of the world has tons of belly fat as well. Whenever I travel overseas, I've been noticing over time how more and more people are becoming heavier. I have been to South Korea many times, and even in that country, obesity is becoming a problem. But you don't have to go overseas to see it. You can just go to any mall in the U.S. and look around.

Currently, there are approximately about 60 million Americans with pre-diabetes in the United States. A very depressing fact is that two out of every three Americans are overweight. Another depressing fact is that childhood obesity has tripled in the last thirty years. So, why are we failing as a country when it comes to battling obesity? I think the fast food industry, our government, our lack of exercise and the lack of knowledge of healthy eating are all contributing factors.

In a recent 15-year-long study called the Coronary Artery Risk Development in Young Adults (CARDIA), scientists followed 3,000 young adults between the ages of 18 and 30 years. The results showed that people who ate fast food two or more times a week experienced an average weight of ten pounds more than the ones who ate fast food less than once a week. Likewise, CARDIA showed that eating fast food increased the risk of increasing insulin levels (remember high insulin levels are not healthy) and increasing the development of diabetes.[7]

Our government is also involved with this obesity crisis. Since President Nixon's Secretary of Agriculture abolished production limits, corn farmers have been guaranteed a subsidy that provides cash to them—even if the market is flooded with corn. Corn is the basis of the fast food industry. The beef that are used in the fast food industry are fed corn grain instead of grass, sodas are made from high fructose corn syrup and french fries are fried in corn oil.[8]

Also, chicken nuggets are almost made of 60 percent corn. The U.S. government encourages farmers to specialize in corn production with its federal subsidies. So instead of our government encouraging healthy living and better health, we have a system that feeds on itself. The food industry has a source of cheap food and inexpensive oils (corn oil, or vegetable oil that has corn in it), sodas and burgers that are primarily fed by corn. Remember, corn is high in carbohydrates (or sugar) that will raise your insulin levels (not good) and thus promote weight gain or belly fat.

When it costs more to have a salad and one bottled water than it costs to have a burger, fries and a soda with free refills, then there is something wrong with the system. By the way, the heaviest place in the U.S. is not in the South, but a U.S. territory called American Samoa. Unfortunately, they've abandoned their traditional foods for cheap processed foods. So whenever you think of fast food, think of corn—the billion dollar industry.

The fast food industry says it's the consumer's choice, but it's not a fair fight since the fast food industry depends on corn, which is heavily subsidized—not to mention the billions of dollars in fast food marketing. How many commercials have you seen on national television for organic vegetables and grass-fed meats?

Another issue about fast foods is that it's filled with chemicals and preservatives. In my office, I often show patients the burger I bought from a fast food place two years ago. Even though it just sits on a shelf, not refrigerated, it has not yet degraded. The burger is hard as a rock, but there are absolutely no signs of bacteria or fungal growth. To learn more about the bionic burger, I recommend watching the video on YouTube at www.youtube.com/watch?v=mYyDXH1amic.

If you don't believe it, just buy fries and a burger at a fast food place and then a week later see if there is any decay. Have your kids do a science project and see what happens when that burger sits around at room temperature. It's not real food, but something filled with chemicals and preservatives. According to the FDA Total Diet Study, it was found that fast food hamburgers contain 113 different pesticide residues.[9]

Remember, the corn that's the food source for the cattle? That corn has been treated with pesticides and preservatives. I highly recommend watching the documentary, *King Corn*, to learn more about the relationship between the corn industry and our health.

Another disturbing fact is that a chemical called bisphenol A (BPA) has been associated with insulin resistance. BPA is a synthetic chemical widely used in the lining of cans, drink packaging, and plastic consumer products (i.e., plastic water bottles). BPA is also classified as an endocrine disrupter since it has estrogen effects, and it is considered an environmental pollutant—having been found in just-born babies. A recent 2011 study showed that women of varying body weight—from lean to obese—who have polycystic ovary syndrome have been found to have high levels of BPA. The higher BPA levels have been shown in this study to have higher insulin levels, higher testosterone levels and insulin resistance.[10]

BPA has been shown to be toxic to the pancreas, to disrupt insulin production, and to cause insulin resistance. Other chemicals like phthalates and dioxins have also been linked to insulin resistance.[11]

Conclusion

There are two types of belly fat and the worst one is called visceral fat. It surrounds the internal organs and is an active endocrine organ that secretes many hormones—such as adiponectin, leptin, resistin and other chemicals that can "turn on" inflammation in your body. Visceral fat (not the subcutaneous, under the skin, fat) is associated with insulin resistance.

The cascade of events that leads to obesity is due to elevated levels of the hormone insulin. If you have too much insulin, then this will cause you to have more insulin resistance. If you eat a lot of processed foods laden with chemicals, or foods that are high in sugar content, then that turns on the hormone insulin, which will promote more visceral fat.

This visceral fat will produce other hormones (leptin, resistin, adiponectin) and chemicals (cytokines) which will increase more inflammation, which will then cause more deposition of fat on the pancreas, liver, and muscle—and thus lead to more insulin resistance.

The food industry and our government are not helping with our major epidemic of obesity. The good news is you can reverse insulin resistance and obtain a healthy body and mind by following the nutritional plan and the supplements in this book. Also, you need to become more active in physical activity.

Remember, even surgery to remove visceral fat does nothing in terms of reducing insulin resistance. You have to change your lifestyle and choose healthier food options that are free of chemicals and preservatives.

CHAPTER 3 REVIEW

— There are two kinds of fat: subcutaneous fat (under the skin) and visceral fat (surrounding the organs).

— Visceral fat is very dangerous because it is associated with insulin resistance.

— Ever since President Nixon's Secretary of Agriculture abolished production limits, corn farmers have been guaranteed a subsidy that provides cash to them, even when the market is flooded with corn. Corn is the basis of the fast food industry.

— Another disturbing fact is that a chemical called bisphenol A (BPA) has been associated with insulin resistance. BPA is a synthetic chemical widely used in the linings of cans, drink packaging, and plastic consumer products (i.e., plastic water bottles). BPA is also classified as an endocrine disrupter since in is has estrogen effects.

— The good news is that you can reduce your visceral fat by improving your nutrition (lowering insulin levels by eating less refined sugars and eating more vegetables) and by increasing your physical activity.

4

You Cannot Not Choose Your Lifestyle

"I'll tell you one thing, you don't always have to be on the go.
I sit around a lot, I read a lot, and I do watch television.
But I also work out for two hours every day of my life,
even when I'm on the road."
— Jack LaLanne

For the most part, your health is determined by two things: genetics and lifestyle. Your genetics are handed down from your parents and will determine the obvious (such as eye color) and the not so obvious (such as propensity for certain health problems or diseases).

Your lifestyle, unlike genetics, is determined largely by you. Don't eat your vegetables, or eat your vegetables. Smoke, or don't smoke. Handle unprotected radioactive plutonium... well, you get the idea.

Now, when you put the two together—genetics and lifestyle choices—the outcome will either help you or hurt you. For example, if your genes have predetermined that you are prone to develop emphysema, then a lifestyle choice not to smoke will most probably lead to a longer life—when compared to a lifestyle choice of smoking. Just like I said on the first page of the Introduction to this book: Your genes are like a loaded gun, and your lifestyle is the trigger.

Poor lifestyle choices will definitely pull the trigger sooner and more often; and sometimes, unfortunately, whatever lifestyle you choose, that trigger might get pulled no matter what you do.

However, healthy lifestyle choices will help delay, and effectually minimize, the pulling of any genetic triggers.

What it all comes down to is that you cannot avoid making lifestyle choices every day. You get out of bed in the morning, or you don't. You recycle that plastic bottle from lunch, or you don't. You go to your 3:00 meeting, or you join a cult and move halfway around the world.

Obviously, there are many lifestyle choices you make every day. I'm going to focus on the three I see most often in my daily practice.

Choose to be Aware

I'm fortunate in that most of my patients are aware of what their bodies need and how they are changing with age. For example, many of my patients maintain an active lifestyle, and so one of the conditions I'm usually treating is sarcopenia—an age-related condition that leads to progressive loss of muscle mass and muscle strength.

While most other people would simply write off the symptoms of sarcopenia as another part of aging, my patients are aware of these changes, and are looking for a way to stop or reverse them—which I can, by the way, with hormonal balance.

As you age, your body starts breaking down your muscles to compensate for its loss of your anabolic hormones (growth hormone, testosterone, and DHEA). While strength training will only slow down that loss of muscle[1], sarcopenia can be reversed by optimizing your hormones.

As an added benefit, hormonal therapy (such as testosterone) can improve on your insulin resistance. A recent 2011 study showed that testosterone treatment not only improves body composition, but also improves on reducing insulin resistance.[2]

In the Journal of the American Medical Association, there was an article recently on a double-blind, randomized, placebo-controlled study (the gold standard of studies) that showed the use of DHEA (dehydroepiandrosterone) lowered visceral fat (bad fat) and improved on insulin resistance.[3]

In addition, there are other hormones besides testosterone that can improve on insulin resistance and help balance glucose. Some of those hormones are DHEA, thyroid and estrogen. However, you need to be monitored because too much cortisol and progesterone will make insulin resistance worse. To learn more about hormonal balance with bioidentical hormones, you should read my book, *Feel Good Look Younger: Reversing Tiredness Through Hormonal Balance*.

So, by choosing to be aware of your changing health, and by being aware of what your options are, you become an empowered, active participant in your health care.

"Now I am much more aware of my body's healthy potential."

On the recommendation from a good friend, whom Dr. Lee had treated with much success, I saw Dr. Lee about my chronic fatigue—which, at 29, is not normal. After extensive testing (compared with conventional medicine) it was found that I am deficient in progesterone, some essential nutrients and that I also have adrenal fatigue.

After making some lifestyle changes (no dairy), taking some much needed supplements and adding bio-identical progesterone and adrenal hormones to my routine, I am feeling better than I can ever remember.

Dr. Lee listens, lets me ask as many questions as I want, and gives excellent counsel about living a healthier, well-rounded life. Thanks to everything Dr. Lee has taught me, now I am much more aware of my body's healthy potential.

I feel blessed to be his patient, and I can't help but sing his praises to everyone I know.

— Krista Davenport

Choose to Exercise

A very important part of reversing insulin resistance is to become more active. Not only is exercise wonderful for burning extra calories, it also helps the body eliminate many toxins through sweating. I take great pleasure in being outside to feel the wind, snow, wind or rain.

I enjoy snowboarding, hiking, camping, swimming, cycling, running, kayaking and surfing. I've also competed in many triathlons and marathons, and have ridden my bike over 100 miles at a time for many years.

However, the saying is true that too much of any one thing is not healthy, especially when it comes to overexercising—and I have experienced many injuries, some adrenal fatigue and some oxidative damage from too much exercise. One of the worst things you can do to cause premature aging is overexercise. Some examples include burning over 4,000 calories per day, training for more than two hours per day or doing more than one marathons or one Ironman in a year.

By overtraining you will increase oxidative stress, or develop many free radicals that can damage your DNA, weaken your immune system or burn out your adrenal glands. Overexercising is an addiction and I have been an addict for many years; however, since I have kids now, I am learning to enjoy a different chapter of my life.

I still enjoy working out by swimming on a swim team, doing weights, core workouts, some short distance running and cycling. Occasionally, I run a half marathon or do an Olympic distance triathlon just to satisfy my thirst to race. I also get much exercise by coaching my kids' soccer teams.

For some of the people I see in my practice, I don't have to worry about them over-training, and I am happy if they do any type of activity at all; however, I truly believe that where there's a will, there's a way.

I remember this one story of an extremely obese woman who weighed over 500 pounds and could not leave her bedroom due to her weight. Then one day, she decided to do something about it. Because she couldn't go to a gym, she simply lifted her arms and legs as exercise, and eventually she lost a significant amount of weight. The point is that you do not have to join a gym to lose weight, but if you want to join a gym or have a personal trainer, then that's even better.

My advice when exercising is to focus on five key areas: cardio with interval workouts, strength training, balance exercises, flexibility exercises and core exercises. For example, when a new patient says they've been doing an hour on the treadmill but they can't lose any weight, I'll switch them to interval workouts of 20 to 30 minutes, and they'll accomplish weight loss.

I often recommend warming up for ten minutes and then running as fast as you can for one minute, and then walking back to where you started—repeating that five times. To make it easier, wear a watch with a timer and set it to beep once a minute.

Try to run faster each time. If you can get to a track then try to run one lap as fast as you can, and then walk one lap—then repeat that for five times.

"I no longer dread the changes of aging, or feel like decline is inevitable."

I made a commitment that I was going to run my first half-marathon on my 46th birthday. It seemed like a reasonable goal as I had been a runner for over 15 years. But as the training wore on, I began to feel it was an impossible goal. I was getting slower, and longer runs left me exhausted.

In fact, it seemed I had no energy for anything outside of work. I was having problems falling asleep and I no longer felt rested. I had always looked forward to things such as trips and outings, or time spent with my family, but now these activities seemed to exhaust me. It would have been easy for a physician to label me with depression. But I didn't feel depressed, I felt like I was... aging. Sadly, I felt like the best part of my life was behind me, and that this inevitable decline would continue.

Then a colleague suggested I see Dr. Lee. He listened to my story and we began a treatment plan. Through improved nutrition and hormonal balance I immediately felt a change. My training, my energy, my sleep, my whole atti-

tude dramatically improved. It's as if the clock has been turned back ten years. That's ten years of vigorous, energetic life that I feel was given back to me. And best of all, I no longer dread the changes of aging, or feel like decline is inevitable.

— *Rory Hession M.D.*

An important part of exercise is strength training. If you had to pick just two strength training exercises to do regularly, I'd recommend that you do pull-ups and door squats. If you don't have a pull-up bar, then do pushups—with women doing either the toes-down or the knees-down version.

One of my personal heroes has always been Jack LaLanne, who recently passed away at the age of 96. At his peak, he did over 1,000 push-ups in one try. How many push-ups can you do in one minute?

Also, you can incorporate yoga once a week in your exercise routine to help with flexibility. To prevent injuries, you need to stretch before and especially after. Many runners, like me, tend to have tight hamstrings. Yoga will help keep those hamstrings loosened up.

A goal with yoga is to touch your fingers to your toes, or even your palms to the ground. I'm not there yet with my palms to the ground, but I'm trying every day.

As always, if you need help with any of your workouts or need someone to help get you motivated, then I strongly recommend a personal trainer—especially one who focuses on exercises that deal with balance and core strength.

When it comes to really making improvements in your balance and core strength, I recommend—and enjoy using—the BOSU® Balance Trainer. It's a semicircle ball that works on your core muscles (abdomen and pelvic muscles) while it improves your balance. Try standing on it with one leg out, or with your eyes closed. The first time I had to close my eyes and stand on it, I fell off!

The BOSU® Balance Trainer comes with a wonderful DVD that makes it fun and challenging. The workouts only take about ten minutes, and the equipment does not require much floor space.

To give you an idea of how this unique and highly effective training system works, the following are nine of the exercises I like to do with my BOSU® Balance Trainer. For details on these exercise variations, please be sure to watch the BOSU® DVD or visit www.bosu.com.

As always, before beginning any new exercise routine, be sure to check with your physician before you start.

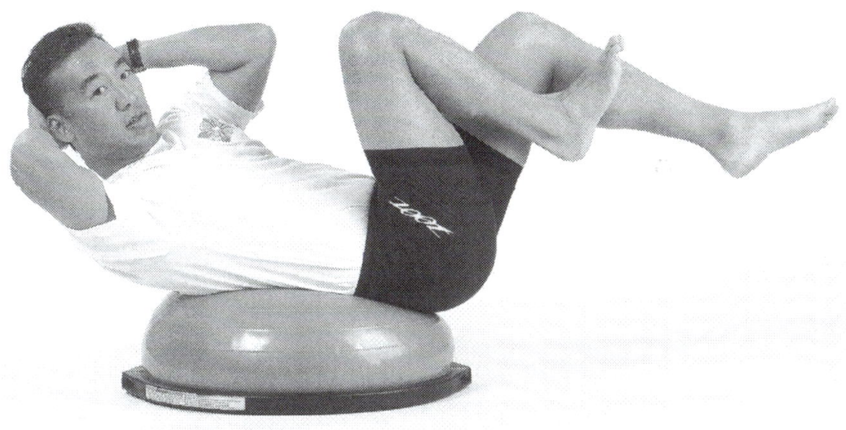

(1) Bicycle Crunches

Point and extend your left elbow toward your right knee, and then point and extend your right elbow toward your left knee. Do as many repetitions as you can until you experience "muscle fatigue," or the feeling that you simply can't do any more repetitions.

For starters, try the simpler version with your feet on the ground instead of in the air.

(2) Side Crunches

Similar to Bicycle Crunches (except that you're on your side instead of back) this exercise works on the internal and external obliques of your core muscles. It's a very unique exercise since you cannot get this range of motion on the ground; however, with the BOSU® Balance Trainer, you get a great way to work on developing these muscles.

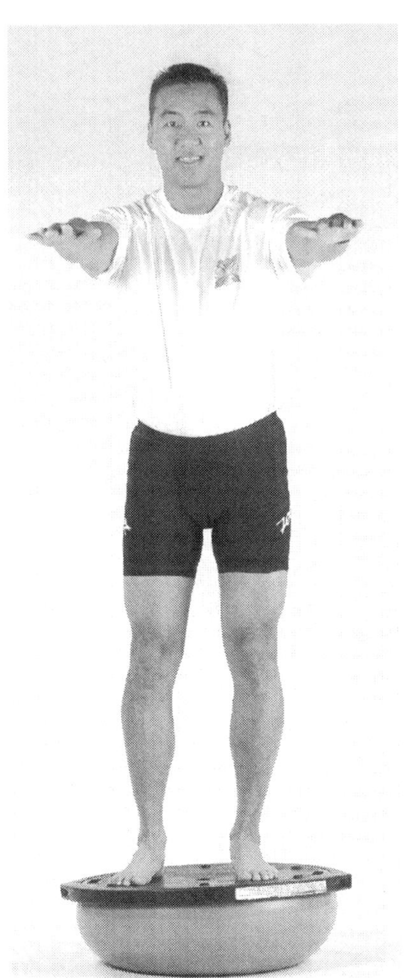

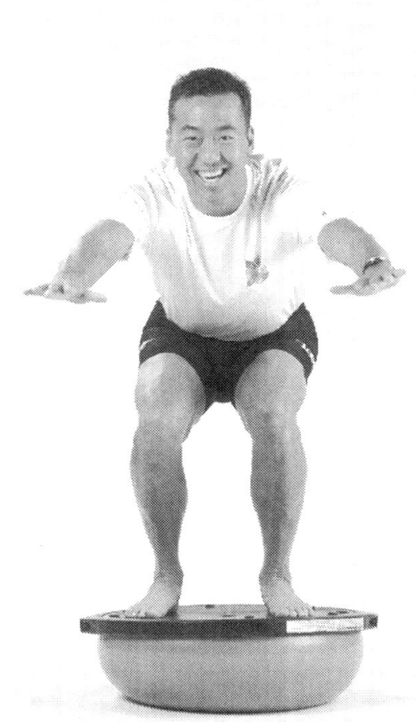

(3) Squats

You get so much more out of squats with your BOSU® Balance Trainer, and it's more challenging!

Start with your arms stretched forward and parallel to the floor. While keeping your back straight and your core muscles firm, squat down to where your upper legs come close to being parallel to the floor, but don't go any lower.

Keeping you back straight and your core muscles firm, return to upright and repeat ten times.

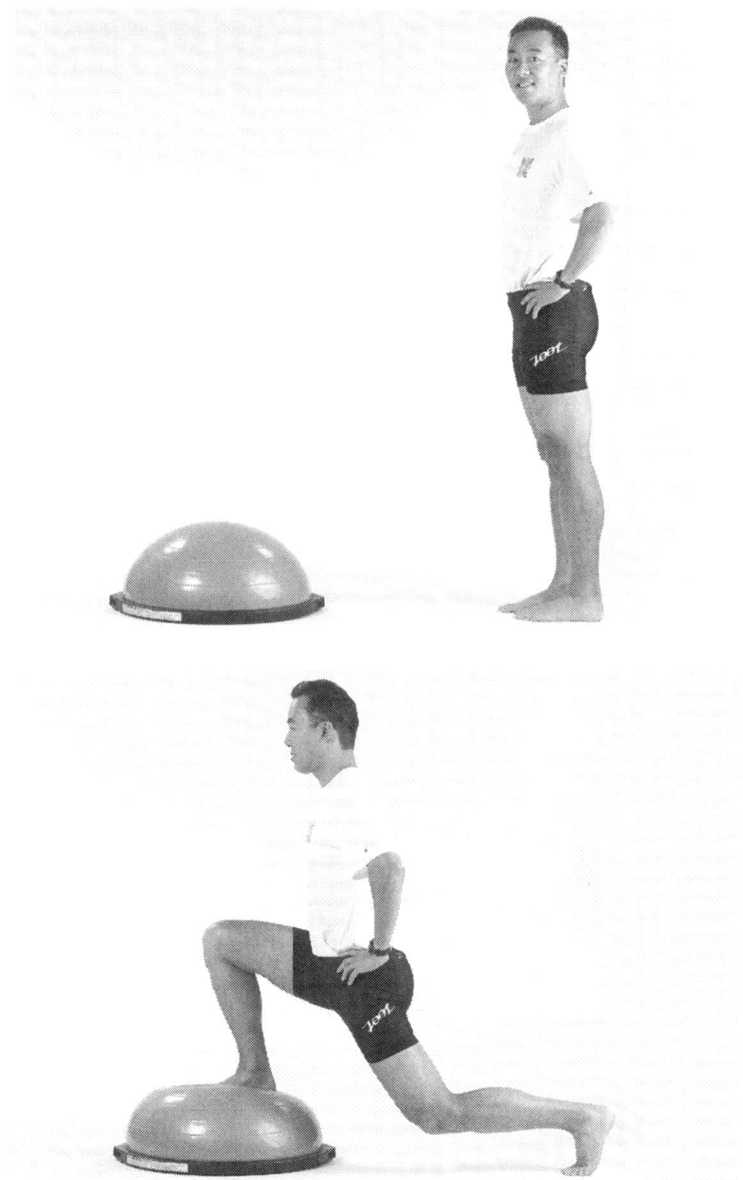

(4) Lunges

Place one foot on the BOSU® Balance Trainer, while keeping your other foot behind you and bent so that your knee is pointing down. Alternate your feet so that both legs—and your core—all get a great workout.

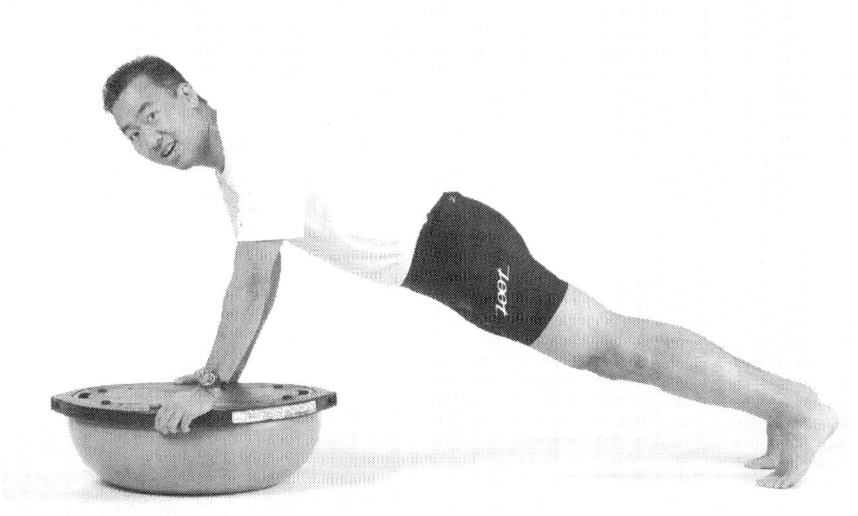

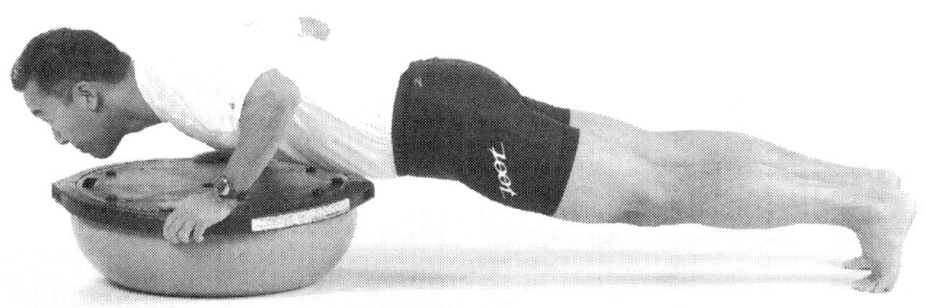

(5) Pushups

Flip the BOSU® Balance Trainer over to do pushups with balance. Keep your back straight, and try to do more than ten at a time. Not only will this work on your chest, but it's great for your core muscles. Work toward being able to do 30 pushups or more.

(6) Dumbbell Curls

You can do this standing on either side of the BOSU® Balance Trainer (round side up, or flat side up). If you want more of a challenge, do it with one foot on the BOSU® Balance Trainer and your other foot held to the side. Do ten curls on each arm, repeating each arm for three times.

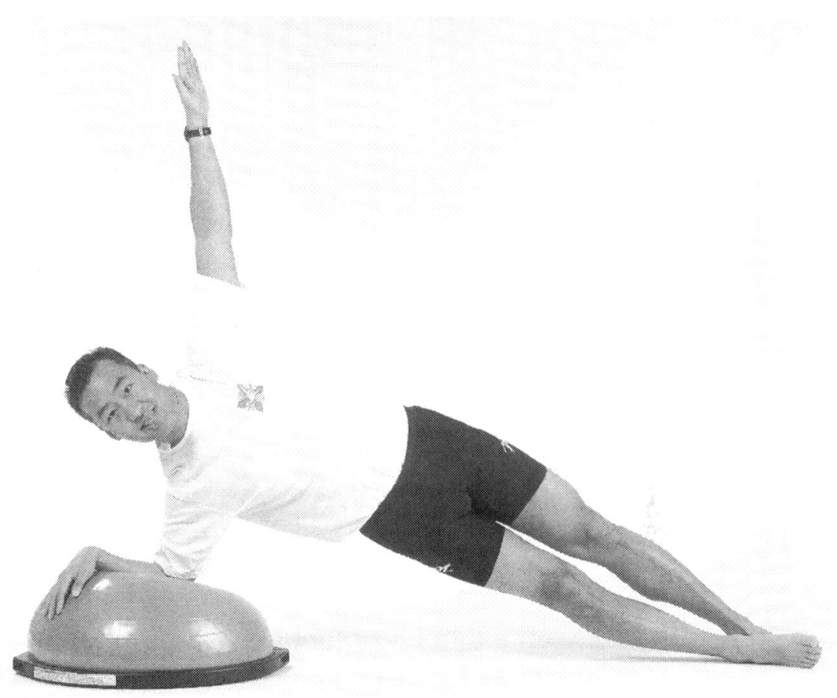

(7) Side Plank

The Side Plank is a great exercise to help shrink any "love handles." It's also great to help strengthen your core. Try to hold for at least ten seconds, or up to one minute, then repeat on the other side.

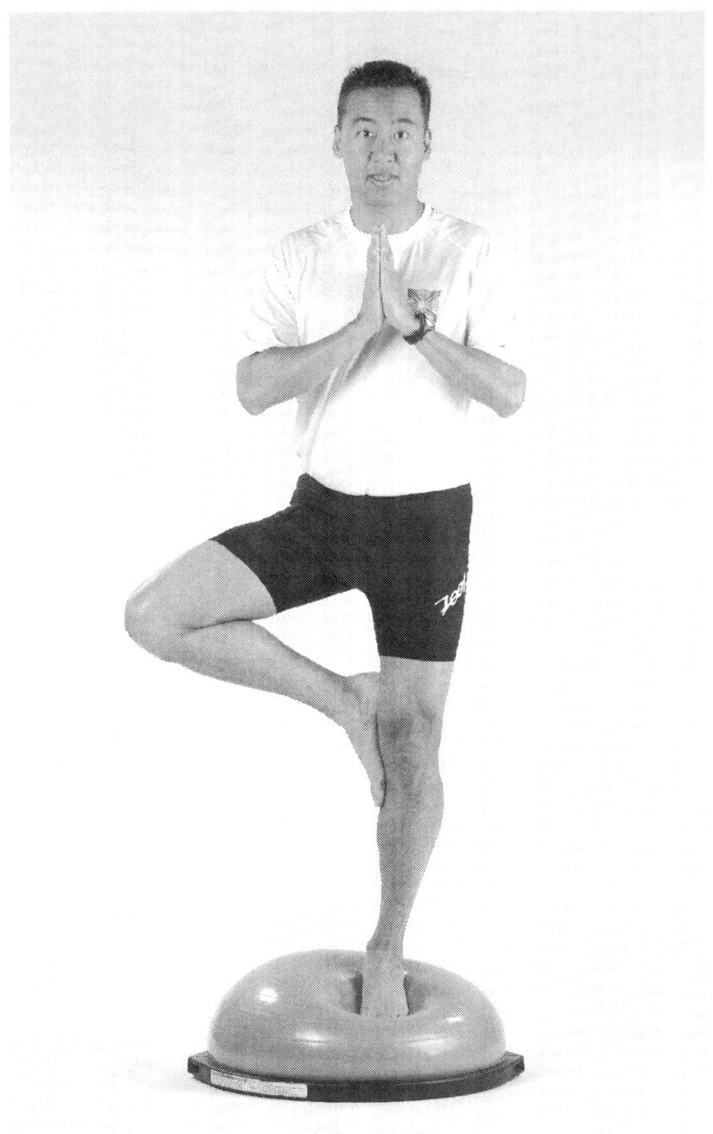

(8) Tree Pose

Balancing on one foot is what makes this a challenging exercise. Begin by standing with both feet on the BOSU® Balance Trainer, then slowly raise one foot barely above the BOSU® Balance Trainer. After you have balance on one foot, then continue to slowly lift your foot to your knee. Try to hold for ten seconds, then alternate feet and repeat.

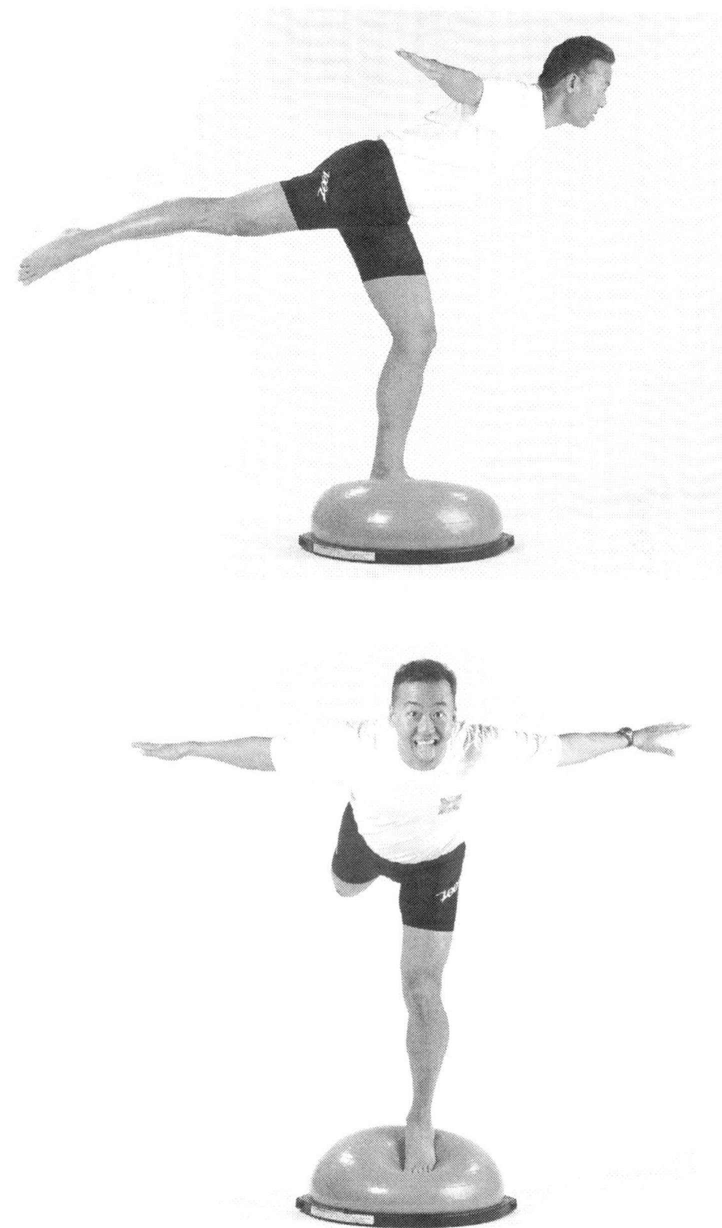

(9) Variation of Warrior Pose 3

Once you've mastered the Tree Pose, go for this BOSU® version of the classic yoga position, Warrior Pose 3. Just for good measure, my personalized version usually includes a Michael Jordan victory face!

Choose Not to Smoke

To achieve a healthy body and mind, you will—without a doubt—have to quit smoking... completely. Smoking will speed up your aging process and increase your risk of lung cancer, heart disease, asthma, stroke and lung disease.

According to the American Cancer Society, smoking causes one in five deaths. Smoking is the single largest preventable cause of disease and premature death. Just by smoking, the body is burdened with the undue process of handling nicotine, carbon monoxide, formaldehyde, arsenic and lead—just to name a few of the toxins.

One of the reasons smoking can cause many problems is that it triggers inflammation, and the markers of inflammation are then elevated—like CRP, TNF and IL-6.

The medication called Chantix® has helped many of my patients to quit smoking, but one must have a desire to quit, as well as a quit date that is set in stone. Also, acupuncture, hypnosis or even laser treatments have helped some of my patients that did not want to stop smoking with Chantix®.

Conclusion

The three lifestyle choices I see every day in my practice—which have significant bearing on your health—are: choosing to be aware of what your body is telling you; choosing not to smoke; and choosing to exercise.

When you think about it, there is a magic pill you can take to lose weight. It has no side effects and it is very inexpensive. It has been around forever, and it has been proven to work. It's exercise.

You must invest in exercise at least 30 minutes every day—and that's beyond work or school. Invest in your body and focus on the five different concepts (cardio with interval workouts, strength training, balance exercises, flexibility exercises and core exercises), and your body and mind will thank you.

I can't emphasize enough the importance exercise has on an active lifestyle when it comes to reducing the most dangerous condition you can have, and that is insulin resistance.

Remember, don't just work out for three months and then quit. You have to do it until you die.

If you are new to exercise, then get a personal trainer and make sure you stretch before and after so that you don't get an injury. Let your body get used to it, and then later you can challenge your body with higher weights, more repetitions or faster intervals.

There is no shortcut to success and you have to make that investment to work out, be active and eat healthy. Enjoy the journey.

CHAPTER 4 REVIEW

— Always exercise, and enjoy it! If you don't enjoy it, find an exercise that you do enjoy.

— The five key areas in exercising are: cardio with interval workouts, strength training, balance exercises, flexibility exercises and core exercises.

— If you are not motivated or you need help, then hire a personal trainer.

— Also, work on flexibility. Your body will thank you as you age.

5

Don't Give Up... There Are Other Options!

"If you're trying to achieve, there will be roadblocks.
I've had them; everybody has had them.
But obstacles don't have to stop you.
If you run into a wall, don't turn around and give up.
Figure out how to climb it, go through it, or work around it."
— Michael Jordan

You've given it your best shot, but you still need some help. Or, just as Laura's story emphasized in the second chapter, you should not give up when there are still other options to be explored.

The core basics for obtaining a healthy body and mind are to have an active lifestyle, reduce your insulin levels by eating less refined sugars, and to eat your largest amount in the morning time. I have seen many of my patients who gave up their wine or alcohol intake (which is high in sugar) and their weight started dropping.

In other cases I have seen my patients easily lose ten pounds or more by making wiser choices in their food selection—or just by exchanging their refined carbohydrates for green vegetables. I often say, "Exchange a grain for a green if you want a healthier body and mind."

In my practice, I'm able to offer other options to people who exercise and do everything else right, but they just can't lose weight. Here are the top "other options" that you can use—temporarily—to help you get over, through or around that wall.

Please know these options are not intended for long time use, and that I always recommend a more active lifestyle, combined with eating less in the evening, to eventually wean you off these options.

"It's amazing how weight just creeps up on you."

Somehow I had gained almost 30 pounds slowly. It's amazing how weight just creeps up on you. I had just adapted, thinking nothing of it. I also did not weigh myself. What I did notice is that I had this bump on my belly where my waist once was slim, and that was really starting to bother me!

The day I finally stepped on the scale I could not believe where I was. Additionally, my blood pressure and blood sugar were elevated and I was having to take medications to address those issues. I sought out Dr Lee to help me.

I wanted a quick fix and I knew he would have the answers. He did have the answers... just not a quick fix as I was hoping. It had taken time to get to where I was, and it was going to take some time to get back to where I really wanted—and needed—to be.

To help reduce my appetite and food intake, he started me on Byetta® and then transitioned to Symlin®. These both really worked to help control my hunger. They also helped with my blood sugar. I did lose some weight, although slowly—probably because I was not ready to give up that red wine I drank every night!

Dr. Lee understood, yet encouraged me to at least limit the wine. After all, the best taste is in the first sips. Then, after reducing my wine, Dr. Lee started me on the HCG Diet.

Wow, what a change in my life. I have lost over 25 pounds in 30 days. For someone who loves food, I was amazed that I could do this, and it wasn't even that hard. The wine did have to go for a while. Although Dr. Lee now allows me one glass a week.

It's an amazing difference in the way I look at food now. I was certain wine and sweets would be the hardest to live without. What I found out is that those were easy to go without on this diet. What I craved was cheese. The human body is so interesting. I am very happy with achieving the weight loss and getting back to where I really needed to be.

And there are wonderful side benefits. My blood pressure has returned to normal and my sugar levels are better. It is so encouraging to see and feel results when you are trying to lose weight. I thank Dr Lee for his support and creativeness to help with my weight loss.

— Brigitte Goersch

Byetta®

For those patients needing extra help, a jump start in their weight loss, or some extra help to lose their belly fat, I like to use Byetta® (exenatide), a medication originally developed to help treat type 2 diabetes. The story behind Byetta® is interesting in that it was developed from the Gila monster, a venomous lizard native to the southwestern United States and northern Mexico. A heavy, slow-moving lizard that measures up to two feet in length, the Gila monster is the only venomous lizard native to the United States, and one of only two known species of venomous lizards found in North America. Though the Gila monster's bite is poisonous, its sluggish nature represents little threat to humans; however, the amazing thing about the Gila monster is that it eats only two to three times a year!

In 1992, Dr. John Eng discovered a hormone in the Gila monster's saliva called exendin-4. It has properties similar to a hormone called GLP-1, a glucagon-like peptide-1 that is believed to turn off the Gila monster's appetite. Humans also produce the GLP-1 hormone in our intestine, but as we age our GLP-1 levels diminish. Plus, the Gila monster's hormone remains effective much longer than the human version, which helps diabetics keep their blood sugar levels from getting too high. Exenatide also slows the emptying of the stomach and causes a decrease in appetite, thereby contributing to weight loss. Recently, I got to meet and have dinner with Dr. Eng. He still works at the Bronx Veterans Administration Medical Center in New York where he made his discovery. He holds the patent on exenatide (Byetta®), but he almost went broke in following his gut instinct on getting his discovery patented. He says he first went to the Veterans Administration to see if they wanted to patent it, but they rejected it since it did not address a veteran-specific ailment. Eventually, Amylin Pharmaceutical became interested in Dr. Eng's discovery and later he was able to get a patent. In April 2005 the FDA approved Byetta® for use by type 2 diabetics. The last time I talked with Dr. Eng, he said he cannot even prescribe Byetta® as a diabetic medication because it is not on the formulary at the Veterans Administration. Yet another shortcoming of our government's health care.

Many of my patients have enjoyed dramatic weight loss results through a combination of Byetta® and lifestyle modification. Byetta® has also been shown to decrease the C-reactive protein (CRP), which is a sign of inflammation of the heart. The glucagon like peptide-1 has even been shown to protect the beta cells of the pancreas that secrete insulin from cytokine induced death. In other words, the hormone GLP-1 has a protective role regarding high levels of pro-inflammatory cytokines.

Although Byetta® is intended for diabetics on certain medications, the use of Byetta® (other than for diabetes) to reverse obesity and reduce inflammation before the onset of diabetes has been successfully used in my practice. I have also found that many obese patients treated with Byetta® have much more energy and significantly reduced adrenal fatigue.

Byetta® comes in two doses: five and ten mcg. I often start patients with five mcg 30 minutes before their largest meal, and later I instruct them to use it one hour before their largest meal. The most common side effect of Byetta® is mild nausea. Usually the nausea will resolve by itself. I often find in my patients that if they're really eager to lose weight, they will tolerate the mild nausea. Byetta® may rarely cause vomiting, and I have only seen that in two patients. Approximately ten percent of patients cannot tolerate Byetta® because of unbearable nausea, and those are usually male patients.

The five mcg, once-a-day dose of Byetta® is the most common dose I have with my patients. If a patient is on that dosage (which comes in a pen with 60 injections), I instruct them to keep their medication refrigerated so it can last for two months—instead of the one month it would last at room temperature. Often, my patients will pay out of pocket for this medication since it is usually not covered on insurance without a diagnosis of diabetes. Sometimes, patients need a five mcg dose of Byetta® twice a day—and, in certain situations, I've even increased the dose of Byetta® to ten mcg twice a day.

I used Byetta® myself for about three months. The reason I started Byetta was because I needed something to help prevent me from snacking while I took my recertification exams in Internal Medicine and in Endocrinology. Unfortunately, when I have to study so intensively for that amount of time, I tend to snack a lot. I also knew that if I gained weight, then my blood sugars and insulin levels would rise, my blood pressure would go up, and my markers for inflammation (like CRP) would become elevated. So, when it was recently time to hit the books and study, I gave up my exercise and exchanged it for Byetta®.

I remember the first time I injected Byetta® and later sat down to enjoy my wife's cooking. Halfway through the meal I told her I was full and could not touch another bite. She was shocked that I didn't finish my plate—and her plate, since I grew up as the "human garbage can." I also did not experience any nausea and I was amazed at how I had this feeling of fullness. I can clearly remember how feeling full—before I finished my plate—was such an alien sensation. In fact, I lost seven pounds while studying for my re-certification exams. After passing the exams, I quit Byetta® and went back to my favorite hobby/activity, which is exercise.

Success with Byetta® comes from the signal that tells you to stop eating when you're full. For example, when you finally realize you're too full to eat one more bite on Thanksgiving Day, then you're already way beyond too full! By the time you get a "full" sensation in your stomach, it usually takes about 20 to 30 minutes for your brain to get the message from your stomach. Byetta® speeds up that process. It is said that by the age of five we start losing our ability to stop eating when we're full. That's when it starts taking about 20 to 30 minutes for your brain to get the "full" message from your stomach. Also, most of us have grown up being told to finish our plates because kids in Africa are dying of hunger (for me, it was all the starving kids in North Korea). A word of advice: if you have children or grandkids, if you teach them to finish their plate they will become "hardwired" to do so when they grow up. It's a hard habit to break, but necessary—especially since the average serving size has increased dramatically in recent years.

"Don't wait for a rude awakening like I did."

One day I found myself in the hospital with palpitations and atrial fibrillation. Thankfully, my wife was at my side, anxious for my well-being and determined to take control of the situation. Afterwards, she accompanied me to each appointment with Dr. Lee—and after every appointment she established ground rules (based on what Dr. Lee advised) for me, and then she ensured that I complied with those ground rules fully.

I lost more than 60 pounds thanks to Dr. Lee's diet, exercise and adjustment of my medications. Dr. Lee has regularly and consistently monitored my lab reports, and made adjustments to my diabetic medications accordingly. His work has allowed me to discontinue my insulin injections, which were increasing my appetite and contributing to my unhealthy weight gain. Dr. Lee also started me on Byetta® to reduce my appetite and help me lose weight.

I feel like I did in college, which was also the last time I weighed this much. I just returned from an active vacation cruise with my wife—who is now planning our next adventure, perhaps to Antarctica.

Don't wait for a rude awakening like I did. Seek Dr. Lee's advice and begin your preventive care NOW!

— *Raymond A. Chouinard M.D.*

Because Byetta® comes in a pen, you will be injecting the medication yourself—which is why I often hear, "I am not going to do the needle." However, the needle on a Byetta® pen is very small, and once we teach a patient to self inject they usually say, "Oh, that didn't hurt." Then, once the needle is in, it's crucial to count to "ten-Mississippi" so you ensure the medication gets into you rather than on the floor. Most of my patients inject into their belly, with their belly button as the center of the clock, with the next injection rotating to the next position on the clock. Start at 12 o'clock and go around the clock by pinching an inch. Or, inject into your thighs or love handles. If someone gets severe nausea with Byetta®, I often have them try injecting halfway through their meal, rather than before eating.

Byetta® should not be used if you have severe renal or kidney failure. Also, it does not replace insulin for a type 1 diabetic (someone who requires insulin for the rest of their life). In addition, you should not use Byetta® if you have gastroparesis (very slow digestion due to a paralysis of the stomach, small intestine and/or colon) or if you're pregnant.

Since August 2008 there has been some concern that Byetta® may cause pancreatitis (inflammation of the pancreas). As of 2010, there have been 36 cases of presumed pancreatitis associated with exenatide; however, 90 percent of those cases had at least one risk factor for pancreatitis.[1]

In the New England Journal of Medicine there has been one case reported of pancreatitis with the use of Byetta®. However, that 44-year-old woman who developed pancreatitis was a type 1 diabetic with gastroparesis. As stated earlier, Byetta® is not indicated for patients with type 1 diabetes and gastroparesis.[2]

However, a recent publication has looked at the rate of pancreatitis associated with Byetta® and noted—in a database of over 786,000 patients—no higher rates of pancreatitis with exenatide when compared to another diabetic medication called sitagliptin. The study found that diabetics, in general, have a higher rate of pancreatitis compared to patients without diabetes.[3]

The advice I give my patients is if they are doing well with Byetta® and have no nausea with it, but then later develop nausea, then I recommend to discontinue their Byetta® and be checked for pancreatitis. I have used Byetta® extensively and have never seen it cause pancreatitis in any of my patients. Actually, Byetta® has been a lifesaver for many of my patients, like in the following case.

When I began treating this woman, she was already on the highest possible dose of insulin and was still gaining much weight. Her overall glucose control was terrible and her average blood sugar with the glucose meter was over 400. She was tired and was having much pain from her excessive weight gain. The consult from her doctor was to fix her diabetes. Immediately, I told her she had severe insulin resistance and that the insulin she was receiving was not only not working, but it was causing her to gain weight.

After doing some more diagnostic testing, which came back negative for Cushing's disease, I gave her the option to stop her 500 units of insulin and try Byetta® while reducing her high intake of refined sugar, integrating more green vegetables into her diet, and to give me a call the next day. She called me the next day and said there must be a problem with her glucose meter because it was reading 120. I told her to get ready for her weight loss. Not only did she lose over 100 pounds, but she also got off of five prescription medications over the next few months. She would sing praises in my waiting room every time she would come for her follow up visit. For her, taking extra insulin was hurting, so Byetta® was her lifesaver.

Symlin®

I also use another medication called Symlin® to help with weight loss. Symlin® is intended for diabetics on insulin. It mimics a hormone called amylin, which is co-secreted with insulin. As we age, amylin, like most hormones, diminishes. The beauty of the hormone amylin is that it helps in weight loss by reducing your appetite. Symlin® works in reducing the appetite by binding to the postrema area of the brain, which controls the appetite.[4]

Symlin®, like Byetta®, requires a daily injection with a very small needle. Many of my patients have successfully lost weight through a combination of Symlin® and lifestyle modification. I have often heard that when you lose weight with Byetta® or Symlin®, it is because you have cut out all the snacking—especially after dinner.

The first case I experienced with Symlin® was an amazing success. A woman was failing her medication with pills and with insulin. I offered her Symlin® and instructed her to reduce her insulin if her blood sugars were dropping. About one month later, I met her while shopping and she told me how her new medicine was helping her lose weight, and that she was off insulin. I was so excited for her! It was amazing how her body was missing the hormone amylin and that, for her, Symlin® was the key to her success.

In a double blind placebo controlled study of 411 obese patients without diabetes, a one-year study on the use of Symlin® looked at whether or not Symlin® can cause weight loss. The doses ranged from 120 mcg three times a day, up to 360 mcg three times a day. Approximately 40 percent of the patients lost ten percent of their weight at the dose of 120 mcg three times a day, and 43 percent lost ten percent of their weight with 360 mcg twice a day, and 38 percent lost ten percent of their weight with the highest dose of 360 mcg three times a day. Also, in conjunction with the study, lifestyle intervention was added for twelve months. The program they used was called LEARN, a well-established and flexible intervention program aimed at making gradual changes in lifestyle.[5]

In another randomized placebo control trial that studied Symlin® for weight loss, 204 obese people (with and without type 2 diabetes) underwent a 16-week trial. Their doses of Symlin® started at 60 mcg three times a day and then titrated to 240 mcg three times a day. About 88 percent of the patients were able to tolerate the highest dose. The most common side effect was nausea, which caused one patient to withdraw—while one patient in the placebo group also withdrew because of nausea. Most of the patients lost about eight pounds and most benefited from the appetite control and had a positive experience with Symlin®.[6]

"Life is beautiful!"

I am a 67 year old woman who had been on Prilosec for my acid reflux for about seven years. After going to Dr. Lee I stopped taking Prilosec. By simply raising the head of my bed and drinking alkaline water, he has taken away my acid reflux and given me a wonderful feeling.

Then, when I told Dr. Lee about wanting to lose weight, he started me on Symlin®. I have already lost 18 pounds and find that I don't feel tired and sleepy any more. Life is beautiful!

— Donna Borders

Although the FDA has approved this medication with the use of insulin only, as you can see, there have been medical studies in which Symlin® was used in patients without insulin. I've used Symlin® in many patients without insulin and have seen some great results. Like any other medication, there is no perfect medication that will produce a 100 percent result. Some of my patients have had no effect on Symlin® whereas about 70 percent have had a great response to it. Symlin® should not be given in anyone with renal or kidney problems. Also, Symlin® should not be given to anyone with gastroparesis (very slow digestion due to a paralysis of the stomach, small intestine and/or colon) or any pregnant women.

Symlin® is easier to use than Byetta® since it does not have to be given one full hour before eating. I often recommend Symlin® at 60 mcg 15 minutes before the day's largest meal. After three days, I usually increase it to 120 mcg before the largest meal of the day. Later, I either increase it to twice a day, or switch to 240 mcg (or even 360 mcg) before the largest meal. The most common side effect is mild nausea and rarely vomiting. If someone is on insulin, then they must reduce their pre-meal insulin by 25 to 50 percent, depending on their overall glucose control.

It is crucial that if someone is on insulin, they must monitor their blood sugars (before and after a meal) and always carry glucose tablets (or some emergency candy) to treat a low blood sugar reaction. Symlin® is contraindicated in anyone who cannot recognize a low blood sugar reaction (hypoglycemia unawareness). Otherwise, Symlin® can produce great results and help you achieve a healthy body.

Victoza®

The new kid on the block is a medication called Victoza® (lirglutide), which is similar to Byetta®. Victoza® is a recently approved medication for type 2 diabetics and is a once-a-day GLP-1 analog—compared to Byetta®, which is a twice-a-day GLP-1 analog.

I've seen great results with Victoza®, but I use Victoza® if my patients have failed Symlin® or Byetta®. Also, there have been over million people on Byetta® and it has had a clean record so far (aside from the pancreatitis incidence). Victoza® does have flexible dosing from 0.6 mg to 1.8 mg a day, and most of my busy patients have found its a once-a-day dosage to be a great benefit. They usually inject Victoza® in the morning and then it's done for the day. However, there is a small risk of a rare thyroid cancer (medullary thyroid cancer) that was found in the rat and mice safety studies. So far, there have been no reported cases of medullary cancer in humans. If you have a family history of medullary thyroid cancer, or have had medullary thyroid cancer, then you will not be allowed to use it. Time will tell if there is any relevance to humans developing this rare type of thyroid cancer.

"I'm feeling healthy, strong, happy and back in control of my life."

I'm 54 years old, a three-year survivor of breast cancer and a patient of Dr. Lee's for the past two-and-a-half years. In 2008, while going through chemotherapy treatments, I gained 20 pounds, became dependent on Ambien® for sleep and Wellbutrin® for anxiety and stress. As an aftereffect of chemotherapy, my heart developed a fast heart rate so I have been taking atenenol to regulate my heart beat. In my first consultation with Dr. Lee, we set three goals: first, we had to get my strength, energy and overall health in better shape; second, we would work on losing the 20 pounds or more that I needed to lose (I have also improved on my diet and am eating more vegetables); and third, we would work on eliminating my need and dependence on Ambien® and Wellbutrin®.

Six months ago, Dr. Lee prescribed Victoza® as an aid for weight loss and to date, I have lost 24 pounds! He also gave me two types of melatonin, and I no longer take Ambien® and recently, I've been able to eliminate Wellbutrin®.

I am so thankful Dr. Lee is my friend and he cares about my well-being. I'm feeling healthy, strong, happy and back in control of my life!

— Nancy Young

Gastric Bypass Surgery

There is also a surgical option for weight loss. It is gastric bypass surgery, and it is a life-changing procedure that can help with weight loss—even if everything else has failed. I have recommended several of my patients for a gastric bypass and have seen wonderful results, and most of them also reversed their type 2 diabetes.

There are many different options of gastric bypass surgery, such as the Roux-en-Y gastric bypass, lap banding or gastric sleeve surgery. A recently published study continued to show improved insulin resistance and GLP-1 responses after eating (desirable results), even two years later.[7]

However, my concern about gastric bypass surgery is that if you don't correct your approach with an active lifestyle, then you can fail gastric bypass surgery. I have seen many patients who have regained most of their weight after their gastric bypass surgery and have then come to see me for help. You can always drink or eat foods that are high in calories that will cause weight gain after gastric bypass surgery. So, it's sometimes not what you are eating, but *what is eating at you* is more of the root issue. Thus, it's important to take care or have closure on the issues that are consuming you. In summary, gastric bypass surgery can fail in the long term—with failure rates ranging from 20.4 to 34.9 percent over ten years after gastric bypass surgery.[8]

HCG

For quite a while, I debated whether or not to include HCG in this book; but after being at the latest Anti-Aging conference, I now know that I need to at least mention something about its pros and cons.

HCG (human chorionic gonadotropin) is a hormone produced in pregnant women. In the early part of pregnancy, HCG is secreted to help increase the production of another hormone called progesterone to help with thickening the uterus (womb where the baby lives) wall with blood vessels to help the fetus grow. HCG has been used in fertility clinics to help women ovulate, and to help men produce more testosterone. Since pregnant women have the highest levels of HCG, their urine is collected to obtain HCG for this use.

A new fad these days is the HCG diet. It is a very low calorie diet combined with the use of HCG. Although I have seen some patients fail on this program, I have also seen some amazing results. One concern I have is the use of HCG and the HCG diet on a type 1 diabetic (a diabetic that depends on insulin). A type 1 diabetic can develop a condition of diabetic ketoacidosis or DKA—a condition where they have excessive ketones (a breakdown product of fat) and not enough insulin to remove the ketones. Therefore, I would strongly advise against the HCG diet if you are a type 1 diabetic.

These days, there are many variations of the HCG diet. A British physician named Dr. Albert Simeons discovered the use of HCG as a treatment of obesity. He reported it in 1954 and used a very low calorie diet of 500 calories per day—even though most people eat more than 500 calories per meal.

It is believed that HCG helps burn fat. The original protocol is that you inject HCG for about one month, along with a 500-calorie diet per day (the diet is very specific on what you can eat and not to eat) and the next month you eat to maintain your weight (800 to 1000 calories a day), then you repeat the monthly cycle with HCG on, then off.

As I mentioned, there are many different variations of this diet—such as under the tongue HCG or HCG that comes in droppers. However, no HCG diet has yet been proven. There have been randomized clinical studies showing it is actually the low calorie diet causing the weight loss. Currently, there is no scientific evidence that HCG causes weight loss, redistributes fat or reduces hunger. Even the FDA has stated that HCG has no benefit in the treatment of obesity.[9-11]

Although the current science does not support it, one cannot ignore the fact that many people have had success with HCG. Perhaps it's the HCG diet (very low calories) and not the HCG itself that is the reason for their success.

"The use of HCG helped achieve my weight loss."

Nearly two years ago, when I was 61, Dr. Edwin Lee was recommended to me by a bioidentical pharmacist. I had been to three other endocrinologists with little results and was seeking a true professional that would be willing to work with me to make my life better. Dr. Lee's initial consultation included an intense history—both medically and personally. I showed Dr. Lee a picture from my early years as a runner in my 30s—energetic, lean and happy with my abilities. Now, having low levels of testosterone, being overweight (even though I ate very little and conservatively), with swollen feet and, most likely, mild depression.

Less than two years later at age 63, I've increased my testosterone levels. I've lost nearly 30 pounds with HCG, my feet do not swell and my diet knowledge has been enhanced. The staff at Dr. Lee's facility are like family. When appropriate, they compliment my progress and welcome me with comfort.

One of the most important concepts I learned from Dr. Lee was to reduce my refined sugars and increase my vegetable intake to lower my insulin levels. In addition, the use of HCG helped achieve my weight loss.

The greatest thing about my association with Dr. Lee's organization—whether I was in panic or just in need of encouragement—is that they are all personally responsive to your needs.

My success is one of many, and even though I see the staff and Dr. Lee two to three times a year now, my support system is in place and I feel good just in knowing they are there for me.

— *Bud Bernier*

Bydureon™

There is one medication I've been looking forward to because I think it will be a blockbuster. It is Byetta®, but in a once-a-week version called Bydureon™. It was supposed to come out in 2010, but on October 20, 2010 the FDA called for more studies to look at the safety of this new medication. The current studies look promising, with less nausea and similar weight loss compared to Byetta® at ten mcg twice a day.[12]

It is hoped that the FDA will soon approve Bydureon™. Once it's available, it will be a great option for weight loss.

Conclusion

There are some incredible new medications—such as Byetta®, Symlin® and Victoza® (both of which are GLP-1 hormones)—that can help reverse insulin resistance.

While gastric bypass surgery is a surgical option for weight loss, you will still need to adopt an active lifestyle and proper diet for continued results.

Currently, there is no scientific evidence that HCG causes weight loss, redistributes fat or reduces hunger; yet, one cannot ignore the fact that many people have had success with HCG. Perhaps it's the HCG diet (very low calories) and not the HCG itself that is the reason for their success.

For those needing some extra help in reducing insulin resistance and losing weight, the medications in this chapter may be the extra push you need. Remember though, these medications are for temporary use and are not intended to replace the combination of an active lifestyle and fewer calories—especially in the evening.

Like I say to my patients nearly every day, "There is theory, and there is reality. I could talk all day on what you need to do in theory; however, if in reality you are starving and eating everything in the house, you may need some help in reducing your appetite." Thankfully, there are medications to help with weight loss, and they are well tolerated without many side effects.

CHAPTER 5 REVIEW

— There are agents that can help achieve weight loss like Byetta®, Symlin, Victoza® and HCG.

— Byetta® is a hormone called GLP-1 that can help reduce insulin resistance, and help with weight loss. Byetta® can reduce your appetite and help with reducing your snacking, especially after eating.

— Symlin® is a hormone called amylin that comes from the pancreas. It helps with reducing insulin resistance via weight loss.

— Victoza® is the new kid on the block that is a longer GLP-1 hormone. A concern of Victoza® is the association of a rare thyroid cancer, but has only been found in rats and in mice during the safety studies.

— HCG with a very low calorie diet of 500 calories can also work in achieving weight loss.

— Bydureon™ is the once a week GLP-1 hormone shot that is coming soon. It will be a long acting Byetta®.

6

Your Weight Loss Secret Weapon is ALCAT

"It is health that is real wealth
and not pieces of gold and silver."
— *Mahatma Gandhi*

In my first book, *Feel Good Look Younger: Reversing Tiredness Through Hormonal Balance,* I devoted most of the first chapter to food intolerances, or delayed sensitivities, and how important it is to properly identify them. At that time, the best method to identify food intolerances was through a blood test called immunoglobulin G (IgG). Soon after writing *Feel Good Look Younger,* I learned of a major breakthrough with another test called ALCAT. Soon, I started using it, and have seen nothing but amazing results.

The company that developed and administers the ALCAT test, Cell Science Systems (CSS), has been around for 25 years. In fact, it was CSS that pioneered and developed the white blood cell testing that revolutionized the field of allergy and sensitivity testing. There is an excellent book, *Your Hidden Food Allergies are Making you Fat,* that fully explains the ALCAT test procedures in great detail. ALCAT stands for Antigen Leukocyte Cellular Antibody Test. Although this is now a somewhat outdated name (due to the many advancements in this testing procedure) the name remains the same.

Over ALCAT's 25 years, there have been numerous improvements. Thanks to one of those new developments last year, CSS was able to reengineer ALCAT, making their food allergies and sensitivities testing even more accurate than an IgG test.

Delayed food sensitivities are very different from acute food allergies, which are immunoglobulin E (IgE) mediated. IgE is a certain class of antibody that is involved in the immune system, and an IgE mediated reaction is when the mast cells release chemicals (such as histamine, leukotrienes and prostaglandins) that will then cause vasodilatation, low blood pressure and swelling of the airways. Immediate treatment is required since this is a life-threatening medical emergency. Epinephrine is the primary treatment to open the closed airway and improve the low blood pressure.

Insect bites and eating peanuts are common causes for an IgE mediated acute allergic reaction. The most common acute food allergy that people recognize is a seafood allergy. If someone with a history of an acute food allergy (IgE mediated) to shrimp happens to eat shrimp, for example, that person is going to suffer from an anaphylactic reaction with the sudden onset and rapid progression of shortness of breath, swelling of the tongue, hives, low blood pressure and swelling that can close the airway.

After doing the ALCAT test on my six-year-old son, I stopped using the IgG testing that I used to perform for detecting delayed food sensitivities. My son was getting sick frequently, and my wife and I noticed that his immune system was not up to par. For several years he would have a constant runny nose and would get frequent sinus infections and upper respiratory infections. After seeing his pediatrician, he would get temporarily better with antibiotic treatments, but then his runny nose would come back, and later so would another infection.

In the past year he started to use a saline nasal rinse to help clear up his nose, but it was only helping him temporarily. Then, after he became sick on two recent family vacations, I decided that he needed to have the ALCAT test, thinking there could be something he is eating that is causing him to have a low immune system. As parents know, when your child gets sick on vacation and you are out of town, it is no longer a vacation.

The two foods on his severe list, which we were shocked to see, were oranges and strawberries. After one week of eliminating his orange juice and strawberries he said, "Mommy my nose is dry." He stopped using his saline nasal rinse, and on our recent summer trip to Alaska we all had a great time. Furthermore, the best news was that he didn't get sick! Since he has followed his elimination diet, he has been healthy and his nose has been dry.

"My opening statement was, 'I am sick of being sick.'"

I came to see Dr. Lee after being recommended to him by a friend who told me how much better he felt after seeing Dr. Lee.

I had suffered with chronic sinus issues all my life, and I would get sinus infections and lose my voice five or six times a year. I went to every doctor under the sun and had every test, but nothing helped. I even had sinus surgery, and I did begin to breath better, but not even that could clear up the congestion. So I went back to my ENT and he recommended I stay on Flonase twice a day and take Zyrtec. That was not the answer I was looking for.

I am 57 years old and work in a fast-paced, high-powered position within my industry, so I am consistently on the go. When I went to Dr. Lee, my opening statement was, "I am sick of being sick." After we discussed my lifelong issues, we put together a hormone/diet/food allergy plan (via my ALCAT test) for me to follow—which I did to the "T."

I have lost 12 pounds so far, have more energy, and have not had another sinus infection.

I recommend for anyone wanting to improve their quality of life—and to truly, finally understand how to feel better—that you should listen to Dr. Lee.

— *Marilyn Vogel*

The ALCAT test I most often use is the 200 Foods Sensitivity Test, since this is a test for what you can control. The ALCAT test can also be used to test for other things such as environmental chemicals, molds, preservatives and additives.

The book, *Your Hidden Food Allergies are Making You Fat*, explains in detail how the test is done. When I explain it to my patients, I start by saying that we draw your blood—which does not have to be after a fasting period—and we send it out to the company that runs the ALCAT test. Then, they collect your entire immune system (white blood cells) and put a small drop of your immune system (white blood cells) in 200 empty cups.

Into the first cup that has your immune system (white blood cells) they add gluten, into the second cup they add cow's milk, into the third cup they add chicken and so on. Next they incubate, or cook, the entire 200 cups to see what happens.

Once that is done, there are only two possible results: one is that nothing happens (peace), or the other result is that the immune system went to war (mild, moderate, severe).

This is different from the IgG testing that, like the ALCAT, tests for the issue of delayed food sensitivity. The IgG is a part of the immune system, and if elevated it may indicate that there is a recent exposure or a delayed food sensitivity. The ALCAT test actually looks at your entire immune system and sees if your immune system has any issue with a particular food—instead of just looking at one part of your immune system, like the IgG.

In addition, with the IgG testing, I sometimes would not get a correlation between the test and the clinical response. For example, one of my teenage patients had the IgG test for delayed sensitivity. Until the results came back, the only advice I could give him for his constant runny nose was to eliminate dairy. After stopping dairy, his nose was dry and he felt significantly better.

Later, his IgG test came back and it said he was negative, or nonreactive, to dairy. So, his IgG blood test showed that he was safe for dairy but clinically he couldn't tolerate it. Shortly after that, I have switched to the ALCAT test.

Leaky Gut

About 2,500 years ago, Hippocrates, the "father of medicine" said, "It appears to me necessary to every physician to be skilled in nature, and to strive to know, if he would wish to perform his duties, what man is—in relation to his articles of food and drink, and to his occupations, and what are the effects of each of them to every one." In modern terms... let food be your medicine, but be aware that certain foods will make you sick or cause you to develop a condition of intestinal hyperpermeability.

Another name for intestinal hyperpermeability is "leaky gut." The current thinking about a leaky gut is that small pieces of undigested food are able to pass through the gut lining into the bloodstream. It's normally the job of the T cells to digest bacteria, but because food does not react with cell walls (as would a bacteria or viral particle) the T cells are ineffective. In response, your immune system calls out the big guns, which are called Natural Killer cells (NK cells). The NK cells are able to track down these food particles and digest them. However, this begins a cascade of immune modulators and signal chemicals that contribute to systemic inflammation. Secondly, the chewing up of the food by the NK cells leaves a large trail of highly reactive free radicals. Free radicals will attack normal tissue and will cause damage. Together these processes lead to systemic inflammation and, ultimately, disease states.

It is believed that this scenario is involved in either starting or contributing to all inflammatory diseases—including autoimmune diseases.

As such, leaky gut syndrome has been associated with inflammatory liver diseases, primary sclerosing cholangitis, autoimmune hepatitis, inflammatory bowel disease and several autoimmune diseases. The theory is that because leaky gut syndrome causes a leakage of bacteria, or toxin (that turns on the immune system) then later develops an autoimmune reaction against an organ such as the thyroid, eyes, kidneys, brain, liver or joints.

To better understand what makes a gut "leaky" in the first place, you need to know about a protein called zonulin. In the late 1990s at the University of Maryland, Dr. Alessio Fasano discovered zonulin, and soon identified it as the "gatekeeper" of your gut.

Fasano explained that our largest "gateway" is the intestine with its billions of cells. Zonulin is what opens those billions of gateway spaces between those billions of cells, allowing some substances to pass through, while keeping harmful bacteria and toxins out. Zonulin is produced in the gut, and if it is elevated, then the tight junctures of your gut will open up even more—allowing harmful bacteria and toxins to pass through. Those opened junctures will not close until your zonulin level goes back down. For testing purposes, zonulin can be measured in your blood.[1]

While zonulin is triggered by any certain foods to which you have a sensitivity, there are other triggers for zonulin—and some of these have dire consequences. For example, stress has been shown to increase your production of zonulin, as have: heavy metals, environmental pollutants and toxins, cosmetics, artificial sweeteners, household cleaners, pesticides and other chemicals. A study with celiac disease patients has shown that gluten increases zonulin, while another unrelated study has proven that a protein similar to gluten (called gliadin) also increases zonulin and leads to a leaky gut as well.[2]

Leaky gut syndrome is also associated with other, more prevalent, conditions such as asthma, arthritis, autism, diabetes and... obesity.

Beating Obesity with ALCAT

For details on weight loss with the use of the ALCAT test, please refer to the book, *Your Hidden Food Allergies Are Making You Fat*, which lists several studies. One study quoted in the book is by the Baylor Medical College and shows that 98 percent of the subjects following the ALCAT plan either lost weight and/or improved their body composition.

Another study in 1995 was presented in Italy at The 14th Mediterranean Day of Esthetical Medicine & Dermatological Surgery. It was a Spanish study, and was designed to determine whether people who could not lose weight on a low calorie diet could achieve weight loss using their results from the ALCAT test.

The results showed that almost everyone in the study lost weight—and they were also noted to have improved skin smoothness, loss of fat from the thighs, improved physical performance and improved digestion.[3]

Also, there were two more recent studies presented in Italy that demonstrated a 97 percent improvement in skin conditions and a 98 percent improvement in digestive problems by following the ALCAT plan.

Specifically, in the study on skin conditions, the aim of the study was to evaluate whether food intolerance is associated with cutaneous (skin) reactions, and then to measure the value of the ALCAT test regarding its diagnosis of food intolerance. An overwhelming 97 percent of the participants, in clinical evaluations, showed either "mild improvement" or "very important improvement" with the ALCAT. Even if the "mild improvement" respondents were somehow possibly a placebo effect, the remaining "very important improvement" respondents were still a two-thirds majority at 66 percent. Only 3 percent showed "no improvement" with the ALCAT.

Similarly, in the study on gastrointestinal symptoms, the aim of the study was to evaluate whether food intolerance is associated with gastrointestinal issues. This time, 98 percent of the participants showed either "mild improvement" or "very important improvement" with the ALCAT. Once again, even if the "mild improvement" respondents were somehow possibly a placebo effect, the remaining "very important improvement" respondents were still a 71 percent majority. Only 2 percent showed "no improvement" with the ALCAT.

More details on these two landmark studies should be published soon. I suspect that if the upcoming data includes the weight of each subject (before and after the study) then the overweight subjects will also show a reduction in weight during the study.[4-5]

In an unrelated overseas study that looked at people who had failed a low-calorie diet, the study showed that after twelve weeks on the ALCAT diet, the subjects' body weights dropped from an average of 91 kilograms (200 pounds) to an average of 74 kilograms (162 pounds). Also, their body fat decreased significantly, from 37 to 27 percent.[6]

"ALCAT got me over that last, seemingly impossible, hurdle."

For me, the ALCAT wasn't so much about losing pounds, but losing body fat and just feeling better overall. Within the first two weeks—without changing anything but excluding the foods that my body had previously been negatively reacting to—my body fat percentage went from 23 to only 18 percent, and that was accomplished along with a weight loss of only eleven pounds!

However, the biggest benefit for me was that ALCAT got me over that last, seemingly impossible, hurdle. To understand what that means, I need to explain that 13 or 14 years ago, I was on a number of medications; but for the last eight years, thanks to Dr. Lee, I'm off all those medications and am now only doing hormone therapy. However, even with all those accomplishments, sometimes in the morning I'd still feel like I needed a little something to get me up—to be the upbeat and positive person that people know me as. Sometimes I'd even feel low, or foggy, or like I needed something to "get up to my normal." That's when I'd drink some coffee and by the time I drove my hour to work, I'd have myself in a positive mood and ready for a great day—with that twinkle in my eye.

Now, after my ALCAT diet, I no longer have a low morning—ever. When I wake up, I'm already at my best—no fog, no tired feeling, no occasional low feelings in the morning. Plus, I've noticed that my focus throughout the day is even better, and I never feel overwhelmed. Thanks to ALCAT, I got over that last hurdle. That, and I'm definitely excited about the loss of my belly fat.

All you have to do is be willing to give up those ALCAT-identified foods for six months before reintroducing them in a rotation diet. Those first seven to ten days were hard; however, without hesitation, I would do it all again to feel as good as I do now!

— *Jason Holland*

An insightful question to ask is, how do food intolerances cause weight gain? Or, another way to ask is, why does the elimination diet help with weight loss? There are several theories on this subject, and more research needs to investigate this issue. My thoughts are that it has to do with several factors that cause weight gain.

First, food intolerance can cause intestinal hyperpermeability (leaky gut) which leads to an overactive immune system. This overactive immune system leads to chronic inflammation and the increased blood markers of inflammation—like interleukin 6 and tumor necrosis factor (not a desirable effect)—which accelerate the risk of gaining weight.

Also, there is a depletion of several key neurotransmitters, like dopamine and serotonin, which will then make you crave sugary foods or more refined sugar. It also leads to a lower level of a fat hormone called adiopenctin (not a good sign) that accelerates your risk for obesity.[7-8]

Then, by eating foods that increase your insulin levels, which in turn increases fat storage, you will gain weight. Simply stated: certain foods can make you (individually, you) fat. To lose weight, you need to find out what those foods are.

As for the neurotransmitter dopamine, this needs to be produced from the foods you eat. It is derived from the amino acid called tyrosine. Your body, including your brain, makes dopamine from tyrosine. Dopamine helps you to increase the feeling of pleasure. Dopamine levels are elevated by certain foods, and drug addictions are also linked to the craving for dopamine release. The release of dopamine can cause constant pleasure-seeking behavior.

This pleasure producing mechanism is referred to as the dopamine reinforcement pathway, which is the basis of any addiction. Since dopamine is triggered by both sugar and processed food, eating junk food creates addictive behavior and overeating

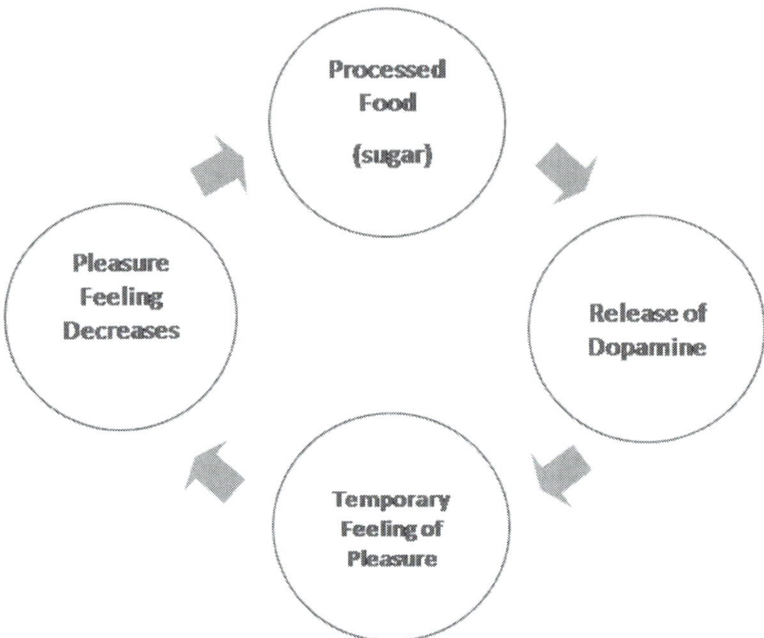

The dopamine reinforcement pathway is the basis of any addiction—including weight gain.

The ALCAT diet is straightforward and simple, yet challenging for some people—due to the lifestyle changes it requires. Your test results will reveal which foods are moderate and severe, which ones you will need to eliminate for six months, and the mild foods that you can rotate individually every four days.

Sometimes though, a patient, for whatever reason, will not follow their ALCAT elimination diet completely. They might do part-time elimination, or selective elimination, on their moderate or severe reactions. Unfortunately, they will never achieve optimal results in this way. For example, one of my patients—a doctor—had an ALCAT test indicate a severe reaction to anchovies; however, he continued taking his fish oil supplements that were made from... anchovies. Thankfully, he finally took my advice to use supplements derived from another source of omega-3 (like from nuts, krill oil, olive oil) and he began to achieve amazing results.

Thus, it is crucial—if you truly want to feel better and achieve an amazing body—that you do this 100 percent. Remember, it will always take total dedication to achieve, and keep, anything worthwhile in life.

Along with the ALCAT elimination diet, you should consider taking a leaky gut regimen that includes: L-glutatmine, digestive enzymes, pre and probiotics, and omega-3 fatty acids. This regimen will help repair your leaky gut.

You should also benefit from doing a liver detoxification. This will accomplish two things. First, by increasing the effectiveness of your liver's own detoxification capabilities, these chemicals will be processed out of the body and will not cause a leaky gut—or at least it will minimize the condition. Second, we know that when you begin the ALCAT elimination diet, the biochemistry of your body is altered enough that your body sheds any toxins that have been stored in fat. Then, a healthy and efficient liver will eliminate those toxins and prevent additional problems.

"Those foods were my own 'personal poison.'"

It has been said, "You are what you eat." However, I have learned that for me the key to optimal wellness depends on what I don't eat! As a breast cancer survivor I pride myself on following a clean nutritious diet of natural foods–salmon, sweet potatoes, asparagus, nuts and colorful fruits and vegetables. Three years ago I developed a cough that gradually escalated from a slight tickle to chronic choking. Gasping for air and stopping conversations mid-sentence became an everyday occurrence. Physically, mentally and financially drained I began the expensive and time consuming journey to find the cause of this distress.

Despite consultations with four specialists, multiple diagnostic procedures and prescriptions lining my kitchen counter I remained symptomatic, until consulting with Dr. Lee! His innovative holistic approach and commitment to a healing partnership have been a prayer answered!

Through extensive hormonal and ALCAT food testing it was discovered that these healthy foods and 90 others were to blame—those foods were my own "personal poison" in that they triggered auto-immunity and induced inflammation and other symptoms. Following Dr. Lee's recommended treatment for adrenal fatigue; hormonal imbalance and leaky gut has transformed my life–in just six short weeks! It is as if someone flipped a switch and turned back the hands of time. I pinch myself and celebrate the joy of this newfound energy, renewed sexual vitality and the fact that there is no more coughing! The balance of all the above gave me yet another gift–slipping into my smaller size wardrobe that had been packed away for years.

As women caring for those around us, we often minimize the symptoms of our own bodies when things seem "off." Each day is a gift to be celebrated and cherished. Your health is an investment in yourself. I encourage others to make the commitment to reclaim the vitality you so deserve. Thank you Dr. Lee for your gift of vision and commitment to wellness and balance. You are a blessing to us all!

— Cathy Bostwick

Another very important point is that you need to rotate your diet and not eat the same foods incessantly. We are creatures of habit and tend to eat the same foods over and over. If you write down all of what you eat for two weeks, then you will probably see that you eat the same breakfast and lunch every day (or, with little variation) while dinner may vary a little, though not as much as it should.

You really need to have variation in eating, and to eat real food, not processed food that comes from a box. The ALCAT test results come with a rotation diet plan. You should retest in six months to see if there is any improvement, or if you will always have an issue with certain foods.

For me, I never liked coffee and I found that I have a moderate reaction to coffee. An interesting fact is that my wife, who loves coffee, also has a moderate reaction, as does our six-year-old son, who has never drank coffee. It may be a genetic issue for my family with coffee. Nevertheless, my wife has given up coffee and is feeling much better.

The ALCAT test also determined that one of my severe reactions were peanuts—which now means that I have to stay away from Thai foods, and that I have to ask what oils a restaurant uses for cooking, since peanut oil is generally used in restaurants.

Also remember (as in my doctor patient example earlier) that some supplements (like omega-3 or fish oils) are derived from certain foods (such as sardines or anchovies). So, if you have a severe or moderate reaction to sardines or anchovies, then you cannot take omega-3 or fish oils that are derived from those foods. Always be cautious in what you consume, whether it is a food or a supplement.

In a similar situation—speaking of supplements—my son's ALCAT solved the mystery of what had been happening with his chewable probiotics. (In trying to help my son improve on his immune system, I was giving him orange-flavored chewable probiotics, but they mysteriously caused stomach pain and even vomiting.)

Probiotics are live microorganisms (in most cases, bacteria) that are similar to the beneficial microorganisms found in our human gut. Consuming probiotics is one of the most important things you can do to help your gut work much better—probiotics help digest your foods better, and they also support general wellness. Examples of foods containing probiotics are yogurt, fermented milk, miso and some soy drinks.

As for solving the mystery of why probiotics were causing my son to experience stomach pain and vomiting, his ALCAT discovered that one of his severe reactions is to oranges. He is even sensitive to orange flavoring, which can cause problems for him. So, thanks to his ALCAT, I switched him from orange-flavored chewable probiotics to probiotics that are not flavored, and all is well.

I really believe that doing the ALCAT test and eliminating the foods that your body does not like will improve on lowering chronic inflammation (a desirable effect)—along with following a nutritional plan that does not raise your insulin levels—are the keys in losing weight and developing an amazing body.

Please note that with the ALCAT—like most things in life—there are other opinions, and there is some misinformation online about ALCAT; however, when all the facts are presented, ALCAT does shine through. I have researched and tested ALCAT thoroughly, I know that it gets results, and I know that it is really helping my patients.

You must also not forget to work out your body on a daily basis to keep it strong, while reinforcing your diet with nutraceuticals (food products), minerals and botanicals—as explained in the next chapter.

Respect your body, and you will be rewarded with the greatest gift in life, and that is good health.

Conclusion

You need to know what foods will make you—and you alone—fat! Remember, not all foods are healthy for everyone. For someone, a certain food may be beneficial, whereas for someone else it may be harmful—like my son and oranges.

Most people have no idea that the foods they like, and are consuming, may be very harmful to them. Certain foods can lead to a leaky gut and thus cause chronic inflammation (not a desirable effect) that cause you to become overweight. Also, a leaky gut can lead to many other conditions like a low immune system, sinus problems, diabetes, ADD and migraines, just to name a few.

There are new medical studies that have shown more significant weight loss results when compared to the weight loss drugs that have been approved by the FDA. In addition, the drugs used for weight loss all have some type of side effect, including death. Fen-phen a drug approved by the FDA was pulled off the market in 1997 due to heart problems and pulmonary hypertension. One terrible case from a side effect of an FDA approved medication was from a 30-year-old woman who wanted to lose a little weight before her wedding but died from taking Fen-phen for only one month. She never made it to the alter.

The best test out there for determining what food sensitivities you have is the ALCAT test. You may call the company (800-872-5228) to find where you can have the test done. This test is not done in every doctor's office since most doctors are not taught in medical school about food sensitivity. Then, once you have the ALCAT results, you need to do a complete elimination of the foods to which you have a moderate and severe reaction. You will need to rotate your safe foods that are provided by ALCAT, and you will also need to have a nutritional plan that does not raise your insulin levels in order to lose weight.

CHAPTER 6 REVIEW

— Certain foods can cause you to become fat, while having absolutely no effect on someone else.

— Not all healthy foods are healthy for everyone.

— To test for your food sensitivities, use the ALCAT test.

— If you have a positive result then you need to eliminate that food for up to six months.

— Take a good probiotic, glutamine and digestive enzymes to help your gut work better.

— Follow a nutritional plan that will not increase your insulin levels.

7

Nutraceuticals, Minerals and Botanicals

"If we could see the miracle of a single flower clearly, our whole life would change."
— *Buddha*

A classic study on preventing diabetes was published in the New England Journal of Medicine, and it compared lifestyle intervention with a medication (called metformin) for preventing diabetes. This landmark diabetes prevention study followed more than 3,000 patients for close to three years. There were three groups in the study, and they were evaluated to determine who did the best. One group was a placebo and was told to do nothing special. The second group took 850 mg of metformin twice a day. The third group exercised for at least 150 minutes a week and followed a diet to lose at least seven percent of their body weight. Physical activity and diet beat out the medication metformin in preventing diabetes.[1] Even though this major study has proven that diet and exercise are more effective, metformin is now the most widely prescribed antidiabetic drug in the world.

The good news is that this study proved proper nutrition and exercise can help reverse insulin resistance. And now that you've read this book so far, you understand how insulin resistance causes obesity, and how it affects not just those with diabetes, but everyone.

In this chapter, nutraceuticals (food products that provide health benefits), minerals and botanicals—as they relate to a diet that reverses insulin resistance—will be discussed. Also, I will reference 92 well-known and published sources of medical data to support these facts. This is an important chapter.

I could have easily written this chapter without any references—and that would have prevented many late-nighters. However, I have a strong passion to raise awareness of the reality that, in order to reduce belly fat, you have to reduce insulin resistance. So, should you desire any additional reading, the references in this chapter are extensive.

"My energy has fully returned."

In 2006 my weight was 200 pounds. Treatment for my severe high blood pressure required three different types of medication at maximum doses. I had experienced a TIA in 2000 and frequently experienced lightheadedness and near fainting episodes.

With treatment from Dr. Lee, which included some nutraceuticals, my weight is now 157 pounds and I no longer take any high blood pressure medication, with my blood pressure being now normal. I am able to enjoy long walks and climbing mountains in western North Carolina without any symptoms. My energy has fully returned and I am again experiencing my former joy of living.

— Dr. H. Dean Shull, Jr.

Nutraceuticals — Fish Oil

Regarding nutraceuticals, there are many that will help with reducing insulin resistance. One that I especially like to use is fish oil, omega-3 (EPA/DHA pharmacy grade). As explained earlier, insulin resistance is a condition of chronic inflammation. EPA/DHA has been shown to reduce chronic inflammation, which is a good thing to do.[2]

In a recent study, omega-3 reduced inflammation by lowering 2 markers of inflammation in the blood: IL-6 and TNF. In addition, the study in healthy older adults using four to five grams of EPA/DHA resulted in lowering insulin resistance and improving on insulin sensitivity.[3]

Animal studies have been used for making many advances in medicine. In understanding how EPA/DHA works on the body there have been many studies on diabetic rats to demonstrate that EPA/DHA increases the GLUT4 receptors in muscles to help allow glucose to enter the muscle cells.[4]

In another rat study, it has been shown that EPA/DHA increases peroxisome proliferator-activated receptor alpha (PPAR-alpha), which is located inside the nucleus of the cell and controls your DNA expression. Increasing PPAR-alpha expression improves on insulin sensitivity. The medication class of fibrates (e.g. TriCor®) and the diabetic medication called pioglitazone (i.e. Actos®) both increase PPAR-alpha expression.[5]

The same study showed that taking EPA/DHA to lower insulin resistance (by the PPAR-alpha pathway) also increased levels of a fat hormone called adiponectin. Higher levels of adiponectin are a good thing to have, and they can reduce insulin resistance.[6]

In review, omega-3 (EPA/DHA) has been shown to reduce inflammation, improve on insulin resistance by working on the PPAR-alpha pathway, increase the hormone adipoenectin, and increase the GLUT4 receptors—making EPA/DHA a much better alternative than taking a prescription medication to improve on insulin resistance.

Besides improving on insulin resistance, fish oil has also been shown to improve on blood pressure, raise HDL cholesterol (high density lipoprotein or "good cholesterol") and lower triglycerides. Although the American diet is high in refined sugars, calories and fat, the type of omega-3 that Americans consume in high amounts is alpha-linolenic acid (ALA), which is found in leafy vegetables, walnuts, soybeans, flaxseed and vegetable oils. Alpha-linolenic acid, which is the first part of the omega-3 pathway, unfortunately does not convert well into the healthy part of omega-3 (EPA and DHA), which is why it's extremely important to supplement your diet with EPA/DHA.[7]

EPA/DHA also has favorable effects in protecting you from heart disease and sudden cardiac death. The reason that EPA/DHA is beneficial is that it reduces the expression of cyclooxygenase-2 and other enzymes involved with increasing inflammation—and with the formation of pro inflammatory markers (cytokines). It also reduces free radicals, which is a good thing for your body.

EPA/DHA also has a positive action on lipid metabolism, lipoprotein particle size (carriers of cholesterol in the body), blood pressure, clotting, inflammatory response, clot formation and protects against irregular heart rhythms.[8]

A recent cardiology journal supports the dietary supplementation that omega-3 be used to protect against heart disease.[9]

Based upon the medical literature, and the results I see daily in my private practice, I recommend supplementing your diet with one to four grams a day of EPA/DHA.

Nutraceuticals — Resveratrol

As one of the hottest "miracle molecules" with much potential, resveratrol is a relatively new supplement, with a long history. Resveratrol is a polyphenol molecule found in grapes, peanuts, cranberries, Japanese giant knotweed and red wine. This connection with red wine has led many to postulate that resveratrol may explain the "French Paradox" of longevity—the French population has a low incidence of heart disease, even though they consume a diet higher in fat than other populations.

Resveratrol lowers the activity of NFKB (the proteins for "turning on" inflammation) and thereby reduces chronic inflammation. Resveratrol reduces the markers of inflammation like TNF and IL-6.[10]

Resveratrol has also been shown to increase life spans in some animal studies by activating the Sirtuin 1 gene, which is more commonly known as the longevity gene. Resveratrol has already been shown to increase longevity in life forms (from fungi and worms to insects and small mammals) by increasing several proteins such as:

SIRT1 (found in humans), Sir2 (found in yeast) and 5' adenosine monophosphate-activated protein kinase (AMPK, an enzyme that plays a vital role in cellular energy).

A group of researchers have determined lower SIRT1 levels induce insulin resistance (bad thing to have) and higher SIRT1 levels increase insulin sensitivity (good thing to have). In another study where mice were overfed to induce insulin resistance and obesity, it was found that resveratrol significantly improved insulin resistance and considerably lower insulin levels were achieved. Besides increasing SIRT1 levels (desirable effect), the researchers also showed that resveratrol lowered levels of an enzyme called protein tyrosine phosphatase — which is a negative regulator of insulin function (another desirable effect).[11-12]

Although the studies in cell cultures and animal models look very promising for resveratrol, there have been very few studies done in humans. Once taken, the concentration of resveratrol peaks in about 60 minutes, and then it's quickly metabolized.

Although there are not yet any human studies showing whether resveratrol improves longevity or provides cancer protection, resveratrol is a flavonoid—and flavonoids already have significant medical data on how they lower blood pressure, improve on insulin sensitivity and improve on lipids.[14] Also, there are studies showing how resveratrol can improve on insulin resistance.[13] (More on this later.)

In a 10,000 plus patient study in Finland over one year, it was noted that with a higher intake of flavonoids there was a lower incidence of type 2 Diabetes, prostate cancer, lung cancer and stroke.[15]

In the highly regarded Iowa Women's Health Study, there were over 34,000 women who were free of heart disease. These women were followed for 16 years and it was noted that foods rich in flavonoids (apples, pears, grapefruit, strawberries and red wine) were associated with less heart disease, stroke and early death.[16]

The debate on whether or not resveratrol can be helpful in reducing insulin resistance is now being addressed by the American Diabetes Association (ADA). They have awarded $600,000 to the Albert Einstein College of Medicine to study resveratrol on glucose metabolism, and on reducing insulin resistance. At the ADA's 70th scientific meeting, there was a small study presented on ten adults with type 2 diabetes who improved their insulin resistance and lowered their post meal blood sugar levels with resveratrol. With the ADA grant, a larger study by the Albert Einstein College of Medicine will be done to confirm the findings of the smaller study.

Also at that ADA meeting, there was another small study (ten adults) presented by the University of Buffalo that showed how resveratrol reduced the body's inflammatory response to a high fat/high carbohydrate meal. And, in another more recent double blind study that was just published, resveratrol in diabetic patients was shown to lower insulin resistance while lowering inflammation.[17]

Resveratrol looks even more promising now that more studies are being conducted on people. I believe the current human clinical trials will only further confirm the benefits of resveratrol.

Nutraceuticals — Alpha-Lipoic Acid

Another amazing nutraceutical is alpha-lipoic acid (ALA). Please be sure to note that alpha-lipoic acid is not the same as alpha-linolenic acid. It can be confusing because both are commonly abbreviated as ALA. To avoid any confusion, I will only refer to these nutraceuticals by their full names.

The history of alpha-lipoic acid is interesting. It started in the 1930s when scientists noticed that alpha-lipoic acid was an important factor for growing several different bacteria.[18] From the 1950s through the 1980s, alpha-lipoic acid was known to be a very powerful antioxidant. It was also noted that alpha-lipoic acid was involved with energy production and glucose metabolism. What I find fascinating about alpha-lipoic acid is that there are case reports of alpha-lipoic acid helping patients with chronic liver disease. Also there are case reports of successful therapy in patients with metastatic pancreatic cancer.[19-21]

Alpha-lipoic acid is unique as an antioxidant since it functions both in fat and in water. It helps to regenerate a very important chemical called glutathione, which helps the liver to detoxify better. Alpha-lipoic acid is also a fatty acid that is found naturally in every cell in your body. The dietary sources of alpha-lipoic acid include organ meats, potatoes, broccoli and spinach.

Not only is alpha-lipoic acid a great antioxidant, it also helps with glucose metabolism and energy production. Alpha-lipoic acid prevents glycosylation, a process where glucose is attached to a protein. Alpha-lipoic acid helps with energy production by being involved in the Krebs cycle as a coenzyme. Our cells produce energy through the Krebs cycle.

Alpha-lipoic acid has also been shown to improve on insulin sensitivity or improve on insulin resistance. In a Glucose Clamp Study (the gold standard in measuring insulin resistance) alpha-lipoic acid has been shown to improve on insulin sensitivity.[22]

There are actually many studies that prove alpha-lipoic acid helps with lowering blood sugars in diabetes, and with a complication in diabetes called diabetic neuropathy. Diabetic neuropathy is a condition where the nerves are damaged from chronic high blood sugars, oxidative stress, chronic inflammation, excessive free radicals and the production of advanced glycation end-products (AGE, sugar coated protein that has altered its function). The production of AGE is the result of chronic inflammation, which will result in damage to any nerve that is involved—from your brain to your toes. A nerve is like a fragile wire in the body, and if that wire gets damaged then it is very difficult to reverse the damage.[23]

Some examples of neuropathy can present themselves with a burning sensation, extreme sensitivity to touch, pain, erectile dysfunction, urinary incontinence, impaired sense of position and weakness of a muscle. Four large clinical trials (ALADIN I, ALADIN III, SYDNEY and NATHAN II) studied intravenous alpha lipoic acid at 600 mg and showed that it significantly helped reduce symptoms of neuropathy, and that it was safe to use.[24]

Orally administered alpha-lipoic acid has also been shown to help with diabetic neuropathy.[25]

With insulin resistance, there is a complication of endothelial dysfunction, or damage to the flexibility of the blood vessels. In a medical study that used 300 mg alpha-lipoic acid alone—and in combination with a certain blood pressure medication—alpha-lipoic acid (which decreases inflammation through the reduction of markers in the blood called IL-6 and PAI-1) was shown to significantly improve on the flexibility of blood vessels by itself, and when combined with the blood pressure medication.[26]

This is an important finding since you want more blood flow and oxygen delivery when you need it. If you don't get enough oxygen to a certain tissue, then it will die off.

The last point on alpha-lipoic acid is the improvement of glucose uptake in an insulin resistant state. Just recently, alpha-lipoic acid has been shown to improve insulin resistance by increasing certain heat shock proteins, which then blocks certain enzymes, which then improves on glucose uptake in the cells. In insulin resistance the cells become resistant for insulin to work, which makes it difficult for glucose to come into the cell. Alpha-lipoic acid helps glucose come into the cell in an insulin resistant state.[27]

In addition to helping glucose, alpha-lipoic acid increases the GLUT4 receptors for glucose to come into the cells.[28]

Alpha-lipoic acid is an amazing nutraceutical that helps to improve on insulin resistance and glucose uptake, decrease inflammation, improve on the production of glutathione (for the liver to detoxify better), improve on energy production and is a powerful antioxidant. Alpha-lipoic acid is well tolerated and the most common side effect is upset stomach or nausea (usually dose dependent).

The dose that has clinical data for alpha-lipoic acid ranges from 300 to 1200 mg a day. The optimal dose still needs to be determined, but I would recommend a dose of 300 mg to 1000 mg a day to help reduce insulin resistance.

Nutraceuticals — Coenzyme Q10

The last nutraceutical I will cover is Coenzyme Q10 (CoQ10), otherwise known as ubiquinone. More than 50 years' worth of studies have looked at the benefits of this amazing supplement. It was first discovered in 1957 at the University of Wisconsin in the heart of a cow. CoQ10 is found in certain foods and the highest concentration is in fish such as sardines and mackerel. In general, meats, fish, nuts and some oils are the richest sources of CoQ10. Other sources are from vegetables like broccoli and spinach.[29]

Coenzyme Q10 has a unique structure. It is a fat-soluble substance with two parts to it. The "tail" part attaches to the inside of the cell, and the "head" part (Quinone) of CoQ10 is involved with transferring electrons for energy production. CoQ10 is involved in producing energy in your body. CoQ10 specially works inside your mitochondria cells to help produce more energy. The "Q" in CoQ10 stands for Quinone and the "10" stands for the tail length. Every vital organ we have needs CoQ10 to function properly.

Since CoQ10 was discovered, it has been noted that the heart has a higher demand for CoQ10. Accordingly, CoQ10 has been used extensively across the world for the treatment of congestive heart failure. A review of eight clinical studies showed that CoQ10 improved cardiac output, or cardiac function.[30]

Another review of eleven clinical trials that used CoQ10 in heart failure also showed a marked improvement of heart function.[31]

Recently, there was a published study showing that if you have a low levels of CoQ10 in your blood, then you are at a higher risk of dying earlier if you have heart failure.[32]

The most common causes for low CoQ10 levels are the cholesterol medications called statins. Some common examples of statins are Zocor®, Lipitor®, and Crestor®. Although most conventional doctors know that statins have the side effect of myopathy (muscle pain), they are not aware that statins block the production of CoQ10 by blocking the production of farnesyl pyrophosphate.[33]

Besides being involved with energy production, CoQ10 is also a very strong antioxidant. In a recent study where type 2 diabetic patients were given 200 mg of CoQ10 daily over twelve weeks, endothelial dysfunction (damage to the flexibility of the blood vessels) improved. The study also noted that CoQ10 reduced the markers of inflammation.[34]

Another study showed that the use of Coq10 at 200 mg a day helped lower blood sugars of the subjects, and lowered their three-month glucose average blood test (called the hemoglobin A1c). The study also showed that Coq10 helped lower blood pressure.[35]

Another recent study on CoQ10 looked at twelve clinical trials (three randomized controlled trials, one crossover and eight open labeled studies). CoQ10 was shown to lower blood pressure by 17 mm Hg on the systolic blood pressure (top number) and by 10 mm Hg on the diastolic blood pressure (bottom number).[36]

CoQ10 can also lower insulin resistance. In an eight week study with CoQ10, fasting glucose and insulin levels were lowered—and, two-hour insulin and glucose levels were also lowered. In the study it was mentioned that CoQ10 might provide protection to the beta cells of the pancreas (the cells that make insulin), liver cells and endothelial cells.[37]

In a recent six-month study (randomized placebo controlled) that used a combination of vitamin C (500 mg), vitamin E (200 IU), CoQ10 (60 mg) and selenium (100 mcg), 70 patients who had risk factors for heart disease showed that the combination helped lower glucose, insulin resistance and the markers of inflammation. It also showed that the antioxidants improved the elasticity of small and large arteries (a desired result).[38]

Another study has shown that CoQ10 is able to lower inflammation by lowering TNF (Tumor Necrosis Factor—a bad chemical in your blood).[39]

Currently there is debate on which type of CoQ10 should be used. CoQ10 comes in two flavors. One is called ubiquinol and the other is ubiquinone. The difference is that ubiquinone picks up electrons and then becomes ubiquinol. Ubiquinol then releases its electrons and becomes ubiquinone again. Ubiquinol can become ubiquinone and vice versa. The medical studies so far have generally been done on ubiquinone. The dose that I would recommend in addressing insulin resistance is between 100 to 300 mg a day of ubiquinone. It is usually very well tolerated, although some patients may have minor stomach issues or dizziness. Also, it can thin the blood so you will need to have your blood thinner (warfarin) adjusted.[40]

"I had persistent 'brain fog.'"

At 43 years of age, I found myself crying uncontrollably in Dr. Lee's office. In the middle of early menopause and having problems with the absorption of my current thyroid medication I was unable to function. I had persistent "brain fog" and was having trouble caring for my husband and four boys.

In less than a year, Dr. Lee was able to turn everything around by "tweaking" my hormone replacement, changing my thyroid medication and providing the right nutraceuticals and supplements for me. With every visit Dr. Lee listens to my concerns and I never feel rushed. If I ever have any questions after I leave his office I know I can call and Dr. Lee will call me back personally. I really value that.

Today, I am back on my exercise routine, eating clean and have easily weened myself off an antidepressant. With the help of a compassionate Dr. Lee, I feel great, and we are a happy family again.

— Elizabeth Moran

Minerals — Magnesium

Magnesium is a crucial mineral that is required for every living organism on earth. For example, if plants have magnesium deficiency then the leaves will begin to turn yellow. Magnesium in the body helps with contraction and relaxation of muscles, is involved in energy production, contributes as enzymes and helps with the production of protein. Dietary magnesium comes from dark, green, leafy vegetables. Other foods with magnesium are bananas, apricots, avocados, almonds, cashews, peas, tofu, brown rice and millet. Magnesium is crucial to your diet; however, depleted farming soils are resulting in diminishing levels of magnesium in our current foods. Recent dietary surveys have shown that the average magnesium intake in western countries is often below the recommended dietary allowance (RDA) of 420 mg for men and 320 mg for women.[41]

Magnesium is a very important mineral in your body. It's necessary for more than 300 different types of biochemical reactions, it helps maintain normal muscle and nerve function, it keeps heart rhythm steady, it keeps bones strong and it's involved in energy metabolism and protein synthesis.

About 60 percent of your magnesium is in our bones. As for the rest, about 20 percent is in your skeletal muscles, 19 percent in other soft tissues and less than one percent in your extracellular fluids (blood) or outside of the cells.[42]

As you can see, very little magnesium is in your blood and most is in our bones, muscles or other soft tissues. The reason most physicians are not diagnosing low magnesium is that they are not doing the correct test because they have not been educated about red blood cell magnesium or mononuclear (special white blood cell) magnesium. I prefer the red blood cell magnesium test, which happens to be very affordable. Most doctors check for blood (serum) magnesium; however there is a poor correlation between (blood) serum and red blood cell magnesium.[43]

It's still debatable as to which method is the best for measuring the total body content of magnesium; although, since the 1980s, red blood cell magnesium, mononuclear cell (special white blood cell) magnesium and muscle magnesium have been used for determining intracellular magnesium concentration.

A recent study of 246 geriatric patients showed that all of them had normal serum (blood) magnesium; however, 57 percent of them had low red blood cell magnesium. Also, there was a trend that the people with low red blood cell magnesium had a higher rate of high blood pressure, high cholesterol, diabetes, B12 deficiency and heart disease.[44]

"I had suffered for years with multiple health problems."

When my cortisol level came back high, my family doctor recommended that I go see Dr. Lee. I'm so glad that I did because it has improved my quality of life. Before Dr. Lee, I had suffered for years with multiple health problems. I had seen many doctors and been hospitalized multiple times, but no one believed me because I was only 26 years old. The vast majority of them believed it was in my head, that I was just depressed and anorexic.

The truth was that I was depressed, but I was also having diarrhea several times a day and got nauseous every time I ate. It was horrible—and depressing! I was exhausted, my hair was thinning and falling out and I had gotten down to 92 pounds. Even though I'm only 5'1," that is still way too thin.

Dr. Lee diagnosed me with leaky gut, adrenal fatigue and a progesterone deficiency. I was also very malnourished due to my condition and needed vitamin D, B12, magnesium, iron and other vitamins and minerals. Dr. Lee put me on several supplements including UltraInflamX®. Within six weeks I noticed a huge difference. I had gained 15 pounds and was eating great!

Now that my gut is on the mend, Dr. Lee is working with me to get everything else in order. I am extremely grateful for Dr. Lee and his integrative, holistic care of me. I am really looking forward to the whole me being healthy and feeling youthful.

— Misty Sons

If you want to know if you have low magnesium then request a red blood cell magnesium level. It does not make sense to check a serum (blood) magnesium level since only one percent of your magnesium is in your serum (blood) and 99 percent is in your cells. Again, there is a poor correlation between serum (blood) and red blood cell magnesium. I suspect that it will take another decade before this will be an accepted practice in conventional medicine. Also, there will be other studies presented that show low red blood cell magnesium is linked to insulin resistance.

Just recently, with one of my patients and his wife, I was explaining the best regimen for optimizing his diabetes. We talked about avoiding alcohol since it has sugar and to use a new glucagon-like peptide medication to help with his blood sugars. When I got to the subject of adding magnesium to his regimen his wife did not want him to take another supplement. Unfortunately, there are difficult patients who are not receptive to optimizing their nutrition, or feel that taking "recommended supplements" is just too much trouble. Yet, there are people who unquestioningly take handfuls of prescription pills every day.

As for blood sugars, if you have low magnesium then your blood sugars will be higher. Also, low magnesium will prevent your insulin from working correctly.[45]

In a study comparing serum (blood) magnesium levels to special white blood cell (mononuclear) magnesium levels, it was shown that mononuclear magnesium levels are much better for detecting deficiencies of magnesium. Also, it showed that low magnesium is common among people with metabolic syndrome and insulin resistance.[46]

A recent double-blind, randomized, placebo-controlled study (gold standard) looked at subjects with normal magnesium levels (but with insulin resistance) who took 365 mg of magnesium aspartate hydrochloride a day for six months.

At the end of the study, magnesium significantly improved on insulin resistance, and it improved on fasting glucose levels. This study emphasized the use of optimizing magnesium to prevent insulin resistance and, subsequently, type 2 diabetes.[47]

In a classic 1993 study, it was shown that magnesium deficiency produced insulin resistance. This study also showed that if you had low magnesium, then you also had higher markers for: inflammation, blood vessel disease, aldosterone and thromboxane A2.[48]

Another double-blind, randomized, placebo-controlled study (gold standard) of diabetics with complications of neuropathy (nerve damage), and with heart disease, showed that they also had low magnesium levels. There was no correlation between blood (serum) magnesium versus intracellular magnesium. The method of study was based on the special white blood cell mononuclear cells. Also in the study, it showed that the diabetics required a much higher dose of magnesium oxide (401 mmol a day versus 20 mmol a day) to normalize their magnesium deficiency.[49]

Another interesting study showed if you consume less than the recommended daily allowance for magnesium, then you have a higher level of C-reactive protein (CRP), which is a marker of inflammation and is associated with an increased risk of heart disease. It was also noted that if you are over 40 years of age, with a body mass index of less than 25, and consume less than 50 percent of the recommended daily allowance for magnesium, then you are 2.24 times more likely to have an elevated CRP.[50]

The larger studies that correlate low magnesium with type 2 diabetes are the Women's Heart Study, the Nurses' Health Study, the Health Professional Follow-up Study, the Iowa Women's Health Study and the Honolulu Heart Program.

Based on data from 39,345 women—and a six year follow up—the Women's Heart Study reported a significant relationship between low dietary magnesium intake and a higher risk of developing diabetes.[51]

The Nurses' Health Study (85,000 women were followed for 18 years) and the Health Professional Follow-up Study (42,000 men were followed for twelve years) demonstrated that a magnesium rich diet reduces the risk of developing diabetes by 34 percent in women, and 33 percent in men.[52]

The Iowa Women's Health Study and the Honolulu Heart Program showed that a diet low in magnesium increases the risk of diabetes.[53]

I hope these findings will persuade you to increase your leafy, green vegetables (the best source of magnesium) and to supplement your diet with extra magnesium.

Just recently, I talked with a patient who says her doctor does not understand why she has low magnesium with a "normal" blood (serum) magnesium. She also showed the doctor that her red blood cell magnesium was very low, but was told that is not the standard way to measure magnesium level. Remember, there is a poor correlation of blood (serum) magnesium versus intracellular magnesium or red blood cell magnesium. She then asked her doctor to please do some research on the subject of magnesium deficiency, and on using red blood cell magnesium, but was told by the doctor that he did not have the time to do it. This is exactly the type of attitude that will prevent any improvement of our current medical system. All the doctor needed to do was go to www.pubmed.com and read the data that is out there.

The data (including the gold standard studies—double-blind, randomized, placebo-controlled) is overwhelming that magnesium is helpful for diabetics, and with insulin resistance. However, it is rarely talked about in conventional medicine, or even endocrinology.

Magnesium also has a huge role in helping with migraines, high blood pressure, heart disease, asthma, osteoporosis, strokes, depression, infertility and much more. There are several great books written on magnesium and its vital role in your health. Most likely you do have some degree of magnesium deficiency and can benefit from adding it to your regimen. The only reason you do not want to use magnesium would be if you have severe kidney failure. The side effects of taking too much magnesium are nausea, vomiting, low blood pressure, diarrhea or flushing.

There are many kinds of magnesium you can take. I would recommend taking a dose of 300 mg to 1000 mg a day. A double-blind, randomized, placebo-controlled study (gold standard) showed in diabetics that a dose of 1000 mg of magnesium oxide improved glucose control.[54]

Some examples of magnesium sources are magnesium citrate, taurinate, malate, oxide, glycinate and succinate. The combination will impair your absorption of magnesium, so use separate pills and take magnesium at a different time than calcium.

For constipation, I prefer to recommend magnesium citrate. The best way is intravenous magnesium—especially if you are unable to achieve results by taking magnesium pills.

Minerals — Chromium

Chromium is crucial for normal glucose metabolism and for helping reverse insulin resistance. Since the 1950s, studies on chromium have shown it to be beneficial; however, these days, there is controversy over the real benefits of chromium. Some studies have recently concluded that chromium is not helpful; however, it appears that some of those studies had the dosage too low. Some double-blind, randomized, placebo-controlled studies (gold standard) used chromium picolinate in type 2 diabetics and showed that patients with more insulin resistance had a better response to chromium.[55]

In another study—also a double-blind, randomized, placebo-controlled study (gold standard)—it was also shown in type 2 diabetics that 1000 mcg of chromium picolinate a day helps with weight loss, while also improving on insulin sensitivity and glucose control.[56]

Another double-blind, randomized, placebo-controlled study showed that chromium (chromium yeast at 1000 mcg a day) and vitamin C and vitamin E improves blood sugars in type 2 diabetics, and lowers inflammation (oxidative stress).[57]

There are several reasons why chromium improves on glucose metabolism and lowers insulin resistance. One reason is that chromium has been shown to increase your GLUT-4 receptors, thereby allowing more glucose enter into the cells.[58]

Also, chromium has been shown to decrease inflammation markers such as TNF (tumor necrosis factor), CRP (C-reactive protein) and IL-6 (interleukin 6).[59]

Another unique aspect about chromium is that it can bind to insulin, which has been postulated to have a stabilizing effect on insulin.

Chromium has been tested in many forms—such as chromium chloride, chromium nicotinate, chromium proprionate, chromium histidinate and chromium picolinate. The latter form has been used the most in medical studies, but only about one percent of absorbed chromium from chromium picolinate is found in the blood stream. There are new forms of chromium that are improving chromium bioavailability—such as chromium with D-phenyalanine, chromium dinicocysteinate and chromium with biotin.[60]

Hopefully, there will soon be larger studies that will settle the debate about the newer forms of chromium reducing insulin resistance. Until then, in my current practice, I have seen great results with chromium picolinate in doses of 200 mcg to 1000 mcg a day.

Botanicals — Garlic

Botanicals are derived from plants and herbs and are valued for their medicinal or therapeutic properties. Allium sativum (garlic) has been used for its medicinal properties for over a thousand years. It is also used in many Korean foods that I grew up eating.

The joke I heard from a burn surgeon in the U.S. was that when he was in the Korean War, he always got his eyelashes burned off whenever he talked with someone who was eating Korean food, so it sparked his interest in studying burns.

The oils found in garlic have been shown to lower blood pressure and blood sugars so the pancreas does not have to secrete so much insulin. A double-blind, randomized, placebo-controlled study (gold standard) in Australia looked at 50 patients with uncontrolled blood pressure and on blood pressure medications. Both groups showed that 960 mg of aged garlic extract lowered systolic blood pressure by ten mm Hg.[61]

In another double-blind, randomized, placebo-controlled study (gold standard) 600 mg of dehydrated garlic powder were given daily to 60 patients with type 2 diabetes. The four-week study determined that garlic significantly lowered blood sugars, triglycerides, and fructosamine (the marker in the blood for glucose control).[62]

Since garlic from nature contains many organosulfur compounds, amino acids, vitamins and minerals, it is best taken raw. The countries with a high consumption of garlic have been shown to have lower cancer rates. The downside of garlic is bad breath—and burning off other people's eyelashes. So, add some garlic to your cooking and get a healthier body.

Botanicals — Curcumin

Found in turmeric, curcumin is a compound that is known to help reduce insulin resistance. Curcumin is used as a spice in curries and other South Asian and Middle Eastern cuisine. Curcumin has been used since around 2000 B.C. for its medicinal properties, such as an antiseptic for cuts and burns, and as an antibacterial agent. In some Asian countries it is used as a dietary supplement to relieve stomach problems, and it can even help with irritable bowel syndrome.

Regarding the current medical data, curcumin was presented at the 90th annual meeting of the Endocrine Society held in San Francisco. The study was done on rats genetically prone to gain weight that were being fed a high calorie diet. One group of rats was given curcumin and the other group was not given curcumin. The curcumin group had a lower rate of developing diabetes, and less inflammation, when compared to the group that did not eat curcumin.[63]

While there have been many diabetic rat studies showing how curcumin lowered glucose levels and reduced inflammation, there has been only one study showing that curcumin lowered glucose and reduced insulin requirements in human diabetics.[64] More human studies are needed to confirm that this ancient extract of turmeric is also effective in reducing insulin resistance. There have been clinical human trials looking at curcumin in colorectal cancer, and it is known to be safe and well-tolerated—at doses up to 8000 mg per day.

As for other cancer factors, curcumin reduces inflammation—such as the markers of TNF (Tumor Necrosis Factor) and nuclear factor kappa beta (NFKB)—and has been shown to induce cancer cell death, while also reducing the spread of cancer.[65]

So, enjoy your curry because my prediction is that curcumin—the "ancient botanical"—will prove to have significant benefits in reversing insulin resistance in human studies in the future.

Botanicals — Ginseng

Another wonderful botanical is ginseng, which is said to have been used in the Orient for 5000 years now. It is sometimes referred to as the "root of heaven" or the "king of herbs." In the first Chinese book of herbs, *Pen Tsao Ching* by the famous Chinese Emperor Shen Nung, gold and ginseng are described as being vital for eternal youth.

Ginseng has been used for enlightening the mind, increasing wisdom and many other reasons. Ginseng is usually thought of as an Asian plant and has been found to grow in Japan, Korea, Vietnam, China and Siberia. However, ginseng also grows in North America and has been used by Native Americans for centuries.

In a study done in Toronto, Canada it was shown that three grams of North American ginseng reduced blood sugars after eating. The study also showed there was no difference between the three, six or nine gram doses of ginseng.[66]

Twenty type 2 diabetics in a double-blind, randomized, placebo-controlled study took Asian ginseng (two 369 mg capsules, three times a day) for four weeks. The study showed a decrease in insulin resistance according to the participants' HOMA scores (homeostatic model assessment—a mathematical determination of insulin resistance). Also, there were lower fasting insulin levels and lower fasting glucose levels in the ginseng group.[67]

In a double-blind, randomized, placebo-controlled study of Korean ginseng, 19 type 2 diabetics took two grams of Korean ginseng with every meal for twelve weeks. The participants demonstrated a 34 percent decrease in fasting insulin levels and a 33 percent improvement in insulin sensitivity and improvement of glucose levels. This study also showed insulin resistance improvement with Korean ginseng.[68]

Ginseng is known as an adaptogen and is known to have many health benefits, such as improving sexual desire or libido. In a comprehensive review of the medical randomized control studies on Korean red ginseng (doses ranged from 1800 mg to 3000 mg a day), it was found that Korean red ginseng helped in the treatment of erectile dysfunction. The side effects noted in the different studies were mild and included insomnia, stomach discomfort and constipation.[69]

In another study, Korean red ginseng improved on sexual arousal in menopausal women. The 28 women participating in the double-blind, randomized, placebo-controlled study took one gram, three times a day. It was reported that ginseng significantly improved their sex life.[70]

Being an American of Korean descent, I grew up enjoying Korean chicken soup loaded with ginseng, and drinking ginseng tea. Don't forget to add ginseng into your diet.

Botanicals — Green Tea

Green tea is derived from the leaves of the camellia plant, and has been used in China for at least 4000 years. Camellia leaves are steamed, which sets this tea apart from other teas (such as black and oolong) that ferment the leaves.

The secret of green tea is a polyphenol ingredient called EGCG (epigallocatechin gallate). EGCG is a powerful antioxidant that has been shown to help with treating cancer. An Italian study looked at green tea in men with a high risk for prostate cancer. It was a double-blind, randomized, placebo-controlled study that looked at 60 men with high grade prostatic intraepithelial neoplasia (high risk of prostate cancer). The men took 200 mg of green tea catechin three times a day for one year. After one year, less prostate cancer was detected in the green tea group (one cancer in 30 men) compared to the placebo group (nine cancers in 30 men).[71]

Regarding green tea as an antioxidant, there are studies showing that green tea can significantly reduce oxidative stress. The best test to see how healthy you are is to collect a 24-hour urine sample and have it tested for 8-hydroxy-deoxyguanosine (8-OhdG) to determine if you have any DNA damage from oxidative stress. The 8-OhdG is a biomarker of oxidative DNA damage and is a predictor of increased cancer risk. In one randomized control study, 133 heavy smokers were randomized to either drink four cups of green tea, black tea or water.

After four months, the group drinking the green tea had a 31 percent decrease in 8-OhdG (desirable result). No decrease of 8-OhdG was reported in the black tea or water groups.[72]

In another double-blind, randomized, placebo-controlled study, 124 patients with a high risk of liver cancer (due to aflatoxin exposure and the hepatitis B virus) took either 500 mg or 1000 mg of a green tea extract, or a placebo. The green tea group had lower urinary 8-OhdG levels (desirable result) compared to the placebo group.[73]

As for green tea helping reduce insulin resistance, there are some great studies that suggest it does. In a recent study it was reported that green tea delays the onset of type 1 diabetes (autoimmune disease that requires insulin for survival) in non-obese diabetic mice. The study also showed that green tea increased the anti-inflammatory cytokine IL-10 (good blood marker).[74]

Green tea has also been shown (in obese and thin volunteers) to decrease markers of inflammation (such as nuclear factor kappa beta) while increasing a blood marker called interleukin 10 (desirable result).[75]

In a large retrospective study of 17,000 Japanese adults without diabetes, a 33 percent risk reduction for developing diabetes was found in subjects consuming six or more cups of green tea per day—compared to consuming less than one cup of green tea per week. The study also showed that as more green tea was consumed, the risk of developing diabetes became less.[76]

In a double-blind, randomized, placebo-controlled study in Japan, it was shown that green tea improved glucose control with type 2 diabetes, and increased the fat hormone called adiponectin (desirable result).[77]

Although there are some medical studies on green tea, more long-term studies are still needed (especially on standardized green tea products) to help us understand this incredible botanical. Now, don't you want to drink some green tea for its amazing health benefits?

Botanicals — Cinnamon

Cinnamon is a botanical with an amazing history. The history of cinnamon goes back to about 2800 B.C. when it was used throughout Egypt, Rome and China. Cinnamon comes from the bark of the laurel tree and is native to Southeast Asia (mostly Sri Lanka and India).

In Indonesia they call cinnamon "kayu manis" or "sweet wood." The ancient Egyptians used it in embalming mummies for its pleasant aroma and its preservative qualities. The Bible mentions that Moses used cinnamon with cassia, olive oil, myrrh and hemp for the holy anointing oil. In 65 A.D. the Emperor Nero burned a year's supply of cinnamon at his second wife's funeral to express the depth of his grief.

Cinnamon was a very expensive commodity during the fifteenth and sixteenth century, and was highly sought by the Portuguese, Dutch and English for control of the lucrative cinnamon industry. Back then, cinnamon began to be used for culinary and medicinal uses because it masks the smell of spoiling meat by inhibiting growth of the bacteria that spoil the meat. Some of the early medicinal uses of cinnamon were for curing the common cold, treating diarrhea and aiding in digestion. Since the early nineteenth century, the production of cinnamon has spread to other parts of the tropical world.

Currently, cinnamon has been shown to improve insulin resistance, diabetes and lower cholesterol. Cinnamon comes from the bark of certain trees—of which there are about 250 species. One of them, Cinnamomum zeylanicum or verum (Sri Lanka cinnamon), is similar to insulin. This particular cinnamon stimulates the insulin receptor by activating phosphatidylinositol 3 kinase (PI3K).[78]

Cinnamon has also been shown to increase the GLUT-4 receptor for glucose, which allows glucose to enter into your muscle, fat or heart cells.[79] That's how cinnamon helps to lower blood sugars and reduce insulin resistance—by improving on the uptake of glucose and by helping insulin to work more effectively.

In a randomized, controlled trial using cinnamon cassia (Chinese cinnamon), 500 mg was shown to help lower blood sugars in type 2 diabetics. The three-month study used a dose of 1 gram a day with food. The study noted an improvement in the hemoglobin A1c test (glucose averages over two to three months) with cinnamon, compared to the group that did not receive cinnamon.[80]

Another randomized, single-blind placebo-controlled trial of 60 type 2 diabetics used different doses of cinnamon (Cinnamomum cassia) of one, three and six grams a day. All the doses demonstrated an improvement of blood glucose, triglycerides, LDL cholesterol (bad cholesterol) and total cholesterol levels.[81]

Since there have also been studies that did not show the benefits of cinnamon in type 2 diabetics, a well-designed United Kingdom trial was done to determine if cinnamon can really lower glucose and blood pressure in type 2 diabetics. A double-blind, randomized, placebo-controlled study (gold standard) looked at 58 type 2 diabetics who took two grams of cinnamon (Cinnamomum cassia) daily. After twelve weeks, cinnamon had reduced the three-month glucose average blood test scores (hemoglobin A1c) from 8.22 to 7.86, and it also lowered blood pressure. It was also noted in the study that there was no possible influence in body weight, total calorie intake or sodium intake between the group taking cinnamon versus the group that did not take cinnamon. The two-gram dose of cinnamon was also tolerated well.[82]

As for cinnamon improving insulin resistance, a study of 15 patients with polycystic ovary syndrome—and with insulin resistance—addressed the issue. This was a randomized, double-blind, placebo-controlled trial that used 1 gram of cinnamon cassia for eight weeks. At the end of the study, the fasting blood glucose dropped by 16.9 percent and the score for insulin resistance dropped on the HOMA (Homeostatic model assessment—a special mathematical test for measuring insulin resistance by using a fasting insulin and glucose level). This showed a significant improvement in insulin resistance—and was confirmed by the oral glucose tolerance test.[83]

Cinnamon is generally well-tolerated; however, it may thin your blood, so you must be careful if you're on blood thinners. Otherwise, most of the medical studies have generally been done on cinnamon cassia, whereas most over-the-counter cinnamon uses cinnamon zeylanicum or verum. Since the medical studies are showing the benefits with cinnamon cassia, I would strongly recommend adding more cinnamon cassia to your diet.

A great way to enjoy cinnamon every day is to just drop one cinnamon stick in hot water (or even better yet, hot green tea), let it dissolve and enjoy.

Vitamin D

Vitamin D stands by itself since it is not a nutraceutical, food product, mineral or botanical. Actually, vitamin D is now considered a hormone. Vitamin D is one of today's most popular hormones because it has been shown to reduce cancer and heart disease.[84] Also, low vitamin D has been associated with an increase in autoimmune diseases like type 1 diabetes, systemic lupus erythematosus, arthritis and multiple sclerosis.[85]

The role vitamin D plays in cancer is amazing. Vitamin D has even been found to induce death in cancer cells. A study by the National Cancer Institute found that a vitamin D level of 80 nmol/L or higher is associated with a 72 percent risk reduction.[85] In 2007, a double-blind randomized placebo-controlled study using 1,100 IU of vitamin D showed a reduction in all types of cancer by 60 percent within four years.[87]

The three main sources of vitamin D are sunshine, dairy that is fortified with vitamin D, and the ocean or plankton (the chief source of food for fish).

The cause of an epidemic low of vitamin D in the U.S. remains uncertain. One theory is that since vitamin D is a fat soluble hormone, and considering the increasing rate of obesity, the extra belly fat serves as a "storage area" for vitamin D.

Low vitamin D is higher in certain populations like African, American and Hispanic—who also have the highest risk for insulin resistance, type 2 diabetes and heart disease. According to a recent review of the available medical literature, low levels of vitamin D are associated with insulin resistance.[88]

In a study that looked at 126 healthy Californians, it was shown that levels of vitamin D are associated with insulin sensitivity. Those with vitamin D levels less than 20 ng/ml had a higher risk of insulin resistance and metabolic syndrome.[89]

Concerning heart disease, low vitamin D levels have been associated with a higher prevalence of heart failure and death; however, the optimal level of 25 OH vitamin D level is debatable. In a follow-up study, it was noted that higher vitamin D levels may have even helped more.

In a double-blind, randomized, placebo-controlled study of 123 patients with congestive heart failure, it was shown that vitamin D lowered inflammation while increasing the anti-inflammatory cytokine (good blood marker) interleukin 10, and improving on the pumping action of the heart. In the same study, after nine months of vitamin D, the average level was 42 ng/mL. At that time it was noted that the level was probably too low to optimize all the vitamin D dependent functions.[90]

In another study, which followed over 1,700 people (without heart disease) for over five years noted that those with a very low vitamin D level of less than 15 ng/ml had a 62 percent increase for a first incidence of heart attack—especially if they had a history of high blood pressure.[91]

So, are you ready to optimize your vitamin D level?

"I was deficient in vitamin D—even though I live in the 'Sunshine State!'"

I'm a 50 year old mother of twins who is passionate about competing in triathlons. I've been active all my adult life, but have become increasingly involved in triathlons over the last six years. I've steadily improved, have raced all over the U.S., and have been able to compete in three International Triathlon Union Long Distance World Championships in Europe and two Ironman 70.3 World Championships. I've been a USA Triathlon All Ameri-

can, which is a ranking of the top ten percent triathletes of all distances in the country—for the past five years.

When I was starting in triathlon, I developed a fun rivalry with Dr Lee. He's a much better swimmer and would try to help me. I returned the favor by trying to track him down on the run. I've never succeeded, but I've gotten close!

This past fall, I was a little tired and my race results were suddenly much slower. For example, my run, which is my strength, in the Ironman 70.3 World Championship was seven minutes slower than the previous year! I had similar results in both a ten-mile and a half-marathon road race.

My coach suggested I have some blood work done. Dr Lee ran several tests and discovered that I was deficient in vitamin D—even though I live in the "Sunshine State!" I started taking vitamin D and after a few weeks felt like myself again. When I was tired, I couldn't break a seven-minute mile. Three weeks later, I ran a sub-six-minute mile in the middle of a run!

I turned 50 in April and decided to celebrate by competing in Ironman Lake Placid on July 20. The ironman consists of a 2.4 mile swim, a 112 mile bike ride, and a 26.2 mile run. It was quite a celebration as I had the race of my life! In the pouring down rain, I had a good swim and bike and was in tenth place. I then went on to run past 491 other racers, seven of whom were in my age group. I placed third and earned a slot to the Ironman World Championships in Kona, Hawaii in October in my very first ironman!. I also ran fast enough after biking and swimming to qualify for the Boston Marathon.

I am so relieved and excited. I was worried that my speed was gone forever. Dr Lee is my hero, but I still want to crush him in the next race!

— Julie Sands

As most people know, Florida is considered the "Sunshine State," and one way you can get vitamin D is through the ultraviolet rays of the sun. Even with practicing in Florida, I have diagnosed thousands of patients with vitamin D deficiency or insufficiency.

The current debate in medicine is over the ideal level of vitamin D; however, most everyone does agree that today's reference range for vitamin D is way to low. Most doctors are using about 1,000 IU a day of vitamin D, whereas I recommend an average dose of 5,000 IU a day. A quick comment on taking vitamin D is that you can get it as supplement or as a prescription. The most common side effect of too much vitamin D is nausea, vomiting or a kidney stone. Rarely, you can develop renal failure, which is why close monitoring is needed. Most laboratory data use a level of 20 to 100 ng/ml. I am recommending a 25–OH vitamin D level above 65 ng/ml. Higher vitamin D levels can improve on lowering your risk for cancer, and lower levels of vitamin D are associated with insulin resistance. However it is unknown how long it takes before vitamin D can help with insulin resistance, and how vitamin D works. So, more studies need to be done to look into how taking vitamin D improves insulin resistance. I truly believe that the data will support it.

It is an exciting field of science right now—especially since there is hope that a very cheap supplement can significantly help with the epidemic of insulin resistance.

Recommendations — Supplements with Healing Powers

Listed below are some recommendations on minerals, nutraceuticals and vitamin D. These are essential on improving on reducing insulin resistance and achieving a healthy body. These doses may vary for each person, and are intended only as a general guideline. Consult your physician before taking these supplements.

EPA/DHA (omega-3 not omega-6 or 9) one to four grams a day

Alpha-lipoic Acid 300 mg to 1200 mg a day

CoQ10 (ubiquinone) 100 to 300 mg a day

Magnesium glycinate 300 mg to 1000 mg a day

Chromium picolinate 200 mcg to 1000 mcg a day

Vitamin D3 2000 I.U. to 5000 IU a day

Recommendations — Botanicals with Healthy Powers

Listed below are some recommendations for doses; however, you should simply add these wonderful botanicals into your diet. For example: you can buy the supplement lycopene, but it's 100 times better just to eat an organic tomato that has lycopene. So, enjoy garlic, curcumin, ginseng, greet tea and cinnamon in your diet. These doses may vary for each person, and are intended only as a general guideline. Consult your physician before taking these supplements.

Garlic — 600 mg a day

Curcumin — one to three grams a day

Ginseng — three to six grams a day

Green Tea — five to six cups a day

Cinnamon — one to six grams a day

Recommendations — Foods with "Super" Powers

For mega-doses of vitamins and minerals, choose recipes with these "super foods."

Zinc

- Cocoa powder
- Dark chocolate
- Garlic
- Tahini or sesame seeds
- Pumpkin seeds
- Brazil nuts
- Cashews
- Chestnuts
- Oysters
- Crab
- Chickpeas
- Lamb, beef tenderloin

Vitamin D

- Shiitake and button mushrooms
- Mackerel
- Salmon
- Herring
- Sardines
- Tuna
- Eggs

Vitamin C

- Oranges
- Lemons
- Limes
- Grapefruit
- Tangelos
- Tangerines
- Kiwi
- Mango
- Papaya
- Pineapple
- Black currant
- Strawberries
- Blueberries
- Blackberries
- Raspberries
- Cranberries
- Spinach
- Kale
- Turnip greens
- Dandelion greens
- Mustard greens
- Broccoli
- Cabbage
- Celery
- Parsley
- Tomato
- Red bell peppers
- Sweet potatoes

Vitamin E

- Sunflower seeds
- Almonds
- Hazelnuts
- Nut oils
- Lettuce
- Spinach
- Turnip
- Beet greens
- Tomatoes
- Papaya
- Mango

Glutathione

- Asparagus
- Spinach
- Broccoli
- Zucchini
- Peas
- Brussels sprouts
- Okra
- Acorn squash
- Avocado
- Walnuts
- Peaches
- Watermelon
- Walnuts
- Cinnamon
- Cardamom
- Curcumin
- Turmeric

CoQ10

- Fish
- Liver

Omega-3

- Fish—salmon, sardines, anchovies, mackerel, trout, black cod
- Flax seeds or flax oil
- Walnuts or walnut oil

- Olive oil
- Soybeans
- Navy beans
- Kidney beans
- Brussels sprouts
- Cauliflower
- Cabbage

Conclusion

A question I often hear in my practice is, "What supplements should I take?" By the way, there are many health care providers that simply do not believe in taking any supplements, which is why I wrote this chapter—complete with 92 references of scientific data and medical studies that demonstrate the benefits of taking these supplements.

I truly believe that you should start with a simple and basic foundation. One should always start with a pharmacy grade multivitamin, a pharmacy grade omega-3 or EPA/DHA and a human strain probiotic.

Probiotics are live bacteria or microorganisms that help keep your gut healthy. A probiotic helps improve on your gut's intestinal balance between good bacteria and bad bacteria. Also, a probiotic helps with lowering inflammation. Remember, the key in achieving wellness is to lower chronic inflammation.[92]

Most of my patients take 2000 units to 5000 units of vitamin D3 a day. The average dose in one multivitamin has about 200 units of vitamin D, so most people have to take extra supplements. Later, you can add other supplements, such as chromium, CoQ10, alpha-lipoic acid and magnesium.

As for resveratrol, there are new studies that show it reduces insulin resistance. Future studies on its effects on longevity and cancer protection in humans look promising.

Take advantage of the super foods with amazing powers—like curcumin, ginseng, green tea and cinnamon. Some of them have been used for over several thousand years.

As Hippocrates, the father of medicine, once said, "Let food be your medicine," but make sure you know what foods you may be sensitive to!

CHAPTER 7 REVIEW

— Fish oil or EPA/DHA improves on blood pressure, raises HDL cholesterol, lowers triglycerides and improves on insulin resistance.

— Resveratrol looks promising in recent human studies to reduce insulin resistance.

— Alpha lipoic acid is a great antioxidant for decreasing inflammation and improving on insulin resistance.

— Coenzyme Q10 can improve on heart failure, improve on energy and improve on insulin resistance.

— Magnesium is a crucial mineral that's required for every living organism on earth. Plus, it can improve on insulin resistance. If you want to know if you have low magnesium, then request a red blood cell magnesium level.

— Garlic has special oils to lower blood pressure and improve on blood sugars.

— Curcumin has been used for thousands of years. There has been data showing the benefits of curcumin in lowering glucose levels and reducing inflammation.

— Ginseng, known as the "root of heaven" or the "king of herbs," can reduce insulin resistance.

— Green tea that has been used in China for at least 4000 years is an amazing antioxidant that helps patients with prostate cancer and improves on insulin resistance.

— Cinnamon goes back to about 2800 B.C. and was used in Egypt, Rome and China, and has been shown to improve on insulin resistance.

— Higher levels of vitamin D have been shown to improve on insulin resistance and to reduce the risk of having cancer.

8

Phase One of Your Best Investment

"The first wealth is health."
— Ralph Waldo Emerson

It's now time to take that first step toward your best investment, and really change the way you eat. Outlined in this chapter are your first 30 days, with an emphasis on plant-based foods, and healthful foods that are low in refined carbohydrates.

You'll be preparing your food with recipes from this book, or by simple one or two-step instructions. Also remember that when you're short on time, simply substitute your choice of a steamed (fresh or frozen) vegetable for any vegetable recipe in that meal plan.

See Appendix C: Your New Shopping List for a helpful list of items to shop for. You won't need to buy the full list all at once, but it will give you an idea of how your grocery shopping needs to change.

Also, see Appendix D: Miracle Noodle® if you love pasta and are looking for a healthier alternative that you may add to these recipes, or use as substitute for rice. Miracle Noodle® tastes great, is very easy to prepare, has zero calories, is made from plant-soluble fiber, and is very filling.

As you begin Phase One, just keep it easy, set goals along the way, and then reward yourself for reaching those goals—not with food, but maybe with a new pair of shoes, that new golf club or something else you've been promising yourself.

You'll also notice there is an Option A and an Option B for Phase One. Peruse the menus for both options to choose the one you like best.

But before diving into Phase One, let's look at some tips to help ensure your success, and some helpful guidelines for eating out.

Tips for Success

Drink liquids 30 minutes before meals, and one hour after meals.

If you're craving sweets while limiting sugar, try:

- Squares of 70 percent dark chocolate alone or topped with almond or cashew butter.
- Glass of water with 2 slices of lemon, 4 sprigs of mint and 2 sliced strawberries and let it sit for 20 minutes.
- Mint lemonade with stevia (2 lemons (juiced), handful of mint, 1½ cup water and 1 pinch or 2 drops of stevia. Blend with ice. Add strawberries slices for variety.

It's best to eat fruit in the morning, by itself or before a meal.

Don't eat fruit after a meal—wait at least three or four hours.

When eating out, always start with a salad.

Buy seeds raw to avoid pre-roasted ones that have vegetable oils and salt. Roast at home with coconut oil and sea salt to desired taste. Set oven to 300°F and bake for 10 to 12 minutes. Watch nuts so they do not burn.

Savor each bite of food and chew well for better digestion.

If craving chips or tortilla chips, have kale chips or make your own tortilla chips (bake brown rice tortillas for 8 to 10 minutes in olive oil).

Options When Eating Out

Asian Cuisine

- Chinese
    - Choose steamed vegetables with steamed shrimp, fish, or chicken and brown rice.
    - Avoid heavy sauce dishes.
    - Avoid or limit dishes with black bean sauce, sweet and sour sauce, oyster sauces.
- Vietnamese
    - Vegetable or chicken pho.
- Thai
    - Tom yum goong with shrimp.
    - Curry dishes with coconut milk.
    - Sautéed shrimp, chicken, or beef with basil, onions and chilies.
    - Sautéed scallops and shrimp with mushrooms, zucchini and chili paste.
    - Choose dishes with lemongrass, basil, or any other herb, and are sautéed or steamed.
- Japanese
    - Sashimi, seaweed salad, miso soup, cucumber rolls or any roll can be made without rice.
    - Start meal off with miso soup and salad, and eat slowly.

        - Avoid creamy sauces and rolls with cream cheese.

- Steakhouse
    - Salad, fish, high quality meats, steamed or sautéed vegetables (not creamed).
- Italian
    - Fish, marinara sauce, whole wheat pasta, green salad, sautéed vegetables, baked chicken or lemon chicken.
- Middle Eastern
    - Grilled vegetable kabobs, hummus, Greek style salad dressing on the side, grilled fish or lamb. Ask for salad instead of rice.
    - Choose kofta balls (lamb onion skewers) instead of falafel balls.
- Fast Food—(if possible, avoid completely)
    - Grilled chicken sandwich, no mayonnaise, take off one of the buns or make it protein style by wrapping the chicken in lettuce leaves (ask for extra lettuce).
    - When chicken is not an option, get the most basic burger. Avoid burgers with cheese, bacon and double patties. Take off one of the buns or make it protein style by wrapping the burger in lettuce leaves (ask for extra lettuce).
- Dessert
    - The trick when eating out is to bring a dark chocolate bar and have a couple of squares after dinner instead of ordering a high-calorie, high-gluten dessert. The best high-quality dark chocolate bars are Endangered

Species, Dagoba® or Green & Black's® Organic Chocolate.

- For those times when you just can't skip dessert, stop after one or two bites.

Phase One — Option A

Breakfast

Choose one of these options for breakfast. Remember to mix it up so you're not eating the same thing every day!

- 2 egg omelet with choice of 3 vegetables (mushrooms, tomatoes, spinach, peppers, broccoli, etc.)
- *Green Smoothie* (page 281) and handful of nuts (almonds, walnuts)
- Smoothie with 1 fruit and 2 vegetables
- V8® 100% Vegetable Juice—regular or low-sodium—(not V8 Splash® or V8 V-Fusion®)
- Leftovers from previous day

Snacks

Be sure to enjoy one or two of these snacks every day—just remember to try different combinations.

- 1 serving size of organic cacao bar (at least 70 percent cacao)
- ½ cup sliced fruit or one small piece of fruit (avoid grapes and oranges)
- ¼ cup hummus with sliced vegetables (cauliflower, broccoli, etc.)
- ¼ cup nuts (almonds, walnuts, pine nuts, pistachios)
- ½ cup pumpkin or sunflower seeds
- 6 celery and carrot sticks
- Cherry tomatoes

Day 1

Lunch

Vitamix® Vegetable Soup (page 453)

Cabbage-Apple Salad (page 398)

Dinner

Orange-Ginger Salmon (page 348)

Broccoli with Almonds (page 306)

Skillet Zucchini (page 376)

Day 2

Lunch

Green salad with assorted vegetables (tomatoes, pepper, cucumbers, etc.) and a 4-ounce chicken breast—drizzled with olive oil and balsamic vinegar

1 small apple

Dinner

Roast Turkey Breast (page 361)

Spiced Cauliflower (page 380)

Cumin Carrots (page 318)

Green salad—drizzled with olive oil and rice vinegar

Day 3

Lunch

Turkey Salad (page 431—use leftover *Roast Turkey Breast* from previous day) drizzled with olive oil and balsamic vinegar

¼ cup almonds

Dinner

Spaghetti Squash (page 379)

Marinara Sauce (page 344, or if in a hurry, use organic prepared tomato sauce)

Ratatouille (page 360)

Day 4

Lunch

Vitamix® Tomato Onion Cheese Soup (page 452)

Celery sticks with 2 tablespoons organic peanut butter

1 small banana

Dinner

Rosemary Baked Chicken Breast (page 365)

Broccoli with Turmeric and Tomatoes (page 307)

Smothered Mushrooms and Kale (page 377)

Green salad—drizzled with olive oil and rice vinegar

Day 5

Lunch

Radicchio and Spinach Salad with Walnuts (page 414)

1 small pear

Dinner

Grilled Fish with Citrus Marinade (page 329)

Grilled Vegetables (page 334)

Green salad—drizzled with *Basic Vinaigrette* (page 395)

Day 6

Lunch

Oriental Chicken Salad (page 411)

Dinner

Lentil Soup (page 442)

Green salad—drizzled with *Basic Vinaigrette* (page 395)

Day 7

Lunch

Leftover *Lentil Soup* from previous day

Green salad—drizzled with olive oil and rice vinegar

Dinner

Marinated London Broil (page 345)

Quick Skillet Asparagus (page 356)

Creamy Coleslaw (page 401)

Day 8

Lunch

Italian Vegetable Soup (page 441)

Roasted Red Pepper Hummus (page 363)

Sliced vegetables to dip in *Roasted Red Pepper Hummus*

Dinner

Indian-Spiced Salmon (page 335)

Wilted Spinach with Tomatoes (page 388)

Spiced Cauliflower (page 380)

Day 9

Lunch

Green Salad with Strawberry Balsamic Vinaigrette (page 406)

Celery and carrots sticks with 1 tablespoon organic peanut butter

Dinner

Balsamic-Marinated Flank Steak (page 298)

Grilled Portobellos, Peppers and Squash (page 332)

Steamed Broccoli

Day 10

Lunch

Green salad with assorted vegetables and 4 ounces of chicken—drizzled with olive oil and balsamic vinegar

Dinner

Tuscan Minestrone Soup (page 450)

Spinach Strawberry Salad (page 424)—drizzled with olive oil and rice vinegar

Day 11

Lunch

Leftover *Tuscan Minestrone Soup* from previous day

Green salad—drizzled with olive oil and balsamic vinegar

1 small pear

Dinner

Simple Grilled Chicken Breast (page 372)

Simple Steamed Artichokes (page 373)

Cumin Carrots (page 318)

Day 12

Lunch

Fifteen-Minute Vegetarian Chili (page 439)

¼ cup almonds

1 small apple

Dinner

Seared Scallops with Farmers' Market Salad (page 417)

Italian-Style Green Bean Salad (page 407)

Day 13

Lunch

Green salad with assorted vegetables and 4 ounces of sliced chicken breast—drizzled with *Lime-Rice Wine Vinaigrette* (page 409)

1 small banana

Dinner

Indian-Spiced Chickpea and Fire-Roasted Tomato Soup (page 440)

1 cup assorted sliced, raw vegetables

Day 14

Lunch

Leftover *Indian-Spiced Chickpea and Fire-Roasted Tomato Soup* from previous day

Green salad—drizzled with olive oil and rice vinegar

Dinner

Roast Turkey Breast (page 361)

Skillet Broccoli (or Asparagus) with Sesame Seeds (page 375)

Simple Greens and Garlic (page 421)

Day 15

Lunch

Green salad with leftover *Roast Turkey Breast* from previous day

1 small banana

Dinner

Baked Fish with Basil (page 296)

Pan-browned Brussels Sprouts (page 350)

Maple Glazed Root Vegetables (page 343)

Day 16

Lunch

Spinach Walnut Salad (page 425)

1 small pear

Dinner

Asian Beef Stir-Fry (page 293)

Steamed broccoli

Day 17

Lunch

Vitamix® Tomato Onion Cheese Soup (page 452)

Oriental Chicken Salad (page 411)

Dinner

Fifteen-Minute Vegetarian Chili (page 439)

Green salad—drizzled with olive oil and balsamic vinegar

Day 18

Lunch

Leftover *Fifteen-Minute Vegetarian Chili* from previous day

Green salad

Dinner

Savory Meatballs (page 370)

Lemon-Curry Cauliflower and Kale (page 341)

Skillet Zucchini (page 376)

Day 19

Lunch

Vitamix® Vegetable Soup (page 453)

Hummus with sliced vegetables

Dinner

Blackened salmon (use *Blackened Rub for Fish*, page 303))

Lemon-Asparagus Packets (page 340)

Green salad—drizzled with olive oil and balsamic vinegar

Day 20

Lunch

Leftover blackened salmon from previous day

2 cups mixed steamed vegetables

Dinner

Italian Vegetable Soup (page 441)

Green salad—drizzled with olive oil and balsamic vinegar

Day 21

Lunch

Spinach Salad with Strawberries and Pistachios (page 423)

Leftover *Italian Vegetable Soup* from previous day

Dinner

Grilled Glazed Dijon Chicken (page 330)

Grilled Portobello Mushrooms (page 331)

Asian Cabbage (page 295)

Day 22

Lunch

Vitamix® Tomato Onion Cheese Soup (page 452)

Mixed green salad with vegetables sprinkled with 3 tablespoons raw sunflower seeds

½ cup sliced fruit

Dinner

Mrs. Dash® Fish (page 347)

Curried Cauliflower (page 319)

Steamed Brussels sprouts

Sliced tomatoes

Day 23

Lunch

Asian Chicken Salad (page 391)—drizzled with *Lime-Rice Wine Vinaigrette* (page 409)

Dinner

Mediterranean Beef Stew (page 346)

Mixed green salad—drizzled with *Basic Vinaigrette* (page 395)

Day 24

Lunch

Cabbage-Apple Salad (page 398)

Dinner

Easy Minestrone Soup (page 438)

Green salad—drizzled with *Basic Vinaigrette* (page 395)

Day 25

Lunch

Leftover *Easy Minestrone Soup* from previous day

¼ cup almonds

Dinner

Grilled Caribbean Chicken (page 328)

Crispy Kale (page 316)

Steamed broccoli

Day 26

Lunch

Green salad with assorted vegetables and a 4 ounce chicken breast

¼ cup walnuts

1 small apple

Dinner

Peel and eat shrimp

Dressed-Up Asparagus (page 321)

Steamed cauliflower—drizzled with olive oil and sprinkled with Mrs. Dash® seasoning

Day 27

Lunch

Lean turkey burger

Sliced raw vegetables

1 small banana

Dinner

White Bean Soup with Kale and Sausage (page 454)

Green salad—drizzled with olive oil and balsamic vinegar

Day 28

Lunch

Leftover *White Bean Soup with Kale and Sausage* from previous night

Celery and carrot sticks with 1 tablespoon organic peanut butter

Dinner

Baked turkey breast

Baked Zucchini Fries (page 297)

Italian Green Beans (page 336)

Day 29

Lunch

Turkey on green salad with mixed vegetables—drizzled with olive oil and rice vinegar

Dinner

Seared Scallops with Farmers' Market Salad (page 417)

Simple Greens and Garlic (page 421)

Vegetable Stir-Fry (page 387)

Day 30

Lunch

Spinach Strawberry Salad (page 424)

4 ounce chicken breast

Dinner

Grilled Rosemary Steak (page 333)

Grilled Vegetables (page 334)

Green salad—drizzled with olive oil and rice vinegar

Phase One — Option B

Breakfast

Choose one of these options for breakfast. Remember to mix it up so you're not eating the same thing every day!

All Green Smoothie (page 256)

Almond Butter Banana Green Smoothie (page 230)

Almond Butter Peach Soft Serve (page 237)

Banana Chai Smoothie (page 262)

Basil Blueberry Smoothie (page 264)

Basil and Tomato Scrambled Eggs (page 241)

Beginners Green Smoothie (page 265)

Berry Green Smoothie (page 266)

Blueberry Mint Pear Green Smoothie (page 267)

Caramelized Onion and Spinach Frittata (page 243)

Cherry Walnut Smoothie (page 268)

Cilantro Pineapple Smoothie (page 269)

Cinnamon Flourless Crepe (page 244)

Clementine Creamsicle Smoothie (page 270)

Cocoa Mint Smoothie (page 271)

Cocoa Smoothie (page 272)

Coconut Green Smoothie (page 273)

Day 1

Lunch

Turkey Pilgrim Salad (page 430)

Dinner

Sage-Crusted Chicken Tenders (page 366)

Swiss Chard with Shallots (page 384)

Day 2

Lunch

Simple Green Salad (page 420)

Dinner

Salmon Florentine (page 368)

Pizza Roasted Vegetables (page 353)

Day 3

Lunch

Southwestern Salad (page 422)

Dinner

Mexican Chicken Soup with Ancho Chilies (page 443)

Day 4

Lunch

Chicken Salad Collard Greens Wrap (page 312)

Dinner

Mango Shrimp (page 342)

Summer Salad (page 427)

Day 5

Lunch

Jamaican Jerk Chicken (page 338)

Caribbean Kale (page 309)

Dinner

Smoothie of choice

Day 6

Lunch

Leftover *Caribbean Kale* (page 309) with 2 eggs over easy

Dinner

Plantain Encrusted Halibut (page 354)

Chive Mashed Cauliflower (page 313)

Day 7

Lunch

Blueberry Chicken (page 305)

Japanese Raw Rice (page 337)

Dinner

Everything But The Kitchen Sink Salad (page 402)

Day 8

Lunch

Refreshing Watermelon Salad (page 416)

Simple Grilled Chicken Breast (page 372)

Dinner

Pan-Seared Grass-Fed Beef (page 351)

Garlic Butter Roasted Mushrooms (page 322)

Pizza Roasted Vegetables (page 353) with garlic

Day 9

Lunch

Summer Salad (page 427)

Dinner

Orange Juice Scallops (page 349) on a bed of fresh spinach

Day 10

Lunch

Tomato Minestrone (page 448)

Sicilian Collard Greens (page 419)

Dinner

Spicy Grilled Tuna with Salsa (page 381)

Cauliflower Rice (page 311)

Day 11

Lunch

Pan-Seared Grass-Fed Beef (page 351) wrapped in collard greens

Zucchini Noodle Pasta (page 389)

Dinner

Smoothie of choice

Day 12

Lunch

Tropical Fruit Salad with Arugula (page 429)

Dinner

Pesto Filet (page 352)

Poppyseed Brussels Sprouts (page 355)

Day 13

Lunch

Broccoli Apple Chicken Salad with Poppyseed Dressing (page 396)

Simple Grilled Chicken Breast (page 372)

Dinner

Veggie Omelet (page 258)

Day 14

Lunch

Sage-Crusted Chicken Tenders (page 366)

Shirazi Tomato Cucumber Salad (page 418)

Dinner

Thick & Chunky Tomato Soup (page 447)

Day 15

Lunch

Broccoli Apple Chicken Salad with Poppyseed Dressing (page 396)

Dinner

Smoothie of choice

Day 16

Lunch

Sausage, Egg & Vegetable Casserole (page 253)

Side of mixed greens with choice of dressing

Dinner

Stuffed Avocado Salad (page 426)

Day 17

Lunch

Pumpkin Caesar Salad Dressing (page 407) on choice of salad with 2 eggs over easy

Dinner

Blackened Cajun Salmon (page 304)

Roasted Brussels Sprouts (page 362)

Day 18

Lunch

Curried Ginger Raisin Lentils (page 320)

Dinner

Apple Cabbage Salad (page 393)

Kale Chips (page 339)

Day 19

Lunch

Simple Grilled Chicken Breast (page 372) on *Papaya Salad* (page 412)

Salad of choice

Dinner

Turkey Soup (page 449)

Day 20

Lunch

Turkey Pilgrim Salad (page 430)

Dinner

Pesto Filet (page 352)

Zucchini Noodle Pasta (page 389)

Day 21

Lunch

Summer Salad (page 427)

Dinner

Jamaican Jerk Chicken (page 338)

Everything But The Kitchen Sink Salad (page 402)

Day 22

Lunch

Chicken Salad Collard Greens Wrap (page 312)

Dinner

Fennel Avocado Salad (page 403)

Day 23

Lunch

Pan-Seared Grass-Fed Beef (page 351)

Salad of choice

Dinner

Tomato Minestrone (page 448)

Day 24

Lunch

Blackened Cajun Salmon (page 304) on bed of spinach

Dinner

Smoothie of choice

Day 25

Lunch

Pan-Seared Grass-Fed Beef (page 351)

Vegetable Chips (page 386)

Dinner

Zucchini Noodle Pasta (page 389)

Pizza Roasted Vegetables (page 347)

Day 26

Lunch

Sage-Crusted Chicken Tenders (page 366)

Vegetable Chips (page 386)

Dinner

Pumpkin Caesar Salad Dressing (page 413) on choice of salad

Day 27

Lunch

Mango Shrimp (page 342)

Pizza Roasted Vegetables (page 353)

Dinner

Refresh Soup (page 444)

Salad of choice

Day 28

Lunch

Coconut Curry Chicken (page 314)

Dinner

Southwestern Salad (page 422)

Day 29

Lunch

Broccoli Apple Chicken Salad with Poppyseed Dressing (page 396)

Simple Grilled Chicken Breast (page 372)

Dinner

Smoothie of choice

Day 30

Lunch

Creamy Curried Cauliflower Soup (page 436)

Dinner

Salmon Florentine (page 368)

Salad of choice

9

Phase Two of Your Best Investment

"The greatest of follies is to sacrifice health for any other kind of happiness."
— Arthur Schopenhauer

Congratulations on completing your first 30 days! The phase you just finished was low in refined carbohydrates. Now, the second phase is going to be a 30-day reintroduction of whole grains—while still trying to avoid the "white sins," such as pasta, bread, rice and potatoes.

Like before, you'll be preparing your food with recipes from this book, or by simple one or two-step instructions. Also remember that when you're short on time, simply substitute your choice of a steamed (fresh or frozen) vegetable for any vegetable recipe in that meal plan.

As before, see Appendix D: Miracle Noodle® if you love pasta and are looking for a healthier alternative that you may add to these recipes, or use as substitute for rice. Miracle Noodle® tastes great, is very easy to prepare, has zero calories, is made from plant-soluble fiber, and is very filling.

Also, you will again choose either Option A or Option B. If you chose Option A in Phase One and want to switch to Option B (or vice versa) for Phase Two, that's perfectly fine. Just peruse the following menus to decide which option you like best.

In addition, don't forget to set new goals, while being sure to reward yourself for reaching those goals!

Phase Two — Option A

Breakfast

You now have more breakfast options. Choose one for each day for breakfast. Remember to mix it up so you're not eating the same thing every day!

- 2 egg omelet with choice of 3 vegetables (mushrooms, tomatoes, spinach, peppers, broccoli, etc.)
- *Green Smoothie* (page 281) and handful of nuts (almonds, walnuts)
- Smoothie of choice
- V8® 100% Vegetable Juice—regular or low-sodium—(not V8 Splash® or V8 V-Fusion®)
- Leftovers from previous day
- *Blueberry Walnut Oatmeal* (page 242)
- *Apple-Walnut Amaranth* (page 240)
- *Amaranth with Orange-Berry Topping* (page 238)

Snacks

Be sure to enjoy one or two of these snacks every day—just remember to try different combinations.

- 1 serving size of organic cacao bar (at least 70 percent cacao)
- ½ cup sliced fruit or one small piece of fruit (avoid grapes and oranges)
- ¼ cup hummus with sliced vegetables (cauliflower, broccoli, etc.)
- ¼ cup nuts (almonds, walnuts, pine nuts, pistachios)
- ½ cup pumpkin or sunflower seeds
- 6 celery and carrot sticks
- Cherry tomatoes
- 2 *Oatmeal Cookies* (page 462)
- ¼ cup *Trail Mix* (page 466)
- 2 cups air-popped popcorn

Day 1

Lunch

Vitamix® Vegetable Soup (page 453)

Cabbage-Apple Salad (page 398)

Dinner

Orange-Ginger Salmon (page 348)

Cruciferous Couscous (page 317)

Skillet Zucchini (page 376)

Day 2

Lunch

Black Beanofritos (page 302)

1 small apple

Dinner

Roast Turkey Breast (page 361)

Spiced Cauliflower (page 380)

Cumin Carrots (page 318)

Green salad—drizzled with olive oil and rice vinegar

Day 3

Lunch

Turkey sandwich (use leftover *Roast Turkey Breast* from previous day) made with two slices 100 percent whole wheat bread, sliced tomatoes, spinach and mustard or organic mayonnaise

½ cup sliced fruit

Dinner

Garlic Chickpeas and Pasta (page 323)

Green salad—drizzled with olive oil and balsamic vinegar

Day 4

Lunch

Vitamix® Tomato Onion Cheese Soup (page 4452

Celery sticks with 2 tablespoons organic peanut butter

1 small banana

Dinner

Rosemary Baked Chicken Breast (page 365)

Steamed green beans

Sweet Potato Fries (page 383)

Green salad—drizzled with olive oil and rice vinegar

Day 5

Lunch

Radicchio and Spinach Salad with Walnuts (page 414)

1 small pear

Dinner

Grilled Fish with Citrus Marinade (page 329)

Grilled Vegetables (page 334)

Green salad—drizzled with *Basic Vinaigrette* (page 395)

Day 6

Lunch

Oriental Chicken Salad (page 411)

Dinner

Lentil Soup (page 442)

Green salad—drizzled with *Basic Vinaigrette* (page 395)

Day 7

Lunch

Leftover *Lentil Soup* from previous day

Green salad—drizzled with olive oil and rice vinegar

Dinner

Marinated London Broil (page 345)

Quick Skillet Asparagus (page 356)

Creamy Coleslaw (page 401)

Day 8

Lunch

Italian Vegetable Soup (page 441)

Roasted Red Pepper Hummus (page 363)

Sliced vegetables to dip in *Roasted Red Pepper Hummus*

Dinner

Indian-Spiced Salmon (page 335)

Wilted Spinach with Tomatoes (page 388)

Spiced Cauliflower (page 380)

Day 9

Lunch

Sweet Potato Soup (page 445 for Option A, page 446 for Option B)

Celery and carrots sticks with 2 tablespoons organic peanut butter

Dinner

Balsamic-Marinated Flank Steak (page 298)

Grilled Portobellos, Peppers and Squash (page 332)

Steamed broccoli

Day 10

Lunch

Green salad with assorted vegetables and 4 ounces of sliced chicken breast—drizzled with olive oil and balsamic vinegar

Dinner

Tuscan Minestrone Soup (page 450)

Spinach Strawberry Salad (page 424)—drizzled with olive oil and rice vinegar

Day 11

Lunch

Quinoa with Corn and Peppers (page 358)

Green salad—drizzled with olive oil and balsamic vinegar

1 small pear

Dinner

Simple Grilled Chicken Breast (page 372)

Simple Steamed Artichokes (page 373)

Cumin Carrots (page 318)

Day 12

Lunch

Fifteen-Minute Vegetarian Chili (page 439)

¼ cup almonds

1 small apple

Dinner

Seared Scallops with Farmers' Market Salad (page 417)

Italian Green Beans (page 336)

Day 13

Lunch

Green salad with assorted vegetables and 4 ounces of sliced chicken breast—drizzled with *Lime-Rice Wine Vinaigrette* (page 409)

1 small banana

Dinner

Indian-Spiced Chickpea and Fire-Roasted Tomato Soup (page 440)

1 cup assorted sliced raw vegetables

5 "ak-mak Bakeries" crackers, or other 100 percent organic whole wheat crackers

Day 14

Lunch

Leftover *Indian-Spiced Chickpea and Fire-Roasted Tomato Soup* from previous day

Green salad—drizzled with olive oil and rice vinegar

Dinner

Roast Turkey Breast (page 361)

Cruciferous Couscous (page 317)

Steamed Brussels sprouts

Day 15

Lunch

Black Beanofritos (page 302)

1 small banana

Dinner

Baked Fish with Basil (page 296)

Pan-browned Brussels Sprouts (page 350)

Maple Glazed Root Vegetables (page 343)

Day 16

Lunch

Spinach Walnut Salad (page 425)

1 small pear

Dinner

Asian Beef Stir-Fry (page 293)

Steamed broccoli

Brown rice

Day 17

Lunch

Vitamix® Tomato Onion Cheese Soup (page 452)

Oriental Chicken Salad (page 411)

Dinner

Fifteen-Minute Vegetarian Chili (page 439)

Green salad—drizzled with olive oil and balsamic vinegar

Day 18

Lunch

Leftover *Fifteen-Minute Vegetarian Chili* from previous day

5 "ak-mak Bakeries" crackers, or other 100 percent organic whole wheat crackers

Green salad—drizzled with olive oil and rice vinegar

Dinner

Savory Meatballs (page 370)

Quinoa with Roasted Garlic, Tomatoes and Spinach (page 359)

Skillet Zucchini (page 376)

Day 19

Lunch

Vitamix® Vegetable Soup (page 453)

Hummus with sliced vegetables

Dinner

Blackened salmon (use *Blackened Rub for Fish,* page 303)

Lemon-Asparagus Packets (page 340)

Roasted Sweet Potatoes (page 364)

Green salad—drizzled with olive oil and balsamic vinegar

Day 20

Lunch

Leftover salmon from previous day

2 cups mixed steamed vegetables

Dinner

Garlic Chickpeas and Pasta (page 323)

Green salad—drizzled with olive oil and balsamic vinegar

Day 21

Lunch

Spinach Salad with Strawberries and Pistachios (page 423)

Italian Vegetable Soup (page 441)

Dinner

Grilled Glazed Dijon Chicken (page 330)

Grilled Portobello Mushrooms (page 331)

Asian Cabbage (page 295)

Day 22

Lunch

Sweet Potato Soup (page 445 for Option A, page 446 for Option B)

Mixed green salad with vegetables—sprinkled with 3 tablespoons raw sunflower seeds

½ cup sliced fruit

Dinner

Mrs. Dash® Fish (page 347)

Curried Cauliflower (page 319)

Steamed Brussels sprouts

Sliced tomatoes

Day 23

Lunch

Asian Chicken Salad (page 391) drizzled with *Lime-Rice Wine Vinaigrette* (page 409)

Dinner

Mediterranean Beef Stew (page 346)

Mixed green salad drizzled with *Basic Vinaigrette* (page 395)

Day 24

Lunch

Cabbage-Apple Salad (page 398)

Dinner

Easy Minestrone Soup (page 438)

Green salad drizzled with *Basic Vinaigrette* (page 395)

Day 25

Lunch

Leftover *Easy Minestrone Soup* from previous day

¼ cup almonds

Dinner

Grilled Caribbean Chicken (page 328)

Crispy Kale (page 316)

Steamed broccoli

Day 26

Lunch

Green salad with assorted vegetables and 4 ounces of chicken breast

¼ cup walnuts

1 small apple

Dinner

Peel and eat shrimp

Dressed-Up Asparagus (page 321)

Steamed cauliflower—drizzled with olive oil and sprinkled with Mrs. Dash® seasoning

Day 27

Lunch

Lean turkey burger on a 100 percent whole wheat hamburger bun

Sliced raw vegetables

1 small banana

Dinner

White Bean Soup with Kale and Sausage (page 454)

Green salad—drizzled with olive oil and balsamic vinegar

Day 28

Lunch

Leftover *White Bean Soup with Kale and Sausage* from previous night

Celery and carrot sticks with 1 tablespoon organic peanut butter

Dinner

Baked turkey breast

Baked Zucchini Fries (page 297)

Italian Green Beans (page 336)

Day 29

Lunch

Turkey on green salad with mixed vegetables—drizzled with a dash of olive oil and rice vinegar

Dinner

Seared Scallops with Farmers' Market Salad (page 417)

Simple Greens and Garlic (page 421)

Vegetable Stir-Fry (page 387)

Day 30

Lunch

Spinach Strawberry Salad (page 424)

4 ounce chicken breast

Dinner

Grilled Rosemary Steak (page 333)

Grilled Vegetables (page 334)

Green salad—drizzled with olive oil and rice vinegar

Phase Two — Option B

Breakfast

You now have more breakfast options. Choose one for each day for breakfast. Remember to mix it up so you're not eating the same thing every day!

Day 1

Lunch

Coconut Curry Chicken (page 314) with brown rice

Dinner

Turkey Soup (page 449)

Day 2

Lunch

Mediterranean Quinoa Salad (page 410)

Simple Grilled Chicken Breast (page 372)

Dinner

Curried Ginger Raisin Lentils (page 320)

Ginger & Garlic Broccoli Salad (page 405)

Day 3

Lunch

Apple Cabbage Salad (page 393) with turkey

Dinner

Beef & Quinoa Meatballs (page 300)

Zucchini Noodle Pasta (page 389)

Day 4

Lunch

Pesto Filet (page 352)

Sage Cranberries & Butternut Squash with Caramelized Onions (page 367)

Dinner

Smoothie of choice

Day 5

Lunch

Stuffed Avocado Salad (page 426)

Simple Green Salad (page 420)

Dinner

Pan-Seared Grass-Fed Beef (page 351) wrapped in lettuce leaves

Simple Sweet Potato (page 374)

Day 6

Lunch

Quinoa Stuffed Bell Peppers (page 357)

Dinner

Salmon with Buckwheat Noodles (page 369)

Day 7

Lunch

Black Bean Sweet Potato Burger (page 301)

Vegetable Chips (page 386)

Salad of choice

Dinner

Turkey Pilgrim Salad (page 430)

Day 8

Lunch

Fennel Avocado Salad (page 403) with *Garlic Avocado Dressing* (page 404)

Simple Grilled Chicken Breast (page 372)

Dinner

Mexican Chicken Soup with Ancho Chilies (page 443)

Day 9

Lunch

Thai Chicken Peanut Butter Pasta (page 385)

Dinner

Veggie Omelet (page 258)

Sweet Potato Fries (page 383)

Day 10

Lunch

Jamaican Jerk Chicken (page 338)

Ginger & Garlic Broccoli Salad (page 405)

Dinner

Vegetable Soup (page 451)

Day 11

Lunch

Everything But the Kitchen Sink Salad (page 402)

Steamed Vegetables

Dinner

Buckwheat Soba Noodles with Chicken (page 308)

Day 12

Lunch

Spicy Grilled Tuna with Salsa (page 381)

Sicilian Collard Greens (page 419)

Dinner

Smoothie of choice

Day 13

Lunch

Pan-Seared Grass-Fed Beef (page 351)

Goat Cheese Swiss Chard with Rice (page 324)

Dinner

Southwestern Salad (page 422)

Day 14

Lunch

Tropical Fruit Salad with Arugula (page 429)

Simple Sweet Potato (page 374)

Dinner

Plantain Encrusted Halibut (page 354)

Coconut Rice (page 315)

Day 15

Lunch

Chicken Salad Collard Greens Wrap (page 312)

Dinner

Sage-Crusted Chicken Tenders (page 366)

Zucchini Noodle Pasta (page 389)

Day 16

Lunch

Broccoli Apple Chicken Salad with Poppyseed Dressing (page 396)

Dinner

Salad of choice with *Tahini Dressing* (page 428)

Balsamic Roasted Apple Butternut Squash (page 299)

Day 17

Lunch

Blueberry Chicken (page 305)

Cauliflower Rice (page 311)

Dinner

Smoothie of choice

Day 18

Lunch

Sweet Potato and Goat Cheese Frittata (page 255)

Dinner

Orange Juice Scallops (page 349)

Chive Mashed Cauliflower (page 313)

Day 19

Lunch

Fennel Avocado Salad (page 403)

Sweet Potato Fries (page 383)

Dinner

Salmon Florentine (page 368)

Day 20

Lunch

Butternut Squash and Kale Salad (page 397)

Simple Grilled Chicken Breast (page 372)

Dinner

Tomato Minestrone (page 448)

Day 21

Lunch

Sweet Lentil Brussels Burger (page 382) on favorite bun

Side Salad

Vegetable Chips (page 386)

Dinner

Summer Salad (page 427)

Day 22

Lunch

Everything but the Kitchen Sink Salad (page 402) with chopped, hard-boiled eggs

Dinner

Salmon with Buckwheat Noodles (page 369)

Day 23

Lunch

Caramelized Onion and Spinach Frittata (page 243)

Dinner

Southwestern Stuffed Sweet Potato (page 378)

Steamed Broccoli

Day 24

Lunch

Pumpkin Caesar Salad Dressing (page 413) on choice of salad

Dinner

Sesame Noodles (page 371)

Pesto Filet (page 352)

Day 25

Lunch

Quinoa Stuffed Bell Peppers (page 357) with ground chicken added

Steamed Vegetables

Dinner

Thick & Chunky Tomato Soup (page 447)

Day 26

Lunch

Coconut Curry Chicken (page 314) with brown rice

Dinner

Smoothie of choice

Day 27

Lunch

Salad of choice topped with *Pan-Seared Grass-Fed Beef* (page 351)

Dinner

Apple, Almond, Spinach, Quinoa Salad (page 392)

Day 28

Lunch

Leftover *Caribbean Kale* (page 309) with 2 eggs over easy

Dinner

Avocado Coconut Soup (page 433)

Southwestern Salad (page 422)

Day 29

Lunch

Mango Shrimp (page 342)

Caribbean Rice & Beans (page 310)

Dinner

Butternut Squash Soup with Toasted Pecans (page 435)

Day 30

Lunch

Goat Cheese Swiss Chard with Rice (page 324)

Simple Grilled Chicken Breast (page 372)

Dinner

Smoothie of choice

Conclusion

"Your health account, your bank account, they're the same thing. The more you put in, the more you can take out."
— Jack LaLanne

By investing your time and resources in your health, you can achieve optimal health. The hardest thing for most of my patients is to clean up their eating habits and increase plant based foods in their meals—including their breakfast. The key in this book is to lower your insulin levels by avoiding foods that are high in sugar intake or in carbohydrates. This includes foods like bread, pasta, rice, potatoes, corn, sodas, cakes, pancakes, waffles, cereals, ice cream, cookies, candies or other junk foods. If you limit your refined sugars and substitute a grain for a green, then you can easily lower your insulin levels. The one major thing that you can control in your life is what you put into your mouth — or what you feed your body. Respect your body and mind, and in return you will enjoy the benefits of optimal health.

Another major point is to have an active lifestyle. You have to exercise daily, and to understand that exercise is something you do until you die, like breathing. One of my personal heroes that recently passed away at the age of 96 was Jack LaLanne. He was into fitness decades before most Americans realized the benefits of it. In 1936 he opened the first health club and medical community. Back then, people thought he was a "nut" and that weightlifting was harmful to your health—and to your sex drive. I am so glad he did not listen to the medical advice at that time. He is also amazing for his many insights on living healthy.

LaLanne summed up his philosophy about good nutrition and exercise this way: "Living is a pain in the butt. Dying is easy. Living is like an athletic event. You've got to train for it. You've got to eat right. You've got to exercise. Your health account, your bank account, they're the same thing. The more you put in, the more you can take out. Exercise is king and nutrition is queen: together, you have a kingdom."

LaLanne also said in a interview, "In my mind, nothing on this earth is more addictive than refined sugar." Bluntly, he has said that eating too much sugar will KILL you. Unfortunately, he died of a lung complication after heart surgery, but he worked out up to the day before his death.

So enjoy life and make your best investment in working out, avoiding the artificial sweeteners, processed foods and other foods that increase insulin levels. There is so much to do, to experience, to learn and to see in our lifetime. Find your passion, live life to the fullest, and remember to work out every day like Jack LaLanne.

Hope to see you out there exploring this wonderful world in which we live!

Recipes: Breakfast

"Life expectancy would grow by leaps and bounds
if green vegetables smelled as good as bacon."
— Doug Larson

Almond Butter Peach Soft Serve[1]

2 cups peaches, frozen
¼ cup almond milk
2 to 3 tablespoons almond butter
½ tablespoon maple syrup
2 to 3 drops stevia
2 mint leaves, fresh

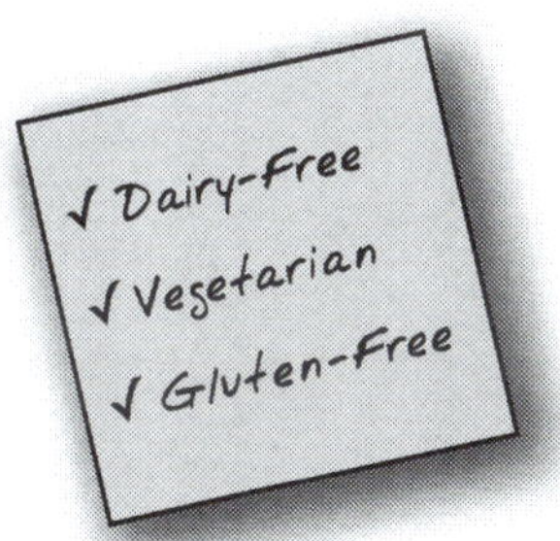

Place peaches, stevia, 2 tablespoons almond butter, and 1 tablespoon almond milk into food processor. Blend until creamy while adding 3 to 4 tablespoons of almond milk until you reach a creamy consistency in the peaches. Taste and adjust flavor with a third tablespoon of almond butter and ½ tablespoon maple syrup. Garnish with fresh mint leaf.

Makes 2 servings (serving size of 8 ounces).

Nutrition per serving: calories 189, fat 10 g, cholesterol 0 mg, sodium 25 mg, carbohydrates 24.72 g, fiber 4.3 g, sugar 20.26 g, protein 5.8 g.

Amaranth with Orange-Berry Topping[2]

1 cup amaranth

3 cups organic plain unsweetened soy, coconut or almond milk

⅜ teaspoon cinnamon

¼ teaspoon sea salt

1 cup mixed frozen berries (5 ounces)

2 tablespoons 100 percent fresh squeezed orange juice

Place the amaranth, milk, ¼ teaspoon of the cinnamon, and ⅛ teaspoon of salt in a saucepan. Bring to a simmer and cook for 20 to 25 minutes, until the liquid is absorbed. Meanwhile, place the berries, orange juice, the remaining ⅛ teaspoon cinnamon and the remaining ⅛ teaspoon salt in a small saucepan. Cook over medium-low heat for 10 minutes while stirring occasionally to break up any large berries. Divide the amaranth into 4 bowls. Top each with 2 tablespoons of the berry topping.

Makes 4 servings (serving size of ¾ cup amaranth and 2 tablespoons berry topping).

Nutrition per serving: calories 239, total fat 3 g, saturated fat 0.7 g, sodium 166 mg, carbohydrates 41 g, fiber 1 g, protein 13 g.

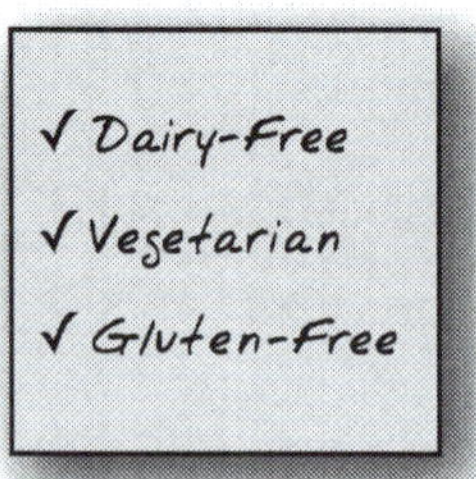

Apple Cinnamon Energy Bars[3]

1 small apple, cored
1 cup dried dates (soak for 1 to 2 hours in water) or ½ cup agave
½ cup cooked quinoa
¼ cup almonds
¼ cup ground flaxseed
2 teaspoons cinnamon
½ teaspoon nutmeg
Sea salt to taste

In a food processor, process all ingredients until desired texture is reached. If you prefer a uniformly smooth bar, process longer. If you would rather have a bar with more crunch and texture, blend for less time. If mixture is to dry add a little water. Remove mixture from processor and put on a clean surface. There are 2 ways to shape the bars: Roll the mixture into several balls, or shape it into bars. To shape into balls, use a tablespoon to scoop the mixture and roll between palms of your hands. To shape as bars, flatten mixture on clean surface with hands. Place plastic wrap over top and roll mixture to desired bar thickness with rolling pin. Cut mixture evenly into 12 bars.

Makes 12 servings (serving size of 1 bar).

Nutrition per serving: calories 71, fat 2.41 g, cholesterol 0 mg, sodium 12.75 mg, carbohydrates 12.3 g, fiber 2.3 g, sugar 8.16 g, protein 1.35 g.

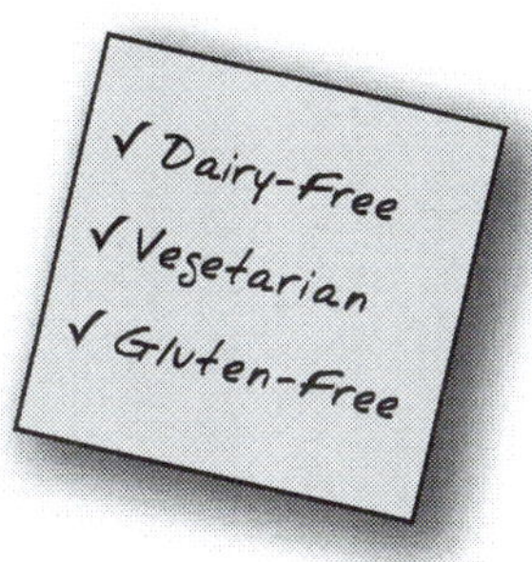

Apple-Walnut Amaranth

1 cup amaranth

3 cups plain soy milk

¼ teaspoon ground cinnamon

1 large apple, skin on, cored and diced

½ cup chopped walnuts

Place the amaranth, soy milk, cinnamon and apple in a medium saucepan. Bring to a boil, stirring frequently. Cover pan and reduce heat to low. Simmer for 25 to 30 minutes until amaranth is soft. Top with chopped walnuts and serve.

Makes 4 servings (serving size of ⅔ cup).

Nutrition per serving: calories 380, total fat 15 g, saturated fat 2.2 g, fiber 10 g, protein 16 g, carbohydrates 48 g.

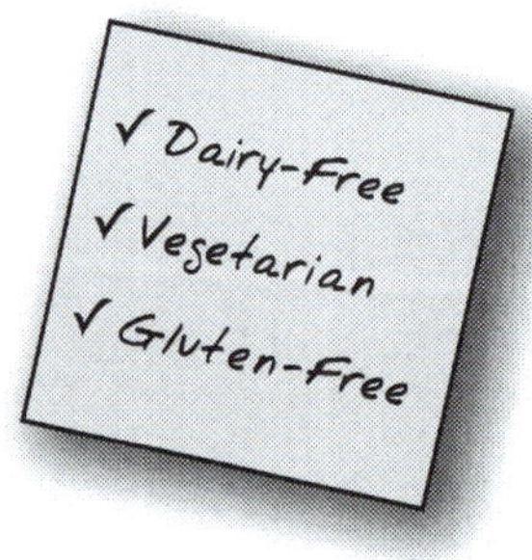

Basil and Tomato Scrambled Eggs

2 eggs
¼ cup chopped tomato
¼ cup chopped onion
1 tablespoon chopped fresh basil

Whisk eggs. Spray skillet with olive oil spray. Add tomato and onions to skillet and cook for about a minute. Add eggs to pan and scramble. Top with basil.

Makes 1 serving.

Nutrition per serving: calories 161, fat 9.05 g, cholesterol 430 mg, sodium 130 mg, carbohydrates 4.05 g, fiber 1.2 g, sugar 0 g, protein 13.23 g.

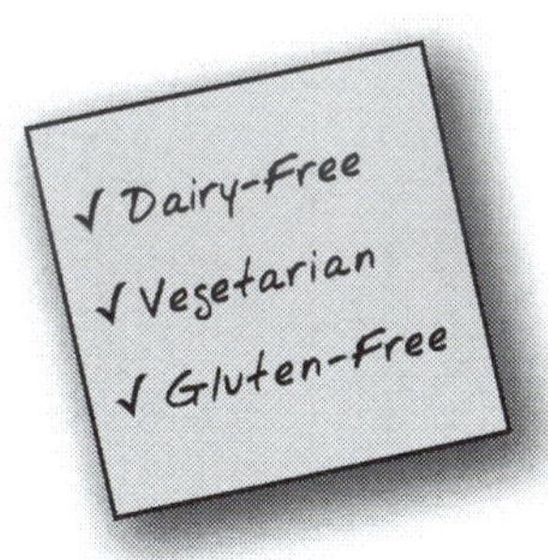

Blueberry Walnut Oatmeal

1 cup water

½ cup Old Fashioned Oats

1 teaspoon cinnamon

½ cup fresh or frozen berries

1 packet stevia sweetener

¼ cup walnuts

Follow instructions for stove top preparation on box of old fashioned oats. Add ½ cup frozen berries, 1 teaspoon cinnamon, 1 packet stevia sweetener and ¼ cup walnuts to oatmeal during the last 2 to 3 minutes of cooking.

Makes 1 serving.

Nutrition per serving: calories 408, total fat 21.7 g, saturated fat 2.2 g, sodium 5 mg, carbohydrates 43.7 g, fiber 8.7 g, protein 9.7 g.

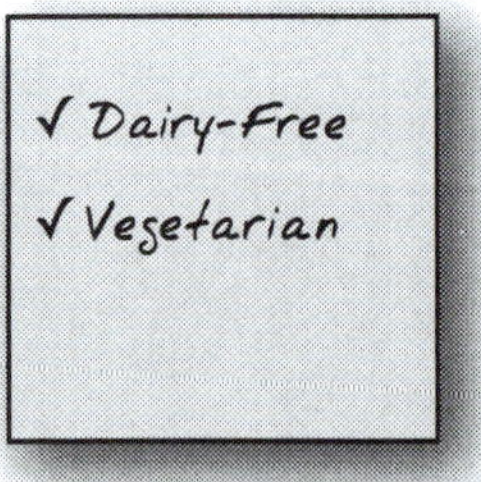

Caramelized Onion and Spinach Frittata[4]

1 tablespoon olive oil
¾ cup yellow onion, julienned
¼ teaspoon thyme
½ teaspoon red wine vinegar
1 cup yellow onions, diced
1 cup red bell pepper, diced
6 cups baby spinach
½ teaspoon dried oregano
16 egg whites, beaten
4 ounces goat cheese, crumbled
¼ cup basil

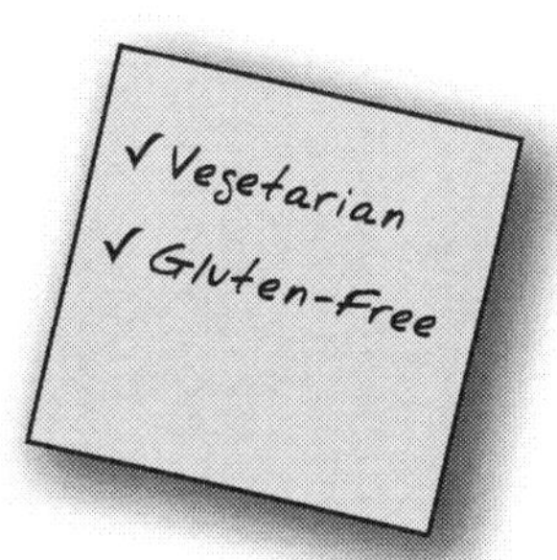

To make caramelized onions: heat olive oil over medium heat. Add the julienned onions and sauté until they are tender and beginning to brown. Stir in the thyme and red wine vinegar and season to taste with salt and pepper. For the frittata: preheat oven to 425°F. In a large, ovenproof, nonstick pan, sauté the onions and peppers in oil until tender. Add the spinach and wilt; make sure to let excess moisture evaporate. Add the oregano and stir to combine everything well. Remove ingredients from the pan and save. Wipe out the pan, reheat and cover generously with pan spray, and add the egg whites. Quickly add the caramelized onions mixture. Push down to equally distribute into the egg whites, but do not stir. Top with the crumbled goat cheese. Finish in the oven until the egg whites are completely cooked. Garnish with basil.

Makes 4 servings.

Nutrition per serving: calories 202, fat 10.41 g, cholesterol 13 mg, sodium 358.75 mg, carbohydrates 7.5 g, fiber 1.05 g, sugar 2.71 g, protein 22.11g.

Cinnamon Flourless Crepe

2 eggs
2 tablespoons coconut milk
2 tablespoons coconut flour or gluten free flour
1 teaspoon vanilla
½ teaspoon cinnamon

Optional: add 1 to 2 scoops of protein powder, mix in with raw eggs

Whip eggs, milk, vanilla and cinnamon in a bowl. It's important to use a small pan and grease it really well (or use a nonstick pan). Pour mixture into pan. Cover and wait to set. Flip to finish cooking. Remove from pan and fill with fresh or baked fruit, almond butter with jelly, or cashew whipped cream. (For cashew whipped cream: blend ½ cup cashews—soaked for 8 hours and drained—½ teaspoon vanilla, ½ cup water and 1 or 2 dates, or 1 tablespoon maple syrup.)

Makes 1 serving.

Nutrition per serving: calories 150, fat 10 g, cholesterol 280 mg, sodium 140 mg, carbohydrates 0 g, fiber 0 g, sugar 2 g, protein 14 g.

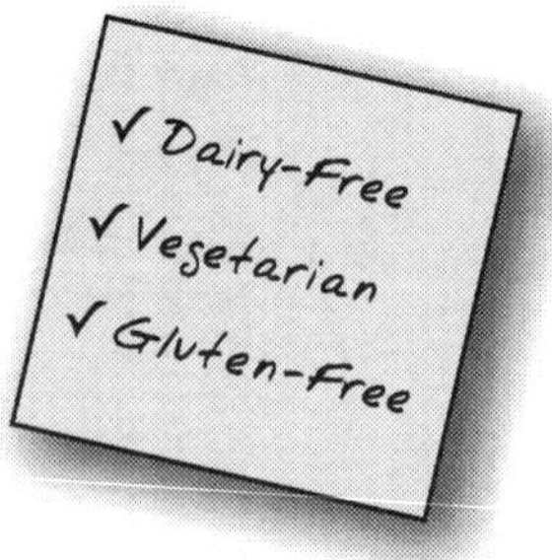

Easy Overnight Oats[5]

⅓ cup oats
¾ cup almond milk
2 tablespoons chia seeds
1 ripe banana, peeled and smashed
¼ teaspoon pure vanilla extract

Mix ingredients together in a bowl and place in the refrigerator overnight. In the morning, add 1 tablespoon nut butter, pure maple syrup or any other additional items. Serve.

Makes 1 serving.

Nutrition per serving: calories 320, fat 9 g, cholesterol 0 mg, sodium 4 mg, carbohydrates 52 g, fiber 11 g, sugar 13 g, protein 9 g.

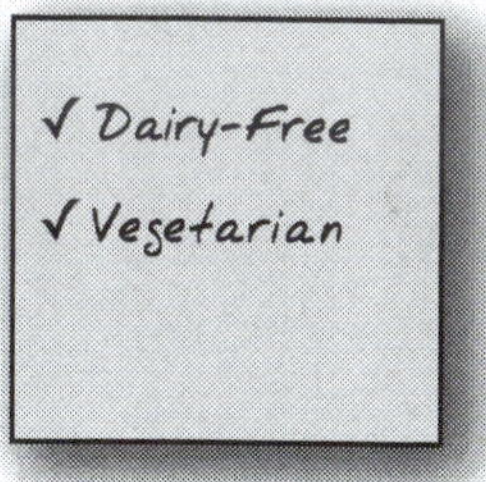

Frittata al Fresco[6]

4 organic eggs
1 teaspoon organic butter
1 to 2 ounces raw goat cheese
¼ cup diced tomatoes
1 tablespoon chopped rosemary or thyme

Preheat oven to 350°F. Whisk eggs thoroughly in a bowl. Heat the butter in a skillet at high heat and add the eggs, then top with goat cheese, diced tomatoes, and herbs. Bake covered in skillet for 10 minutes or until plump and firm. Serve with garden greens.

Makes 2 servings.

Nutrition per serving: calories 206, fat 15.39 g, cholesterol 441.45 mg, sodium 218 mg, carbohydrates 1.625 g, sugar 1.3 g, protein 15.24 g.

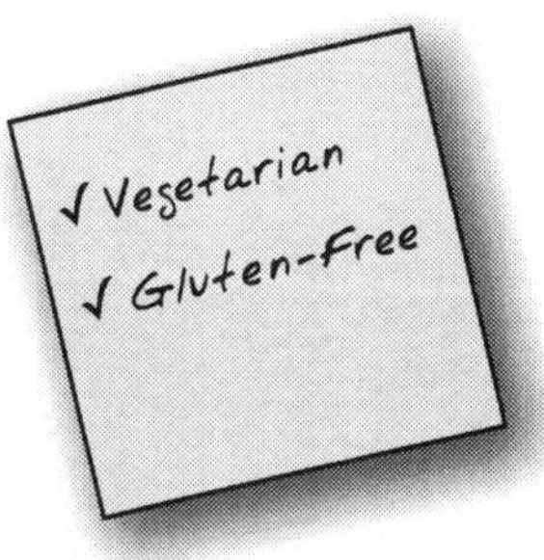

Kiwi Banana Salad

2 tablespoons lime juice
1 tablespoon grapeseed oil
1 tablespoon minced shallot
2 teaspoons rice vinegar
1 teaspoon honey
¼ teaspoon salt
4 kiwis, peeled and diced
2 ripe bananas, cut into thick slices
½ cup diced red bell pepper
2 tablespoons thinly sliced fresh mint
1 pinch of cayenne pepper

Whisk lime juice, oil, shallot, vinegar, honey, salt, and cayenne. Add kiwis, bananas, bell pepper and mint and toss.

Makes 2 to 3 servings.

Nutrition per serving: calories 170, fat 6 g, cholesterol 0 mg, sodium 151 mg, carbohydrates 30 g, fiber 5 g, sugar 1 g, protein 3 g.

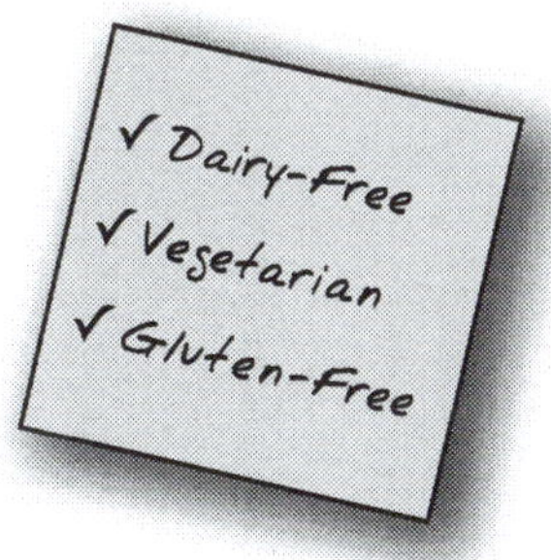

Omega-3 Granola[7]

Dry:
1 cup rolled oats (not instant)
1 cup raw almonds, chopped
¼ cup raw walnuts, chopped
½ cup raw sunflower seeds
2 tablespoons ground flax seeds
2 tablespoons coconut flakes, sweetened
1 teaspoon ground cinnamon
1 pinch of ground nutmeg
¾ teaspoon kosher salt

Optional:
⅓ dried cranberries
⅓ cup raisins
⅓ cup packed brown sugar

Wet:
2 tablespoons honey or grade b maple syrup
1 tablespoon coconut oil
2 tablespoons applesauce
2 tablespoons peanut butter or almond butter

In a medium saucepan over medium heat, add the wet ingredients. Stir well. Bring to a boil and then simmer on low for 5-10 minutes, stirring frequently. In a very large mixing bowl, mix together the dry ingredients. Add the wet mixture (while still warm!) over top of the dry mixture and stir well. It will be very thick and hard to stir, but keep at it until everything is thoroughly combined. Spread onto a pan lined with parchment paper or a nonstick mat and bake in the oven for 45 minutes at 300°F. Remove the pan from the oven every 15 minutes and give the granola a good stir to ensure even baking. Allow to cool for

20-25 minutes on the pan. Stir in dried fruit and toss. Serve with almond milk, goat milk yogurt, or coconut milk yogurt.

Makes 16 servings.

Nutrition per serving: calories 159, fat 10.125 g, cholesterol 0 mg, sodium 3.56 g, carbohydrates 18.01 g, fiber 2.59 g, sugar 5.9 g, protein 3.5 g.

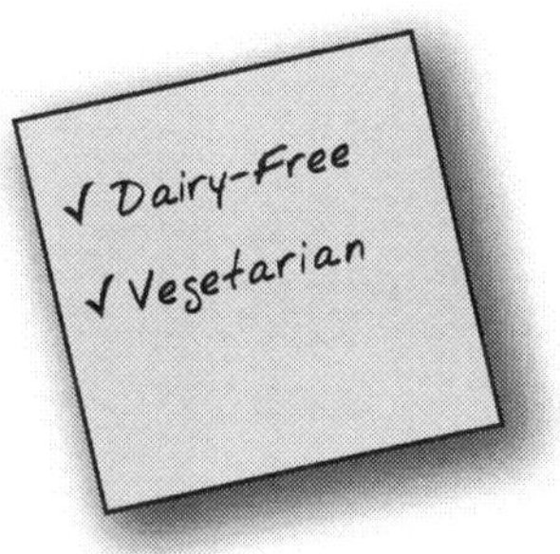

Pumpkin Oatmeal

½ cup oats
¼ teaspoon vanilla
½ teaspoon cinnamon
⅛ teaspoon nutmeg
1½ tablespoons raw honey or maple syrup
⅓ cup canned pumpkin (may substitute apple sauce or sweet potato)
⅓ cup almond milk
1 pinch of salt

Optional:
- 1 tablespoon nut butter
- 2 tablespoons raisins, walnuts, etc.

Preheat oven to 375°F. Combine oats, spices, pumpkin and milk. Pour into small baking pan or ramekin. Cook for 15 minutes, then broil for 3 minutes for a nice crust.

Makes 2 servings.

Nutrition per serving: calories 136, fat 2.365 g, cholesterol 0 mg, sodium 5 mg, carbohydrates 27.23 g, fiber 5.87 g, sugar 10.14 g, protein 3.6 g.

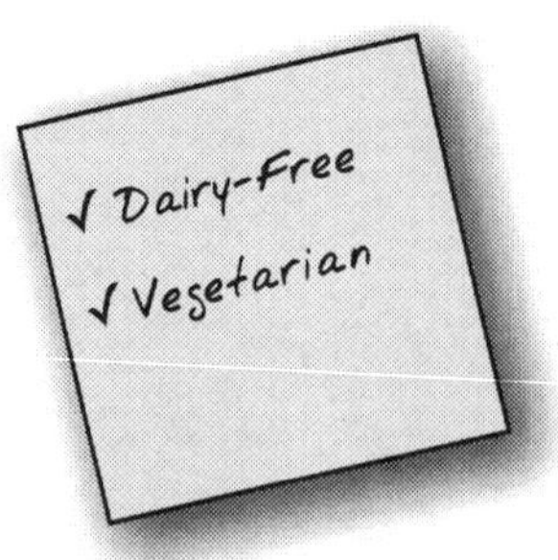

Quinoa Porridge with Apple Compote[8]

½ cup quinoa
½ cup apple juice
½ cup orange juice
1 sweet apple (Gala or Fuji)
¼ cup blueberries

In a saucepan, slowly cook quinoa with juices, stirring occasionally, for about 10 to 12 minutes. Steam the apple. Peel the apple and blend in food processor. Add blueberries and puree lightly (can also steam apple and add to porridge without blending). Top quinoa when ready with fruit compote.

Makes 2 servings.

Nutrition per serving: calories 71, fat 1.08 g, cholesterol 0 mg, sodium 6.88 mg, carbohydrates 31.82 g, fiber 4.05 g, sugar 22.52 g, protein 3.06 g.

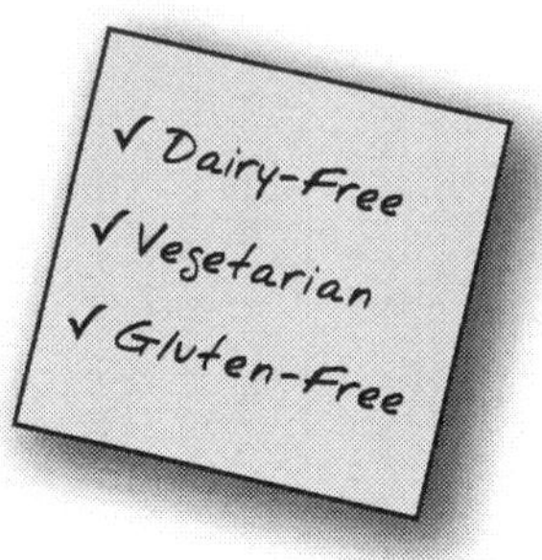

Raw Granola Bars

½ cup raw almond or peanut butter
½ cup raw honey or dates
Choice of: chopped pumpkin seeds, chopped sunflower seeds, flax seeds, dried apple, apricot, raisins, chocolate chips, white chocolate chips, quinoa flakes, puffed rice, chopped toasted walnuts, almonds, coconut

Warm almond butter and honey on stove until melted. Turn off heat and add in pumpkin seeds, sunflower seeds, flax seeds, dried apple, dates, and mini chocolate chips, etc. After mixing in items place in a Pyrex®-like square dish and set to cool in refrigerator or freezer for at least 2 hours. Cut into squares.

Makes 5 to 6 servings (serving size of 1 bar).

Nutrition per serving: varies: calories 204, fat 10 g, cholesterol 0 mg, sodium 0 mg, carbohydrates 29 g, fiber 4 g, sugar 20 g, protein 5 g.

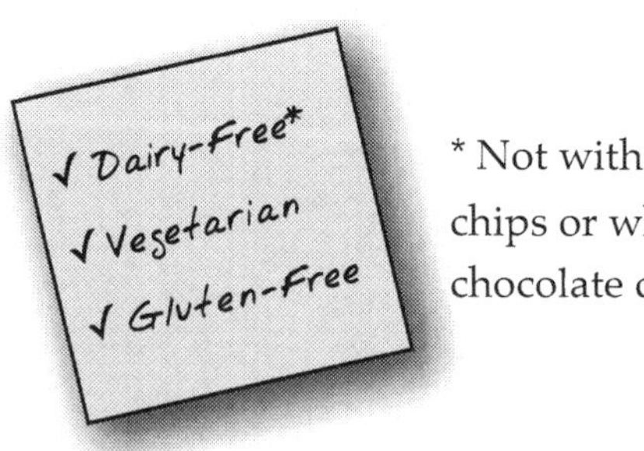

* Not with chocolate chips or white chocolate chips.

Sausage, Egg & Vegetable Casserole[9]

1 pound sweet Italian sausage (or chicken sausage) cut into 1-inch pieces
1 tablespoon olive oil
1½ teaspoons olive oil
½ small head escarole, chopped (or use kale, broccoli rabe or broccoli)
2 zucchinis, thinly sliced
1 small red onion, thinly sliced
1 red bell pepper, chopped
¼ teaspoon salt
¼ teaspoon ground black pepper
7 large eggs
½ cup unsweetened almond milk
¼ cup grated parmesan cheese

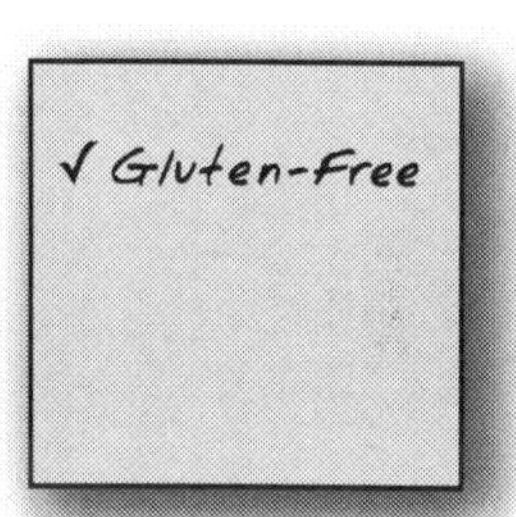

Preheat oven to 350°F. Coat baking dish with cooking spray. Cook sausage in large skillet over medium high heat until half-cooked, 6 to 8 minutes, stirring occasionally. Spread over the bottom of the prepared dish. Discard fat in the skillet. Pour oil into same skillet and stir in escarole, zucchini, bell pepper, onion, salt and ⅛ teaspoon black pepper. Reduce heat to medium. Cook, stirring occasionally, until vegetables are tender and liquid evaporates, 8 to 10 minutes. Let cool for 10 minutes and arrange over sausage. Meanwhile, in large bowl, combine the eggs, milk, cheese and remaining ⅛ teaspoon black pepper. Pour over vegetables. Bake until eggs are set, about 40 to 45 minutes. Cut evenly into 6 squares.

Makes 6 servings.

Nutrition per serving: calories 281, fat 17.9 g, cholesterol 277 mg, sodium 685 mg, carbohydrates 7.1 g, fiber 1.6 g, sugar 2.7 g, protein 23.1 g.

Simple Breakfast Yogurt Cup

½ cup of vanilla Greek yogurt or coconut milk yogurt
¼ cup of muesli or low sugar granola of choice

Optional: berries

Mix muesli or homemade granola into yogurt

Makes 1 serving.

Nutrition per serving: calories 254, fat 3.06 g, cholesterol 0 mg, sodium 66.07 mg, carbohydrates 32 g, fiber 1.97 g, sugar 20 g, protein 12.8 g.

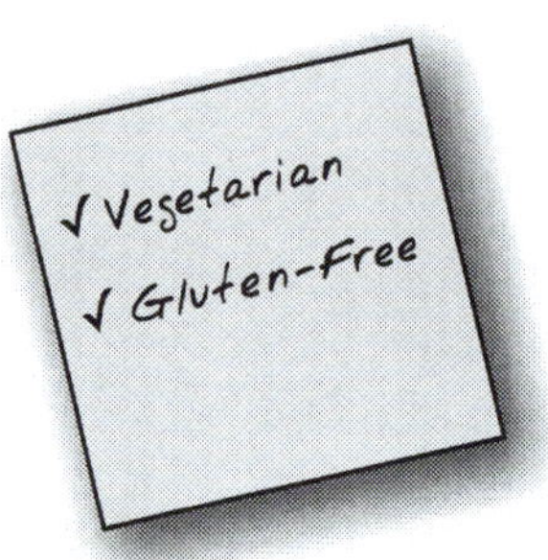

Sweet Potato and Goat Cheese Frittata

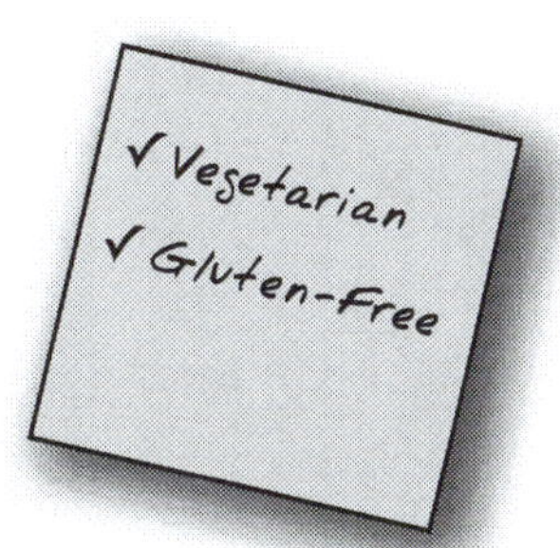

½ sweet potato, peeled (¼ pound)
1 tablespoon butter
1 tablespoon olive oil
3 shallots
1 tablespoon thyme
6 eggs
½ cup unsweetened almond milk
2 ounces goat cheese, crumbled (⅓ cup)
Ground black pepper and sea salt to taste

Preheat oven to 375°F. Steam the sweet potato until barely tender, about 15 minutes. Cut sweet potato into thin rounds—you should have about a dozen slices. Heat butter and olive oil over medium heat in a 10" cast iron skillet. Sauté shallots and the tablespoon of thyme for about six minutes or until soft and just barely browned. Push to the side of the pan and add sweet potato slices. Let them brown on both sides, about two minutes per side. Season with plenty of salt and freshly ground pepper. Beat eggs and milk in a mixing bowl. Remove half of the sweet potato and shallot mixture to a plate. Add half the egg mixture to the pan and distribute the reserved sweet potatoes and shallots over them. Add the remaining egg mixture. Dot the top with goat cheese, the pinch of thyme and a full grind or two of black pepper. Let it cook for about five minutes on the stovetop or until it's just set on the edges (it will still be very runny in the middle). Cook it in the oven for exactly eight minutes and it should be just set throughout.

Makes 4 servings.

Nutrition per serving: calories 215, fat 16.68 g, cholesterol 336.5 mg, sodium 197.5 mg, carbohydrates 4.88 g, fiber 0 g, sugar 1.05 g, protein 11.94 g.

Sweet Potato Pancakes[10]

2 medium sweet potatoes or yams, peeled and shredded (about 4 cups)

2 tablespoons white or brown rice flour (can use wheat flour)

1 dash sea salt

1 tablespoon maple syrup

2 large eggs, lightly beaten

2 to 3 tablespoons coconut oil

Place shredded sweet potatoes in a large mixing bowl. Sprinkle with rice flour and salt. Mix well. Pour in egg and agave and mix until egg completely coats sweet potatoes. Heat 1 tablespoon oil in a large skillet. Working in batches, and using more oil as needed, use ½ cup sweet potato batter to make each pancake. Cook, covered, for 5 minutes on each side, or until lightly browned. Remove to a platter and serve immediately.

They burn easily, so watch them carefully and then serve with maple syrup, almond butter and jelly, or mascarpone cheese.

Makes 5 servings.

Nutrition per serving: calories 270, fat 9 g, cholesterol 85 mg, sodium 340 mg, carbohydrates 43 g, fiber 5 g, sugar 29 g, protein 5 g.

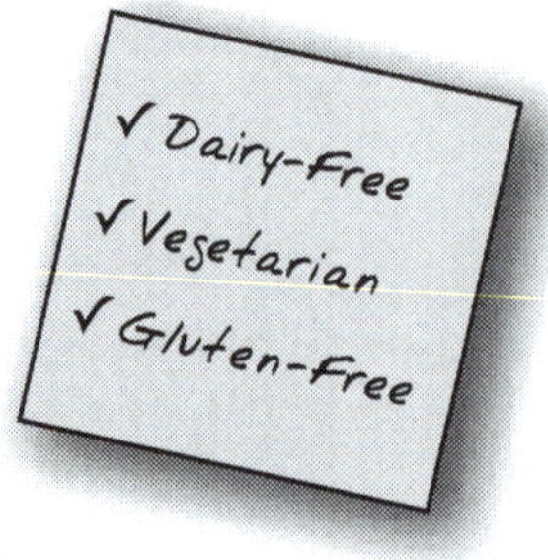

Tropical Quinoa Bars[11]

1¼ cup dry quinoa
2½ cups water
¾ cup full fat coconut milk
3 eggs
3 tablespoons chia seeds (or use sunflower seeds)
1 cup dried unsweetened mango, cut into bite size pieces
½ cup dried unsweetened papaya
¼ cup raw honey
¼ teaspoon sea salt

Optional: ½ cup dried figs

Rinse quinoa by placing in a strainer and running it under water for 1 minute. Transfer to a medium sized saucepan, add water and cover. Bring to a boil, then reduce to simmer for 20 to 25 minutes. Leave lid on while cooking. Once complete, remove lid and set aside. Combine coconut milk, eggs, chia seeds, in a small bowl. Stir and set aside. Preheat oven to 325°F and line 9x13 pan with parchment paper across both sides for easy lifting and set aside. In a large bowl combine quinoa with coconut milk mixture. Stir until fully combined. Add remaining ingredients. Press firmly into prepared pan and bake for 30 to 40 minutes until golden. Remove from oven and allow to cool for 1 hour before cutting

Makes 15 servings.

Nutrition per serving: calories 202, fat 10 g, cholesterol 210 mg, sodium 100 mg, carbohydrates 24 g, fiber 5 g, sugar 11 g, protein 4.5 g.

Veggie Omelet

1 tablespoon chopped onion

1 tablespoon chopped tomato

1 tablespoon chopped bell pepper

1 tablespoon chopped mushrooms

3 egg whites or 2 egg whites and 1 egg

Spray skillet or put a small amount of organic butter into pan. Place vegetable in pan to cook for 1 to 2 minutes. Whisk eggs and place in a nonstick pan and scramble. Top with pepper and fresh basil.

Makes 1 serving.

Nutrition per serving: calories 28, fat 5.2 g, cholesterol 215 mg, sodium 185 mg, carbohydrates 3.96 g, fiber 1.26 g, sugar 0.82 g, protein 15.45 g.

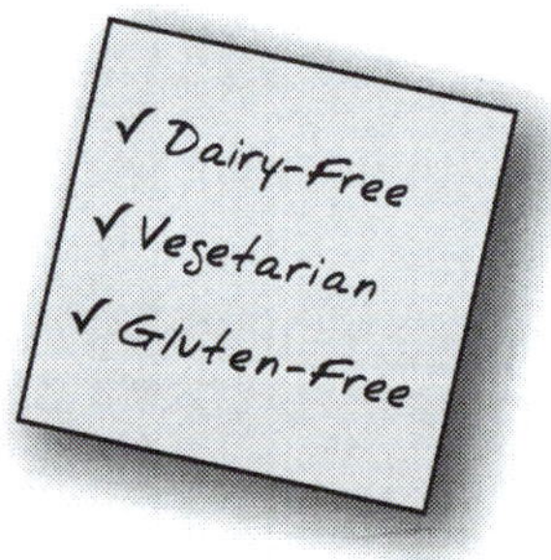

Recipes: Smoothies

"Nothing will benefit human health and increase the chances for survival of life on Earth as much as the evolution to a vegetarian diet."
— Albert Einstein

All Green Smoothie

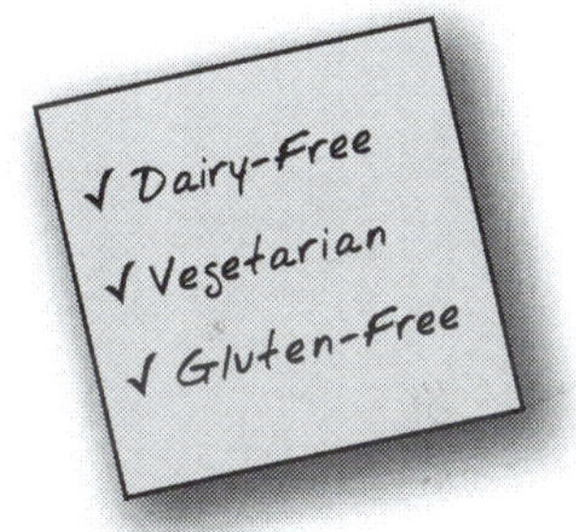

½ cucumber
2 celery stalks
½ avocado
Juice of half a lime
½ granny smith apple
1 handful or romaine lettuce
1 to 2 cups of water, nut milk, or coconut water
½ tablespoon raw honey, 4 drops of vanilla stevia, or 2 Medjool dates
1 pinch of salt
2 to 5 ice cubes

Place ingredients into blender and blend until smooth.

Makes 2 servings.

Nutrition per serving: calories 153, fat 7.1 g, cholesterol 0 mg, sodium 64 mg, carbohydrates 25 g, fiber 6.88 g, sugar 17 g, protein 2 g.

Almond Butter Banana Green Smoothie

1 banana

2 tablespoons creamy unsalted almond butter

1 handful of spinach

1 to 2 cups almond milk

1 teaspoon cinnamon

Optional:

1 to 2 dates

½ tablespoon

Raw honey or 3 to 5 drops of stevia

Place ingredients into blender and blend until smooth.

Makes 2 servings.

Nutrition per serving: calories 221, fat 10.48 g, cholesterol 0 mg, sodium 75.5 mg, carbohydrates 31.53 g, fiber 4.4 g, sugar 19.81 g, protein 6.24 g.

√ Dairy-Free

√ Vegetarian

√ Gluten-Free

Apple Pie Smoothie

1 medium apple, peeled, cored and sliced
6 to 8 unsalted raw walnut halves
1 tablespoon steel-cut oats
1 teaspoon ground cinnamon
1 cup almond milk
½ banana
1 to 2 Medjool dates or stevia to taste

Place ingredients into blender and blend until smooth.

Makes 2 servings.

Nutrition per serving: calories 183, fat 5.63 g, cholesterol 0 mg, sodium 50 mg, carbohydrates 33.74 g, fiber 5.02 g, sugar 15.28 g, protein 2.9 g.

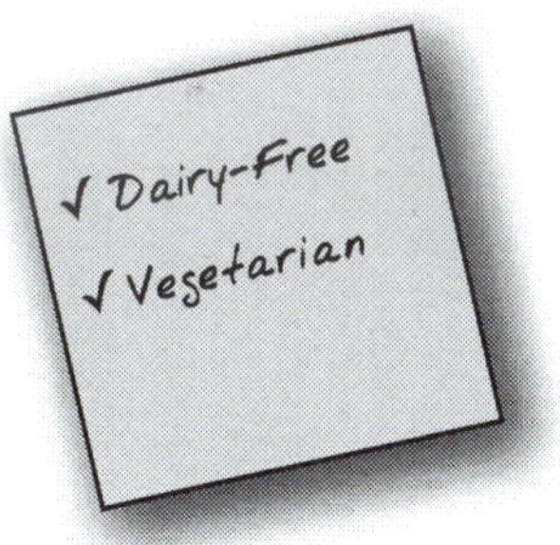

Banana Chai Smoothie

1 teaspoon chai spice (or brew 2 bag of chai tea)
1 ripe banana, best if frozen
1 cup almond milk
1 tablespoon almond or cashew butter
3 to 4 drops of vanilla stevia
2 to 5 ice cubes

Optional: 2 to 3 romaine leaves

Place ingredients into blender and blend until smooth.

Makes 1 serving.

Nutrition per serving: calories 306, fat 11.95 g, cholesterol 0 mg, sodium 151 mg, carbohydrates 38 g, fiber 5 g, sugar 18 g, protein 6 g.

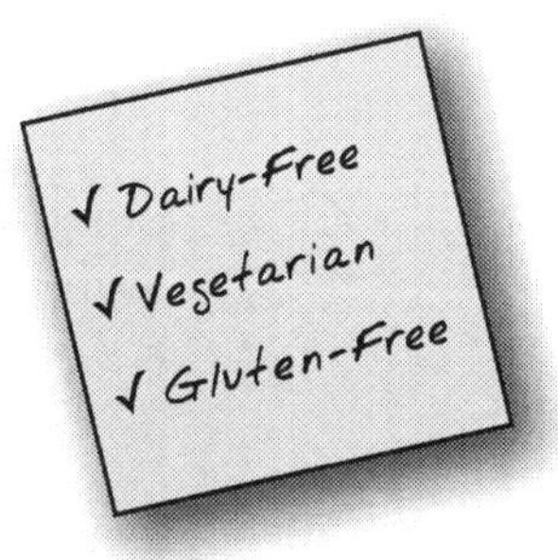

Banana Chocolate Avocado Smoothie

1 medium banana

¼ avocado

1 cup spinach or other greens

2 tablespoons raw organic cacao powder

2 tablespoons milled flaxseed

1 cup almond or coconut milk

1 cup ice

Optional: 1 packet stevia

Blend all ingredients in Vitamix® blender.

Makes 2 servings.

Nutrition per serving: calories 215, carbohydrates 30.1 g, total fat 7.3 g, saturated fat 1.4 g, fiber 10.6 g, protein 7.2 g.

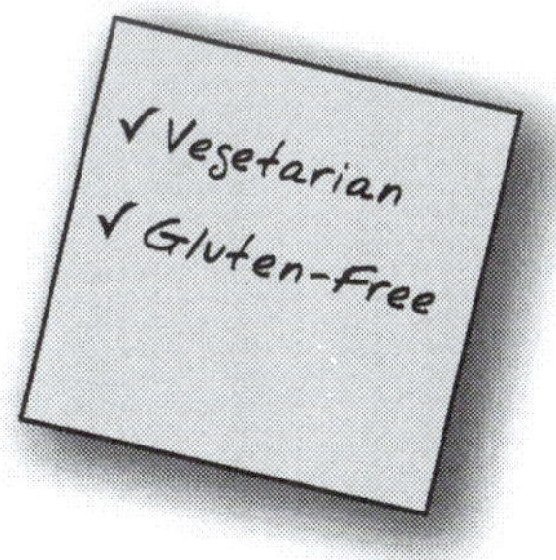

Basil Blueberry Smoothie

½ handful of basil
½ ripe banana or ¼ avocado
1½ cups of water, nut milk, or coconut water
1 cup of blueberries (or mango with a touch of lime)
½ tablespoon raw honey, 4 drops of vanilla stevia, or 2 Medjool dates
2 to 5 ice cubes

Place ingredients into blender and blend until smooth.

Makes 1 serving.

Nutrition per serving: calories 170, fat 3 g, cholesterol 0 mg, sodium 150 mg, carbohydrates 34 g, fiber 6.75 g, sugar 20.3 g, protein 2.74 g.

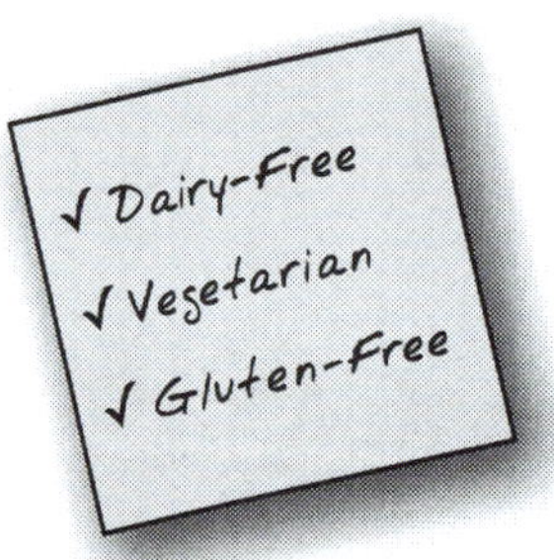

Beginners Green Smoothie

¼ head romaine lettuce
1 ripe banana, best if frozen
1 to 2 cups of water, nut milk, or coconut water
1 teaspoon cinnamon
½ tablespoon raw honey or grade B maple syrup
4 drops of vanilla stevia or 2 Medjool dates
2 to 5 ice cubes

Place ingredients into blender and blend until smooth.

Optional: add 1 scoop of cocoa powder for chocolate green smoothie or 2 tablespoons shredded coconut.

Makes 1 serving.

Nutrition per serving: calories 176, fat 3.7 g, cholesterol 0 mg, sodium 186 mg, carbohydrates 36 g, fiber 4.8 g, sugar 19.6 g, protein 3.1 g.

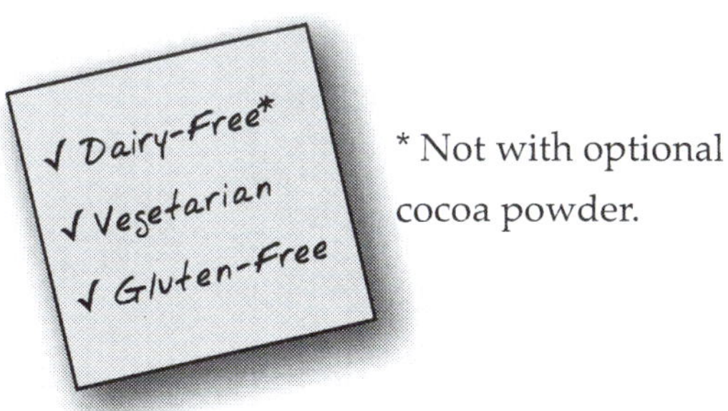

* Not with optional cocoa powder.

Berry Green Smoothie

¾ cup frozen strawberry
¼ cup blueberries
1 handful of spinach
2 romaine lettuce leaves
1 cup liquid of choice (water, coconut water, almond milk, skin milk)
½ tablespoon raw honey, or 4 drops of vanilla stevia
3 to 5 ice cubes

Optional: add banana for creamy texture

Place ingredients into blender and blend till smooth.

Makes 1 serving.

Nutrition per serving: calories 170, fat 2.85 g, cholesterol 0 mg, sodium 172 mg, carbohydrates 35 g, fiber 5.75 g, sugar 24.12 g, protein 4.82 g.

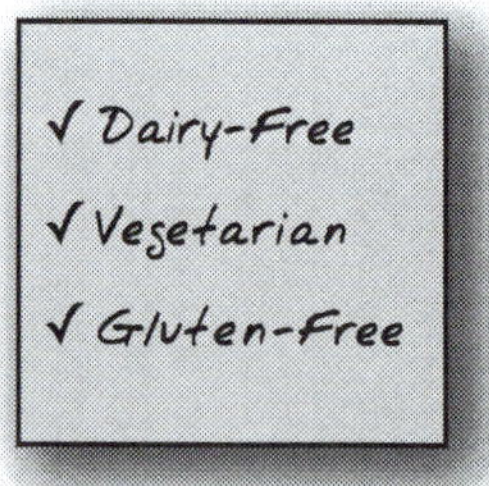

Blueberry Mint Pear Green Smoothie

1 cup of frozen blueberries
½ ripe banana, best if frozen
1 to 2 anjou pears, skin peeled for a creamier smoothie
½ handful of fresh mint leaves
1 to 1½ cups of water, nut milk, or coconut water
½ tablespoon raw honey
4 drops of vanilla stevia or 2 Medjool dates
2 to 5 ice cubes

Place ingredients into blender and blend until smooth.

Makes 2 servings.

Nutrition per serving: calories 180, fat 6.5 g, cholesterol 0 mg, sodium 75 mg, carbohydrates 31 g, fiber 6.5 g, sugar 18 g, protein 3.5 g.

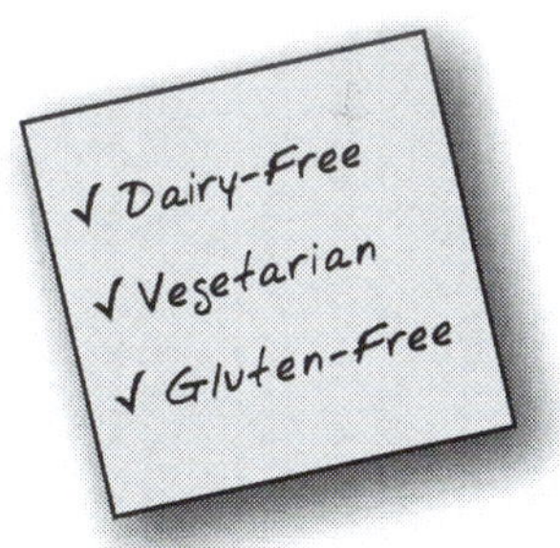

Cherry Walnut Smoothie

1½ cup almond milk
1 cup cherries, frozen
¼ cup walnuts
1 tablespoon raw honey, grade b maple syrup
1 to 2 dates or 4 drops of vanilla stevia
1 teaspoon cinnamon
4 to 5 ice cubes

Optional: add baby spinach or romaine lettuce

Place ingredients into blender and blend until smooth.

Makes 2 to 3 servings.

Nutrition per serving: calories 180, fat 9.25 g, cholesterol 0 mg, sodium 50 mg, carbohydrates 22.13 g, fiber 2.34 g, sugar 18.34 g, protein 5.81 g.

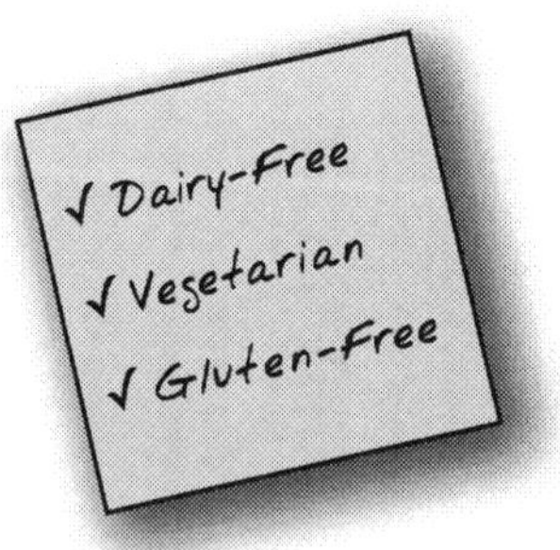

Cilantro Pineapple Smoothie

1 peeled cucumber
¼ cup coconut water
1 cup pineapple
½ tablespoon raw honey coconut sugar
Cilantro
1 teaspoon vanilla
2 leaves of romaine lettuce

Place ingredients into blender and blend until smooth.

Makes 2 servings.

Nutrition per serving: calories 117, fat 0 g, cholesterol 0 mg, sodium 37.5 mg, carbohydrates 29.88 g, fiber 2.3 g, sugar 22.5 g, protein 1.54 g.

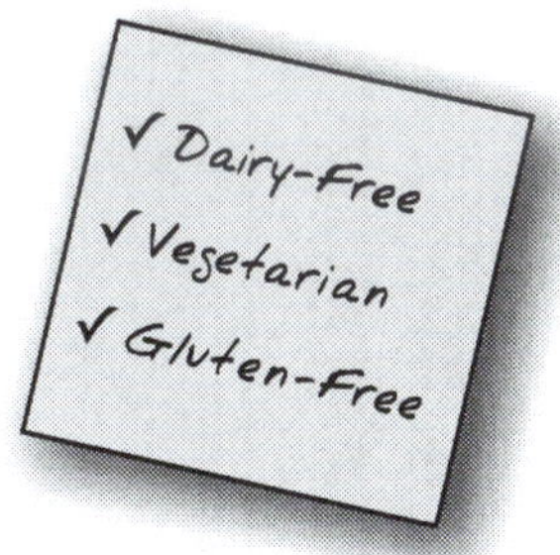

Clementine Creamsicle Smoothie[1]

½ large ripe banana, peeled, sliced and frozen
½ small avocado, flesh scooped out and frozen
2 to 3 clementines, peeled and broken into segments
2 tablespoons coconut milk
1 cup almond milk
1 Medjool date, pitted and chopped
1 teaspoon lemon juice

Optional:
¼ teaspoon almond extract
2 handfuls leafy greens

Place ingredients into blender and blend until smooth.

Makes 2 servings.

Nutrition per serving: calories 172, fat 6.2 g, cholesterol 0 mg, sodium 59 mg, carbohydrates 32.2 g, fiber 5.22 g, sugar 16 g, protein 2.47 g.

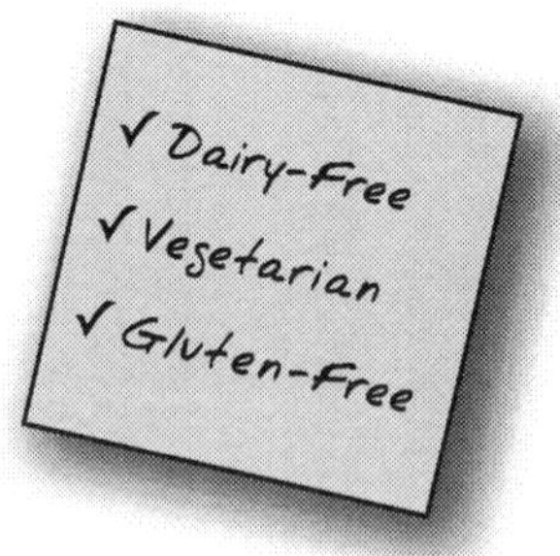

Cocoa Mint Smoothie

1 handful of fresh mint
1 frozen banana
Coconut meat
2 Medjool dates
1 cup almond milk
2 tablespoons cocoa
Add sweetener to taste

Place ingredients into blender and blend until smooth.

Makes 2 servings.

Nutrition per serving: calories 154, fat 3.27 g, cholesterol 0 mg, sodium 51.75 mg, carbohydrates 32.13 g, fiber 4.1 g, sugar 10.95 g, protein 3.09 g.

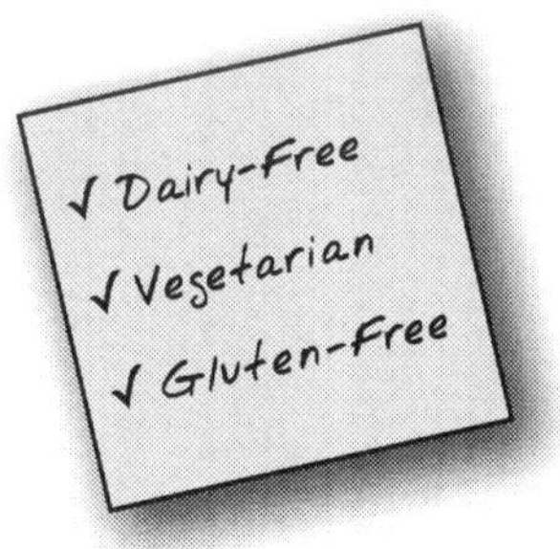

Cocoa Smoothie

2 tablespoons cocoa

1 frozen banana

1 cup of milk (so delicious coconut, almond, skim)

1 Medjool date, honey, stevia to taste

1 teaspoon cinnamon

1 handful of spinach, kale, and romaine

Place ingredients into blender and blend until smooth.

Makes 2 servings.

Nutrition per serving: calories 154, fat 2.39 g, cholesterol 0 mg, sodium 91.25 mg, carbohydrates 33.5 g, fiber 5.42 g, sugar 10.94 g, protein 4.975 g.

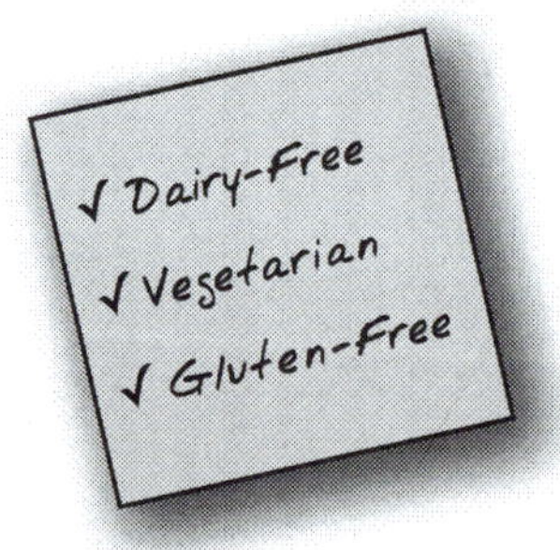

Coconut Green Smoothie

1 young coconut (use meat and water)
1 banana
2 handfuls of baby spinach
1 teaspoon cinnamon
3 to 4 cubes of ice
1 Medjool date (or use 4 drops of stevia for less sugar)

Place ingredients into blender and blend until smooth.

Makes 2 servings.

Nutrition per serving: calories 168, fat 2.35 g, cholesterol 0 mg, sodium 150 mg, carbohydrates 36.28 g, fiber 3.75 g, sugar 14.5 g, protein 2.49 g.

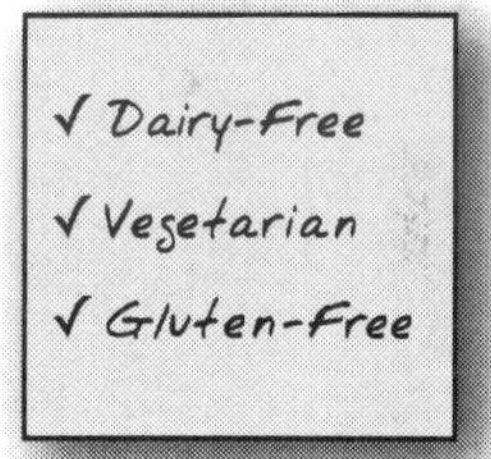

Cranberry Smoothie

½ cup frozen cranberries
½ cup organic spinach
1 teaspoon cinnamon
4 ounces lemon, peeled
1 cup almond or coconut milk
2 tablespoons ground flaxseed (or chia seed)
½ cup cucumber (can use peel if unwaxed)
1 packet stevia sweetener

Place all ingredients in Vitamix® blender with ½ cup ice. Blend for approximately one minute.

Makes 1 serving.

Nutrition per serving: calories 233, total fat 7.7 g, saturated fat 0 g, sodium 168 mg, carbohydrates 34.8 g, fiber 14.6 g, protein 6.5 g.

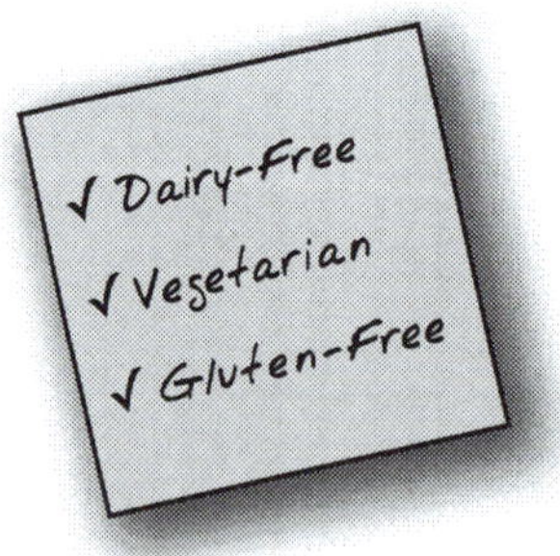

Creamy Green Smoothie

½ banana
1 handful of baby spinach
½ ripe avocado
½ lime
8 ounces water (or nut milk)
3 to 4 drops liquid vanilla or stevia (or ½ tablespoon honey)
5 to 6 ice cubes

Place ingredients into blender and blend until smooth. Add 2 to 3 drops of vanilla stevia for a sweeter smoothie.

Makes 1 serving.

Nutrition per serving: calories 258, fat 16.6 g, cholesterol 0 mg, sodium 252 mg, carbohydrates 26.3 g, fiber 10.3 g, sugar 7.6 g, protein 5.3 g.

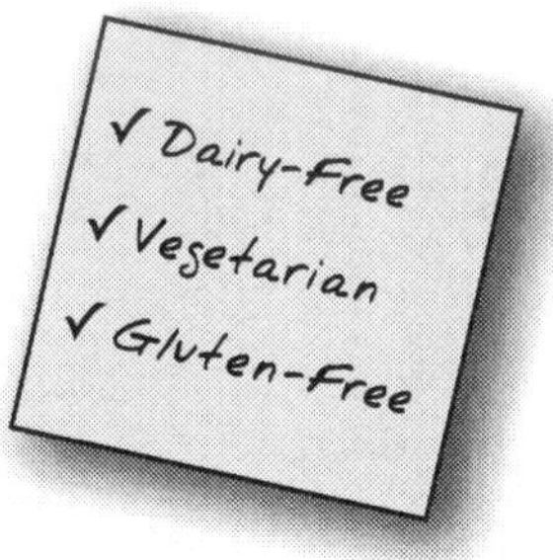

Dark Greens Smoothie

1 bunch of spinach
2 leaves of kale
1 frozen banana
1 cup of almond, walnut or oat milk
1 teaspoon cinnamon
½ tablespoon raw honey, 4 drops of vanilla stevia or 2 Medjool dates

Optional:
1 tablespoon cocoa
1 teaspoon cinnamon

Place ingredients into blender and blend till smooth.

Makes 1 serving.

Nutrition per serving: calories 160, fat 3.2 g, cholesterol 0 mg, sodium 180 mg, carbohydrates 30.2 g, fiber 4.35 g, sugar 13.31 g, protein 6.21 g.

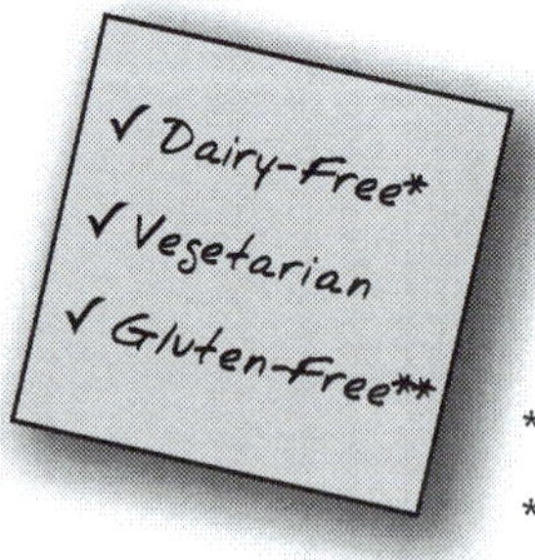

* Not with optional cocoa.
** Not with oat milk.

Dr. Oz's Vitamin C Smoothie

2 oranges
½ cantaloupe
1 cup strawberries
1 tomato

Juice the oranges and combine juice with other ingredients, then blend over ice.

Makes 1 serving.

Nutrition per serving: calories 242, total fat 1.7 g, saturated fat 0.2 g, sodium 33 mg, carbohydrates 51.6 g, fiber 10.5 g, protein 5.5 g.

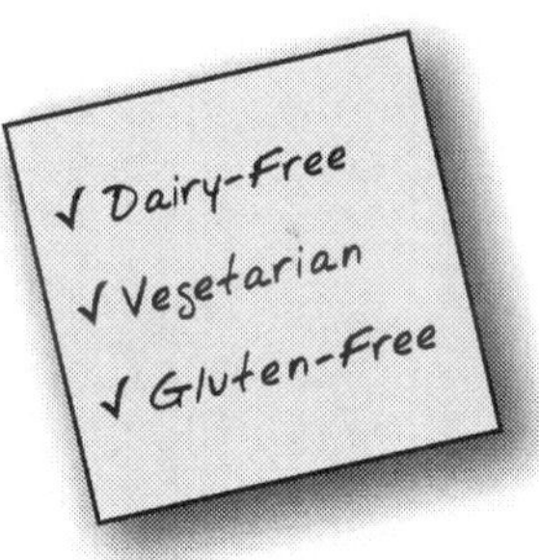

Energy B12 Smoothie

1 scoop spirulina powder (an algae that is high in protein and B12)
1½ cup of vanilla nut milk
¼ cup of fresh coconut meat
1 handful of spinach
½ tablespoon raw honey
½ banana

Optional: for creamier smoothie, add goat milk, yogurt or coconut milk

Place ingredients into blender and blend until smooth.

Makes 1 serving.

Nutrition per serving: calories 241, fat 9.6 g, cholesterol 0 mg, sodium 240 mg, carbohydrates 36 g, fiber 4.5 g, sugar 22.7 g, protein 7.7 g.

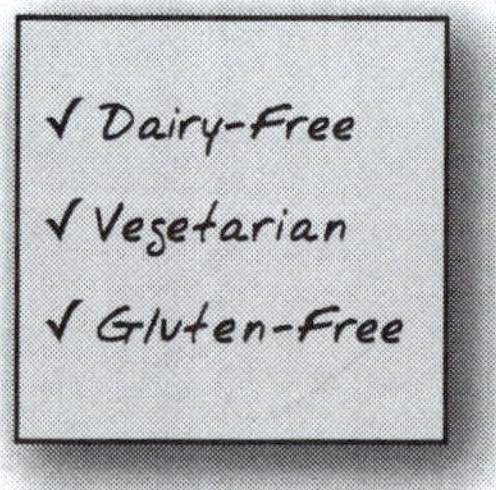

Flaxseed and Fruit Smoothie

½ cup skim milk
½ cup fat-free yogurt
1 cup frozen berries
1 banana
1 tablespoon ground flaxseed
½ teaspoon cinnamon

Combine all ingredients except flaxseed in blender. Blend well. Pour in large glass. Stir in flaxseed.

Makes 1 serving.

Nutrition per serving: calories 266, carbohydrates 53 g.

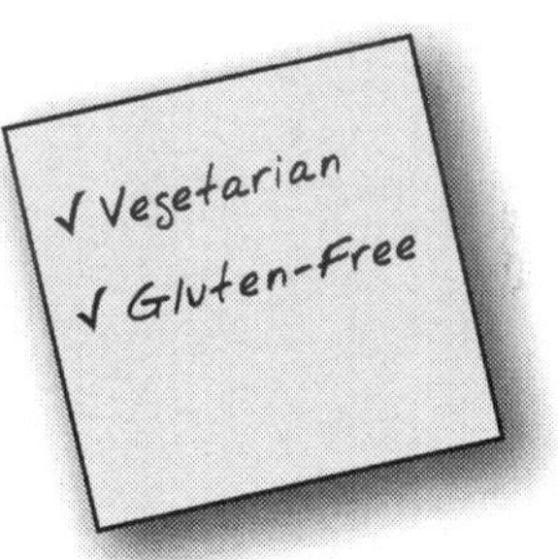

Ginseng Green Banana Smoothie

1 frozen banana
1 teaspoon ginseng
2 to 3 dates, or date paste
1 cup vanilla hemp milk, almond milk, rice milk or coconut water
1 handful of spinach
Variations: add pineapple, peach, avocado mango

Place ingredients into blender and blend until smooth.

Makes 1 serving.

Nutrition per serving: calories 266, fat 2.95 g, cholesterol 0 mg, sodium 51 mg, carbohydrates 60.6 g, fiber 3.5 g, sugar 30.63 g, protein 5.48 g.

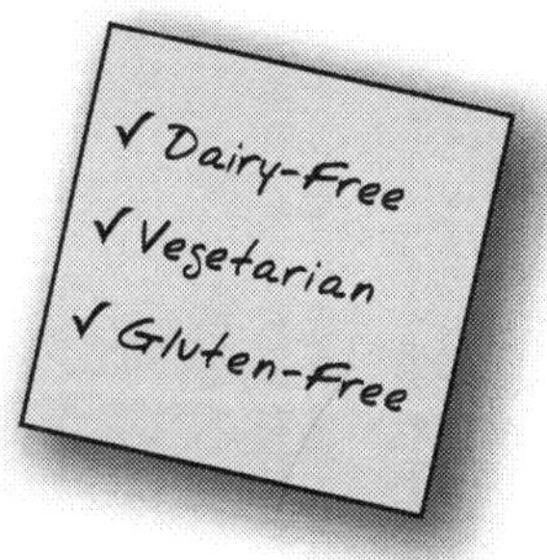

Green Smoothie

1 cup water
2 handfuls spinach
1 apple, sliced, (not peeled)
2 tablespoons flaxseed

Blend in Vitamix® blender for approximately 1 minute.

Makes 1 serving.

Nutrition per serving: calories 151, total fat 5 g, saturated fat 0.1 g, sodium 24 mg, carbohydrates 22.3 g, fiber 7.9 g, protein 4.1 g.

√ Dairy-Free
√ Vegetarian
√ Gluten-Free

Kale Strawberry Peach Smoothie

2 kale leaves
1 pint strawberries
1 small frozen peach
½ tablespoon raw honey, or 4 drops of vanilla stevia
2 cups water

Place ingredients into blender and blend until smooth.

Makes 1 serving.

Nutrition per serving: calories 239, fat 1.12 g, cholesterol 0 mg, sodium 33 mg, carbohydrates 32 g, fiber 10.8 g, sugar 33 g, protein 5 g.

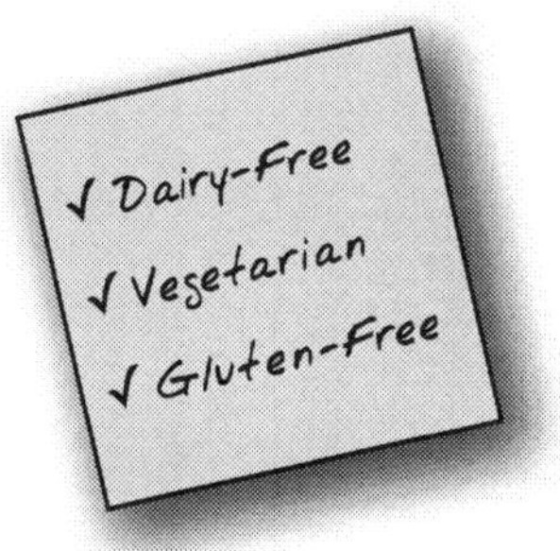

Matcha Green Tea Smoothie

2 to 3 Gala apples, peeled and cored
1 cup vanilla almond milk
1 teaspoon matcha green powder
5 ice cubes
2 to 3 drops stevia or 1 date

Optional: add ½ banana for creamier smoothie

Place ingredients into blender and blend until smooth.

Makes 1 serving.

Nutrition per serving: calories 193, fat 4 g, cholesterol 0 mg, sodium 150 mg, carbohydrates 34 g, fiber 5 g, sugar 28 g, protein 1.4 g.

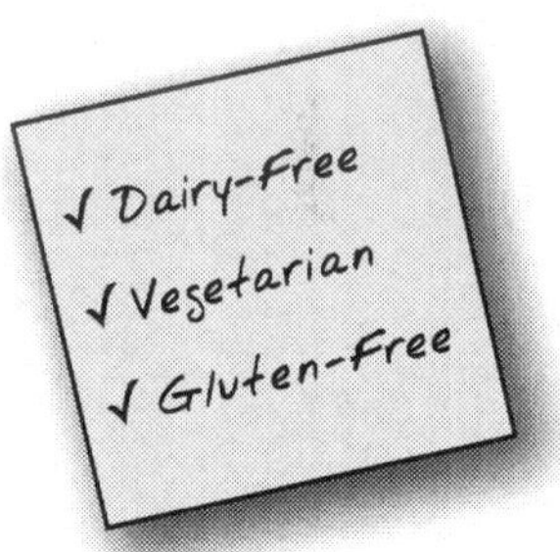

Mint Green Smoothie

½ banana
Juice of ½ lemon
1 to 2 stalks of organic celery
1 handful of mint
2 handfuls of spinach
½ tablespoon raw honey, 2 Medjool dates or 4 drops of vanilla stevia
1½ cup water or almond milk

Place ingredient in blender and blend until smooth.

Makes 1 serving.

Nutrition per serving: calories 167, fat 2.86 g, cholesterol 0 mg, sodium 255 mg, carbohydrates 33.76 g, fiber 6 g, sugar 21.88 g, protein 4.07 g.

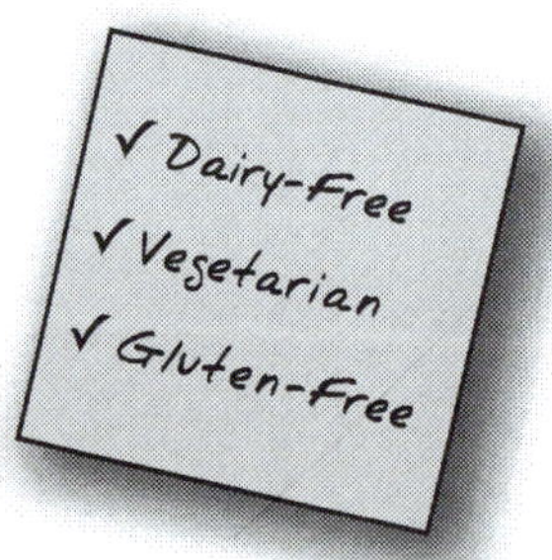

Orange Mango Green Smoothie

½ orange
½ mango
1 bunch of kale, spinach, dandelion greens, or collard greens
1 frozen banana
1 tablespoon raw honey, maple syrup, or 1 date
1½ cups of water, almond milk, or coconut water

Place ingredients into blender and blend until smooth.

Makes 2 servings.

Nutrition per serving: calories 124, fat 0.57 g, cholesterol 0 mg, sodium 15.5 mg, carbohydrates 3 g, fiber 4.2 g, sugar 20.5 g, protein 2.02 g.

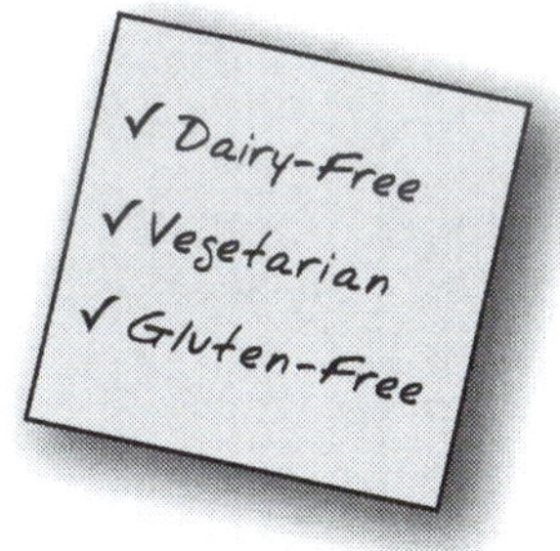

Papaya Fresh Green Smoothie

1 cup chopped papaya
½ cup frozen pineapple
1 tablespoon shredded coconut
1 teaspoon lemon juice
1 cup almond milk
1 handful of spinach
½ tablespoon raw honey or 4 drops of stevia
3 to 5 ice cubes

Optional: add banana for creamy texture

Place ingredients into blender and blend until smooth.

Makes 1 serving.

Nutrition per serving: calories 190, fat 5.35 g, cholesterol 0 mg, sodium 191 mg, carbohydrates 34.75 g, fiber 6 g, sugar 20.87 g, protein 5.07 g.

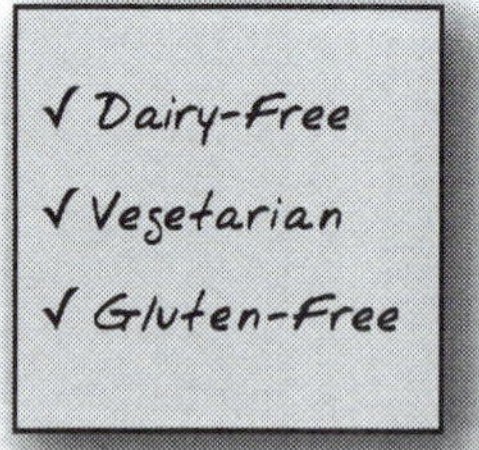

Peach Green Smoothie

½ peach
½ frozen banana
1 handful of spinach (can use kale, dandelion greens or Swiss chard)
1½ cup milk of choice (almond milk or oat milk)
3 to 5 ice cubs

Optional: ½ tablespoon raw honey, or 4 drops vanilla stevia

Place ingredients into blender and blend till smooth.

Makes 1 serving.

Nutrition per serving: calories 175, fat 2.8 g, cholesterol 0 mg, sodium 136 mg, carbohydrates 37 g, fiber 4.3 g, sugar 26.82 g, protein 3.56 g.

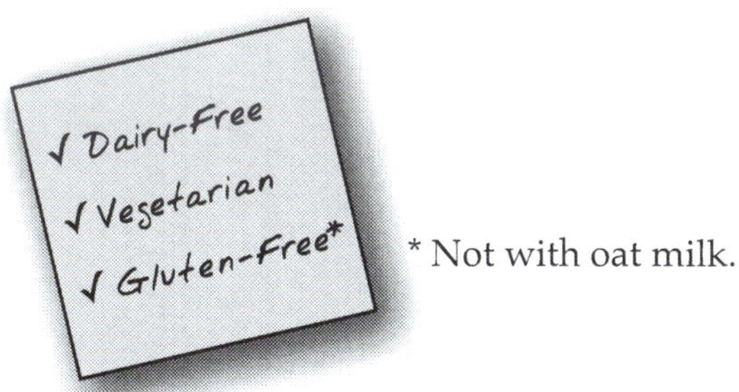

* Not with oat milk.

Persimmon Green Smoothie

½ persimmon
½ frozen banana
1 cup of So Delicious coconut milk
1 handful of spinach (can use kale, dandelion greens or Swiss chard)
1 teaspoon cinnamon
½ tablespoon raw honey, 1 soaked date or 4 drops of vanilla stevia
3 to 5 ice cubes

Place ingredients into blender and blend until smooth.

Makes 1 serving.

Nutrition per serving: calories 187, fat 2.95 g, cholesterol 0 mg, sodium 173 mg, carbohydrates 40 g, fiber 4 g, sugar 26.14 g, protein 4.36 g.

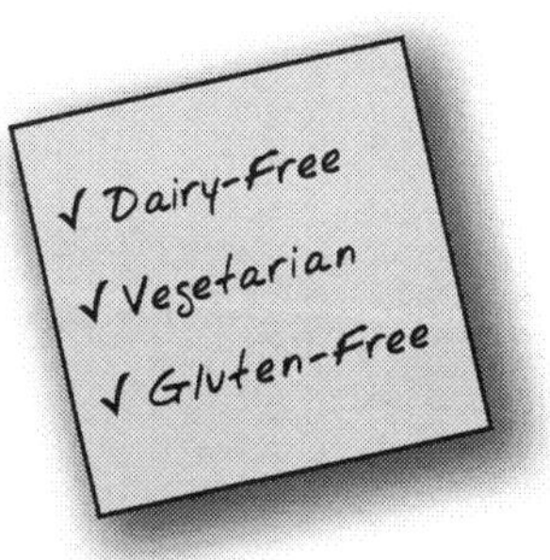

Raspberry Apple Coconut Smoothie

½ cup frozen or fresh raspberries
1 frozen Fuji apple
1 to 2 cups of water, nut milk, or coconut water
1 handful or romaine leaves or spinach
1 tablespoon shredded unsweetened coconut
½ tablespoon raw honey, 4 drops of vanilla stevia, or 2 Medjool dates
2 to 5 ice cubes

Optional: ½ banana for creamy smoothie

Place ingredients into blender and blend until smooth.

Makes 1 serving.

Nutrition per serving: calories 270, fat 3.99 g, cholesterol 0 mg, sodium 205 mg, carbohydrates 58.5 g, fiber 16 g, sugar 36 g, protein 6 g.

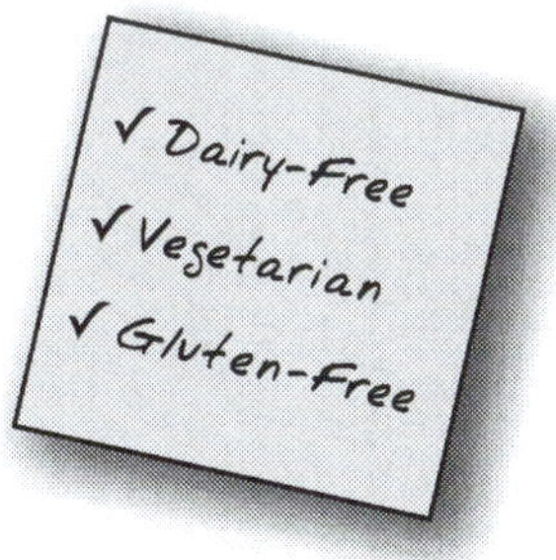

Stomach Soother Smoothie[2]

1 cup cubed papaya
1 cup frozen sliced peaches
1 medium pear
1 tablespoon ground flax seed
1 teaspoon sliced ginger
6 mint leaves
½ cup low fat Greek yogurt, coconut milk yogurt, or almond milk
6 ice cubes

Place ingredients into blender and blend till smooth. Garnish with mint.

Makes 3 servings.

Nutrition per serving: calories 109, fat 2 g, cholesterol 0 mg, sodium 15 mg, carbohydrates 21 g, fiber 4 g, protein 4 g.

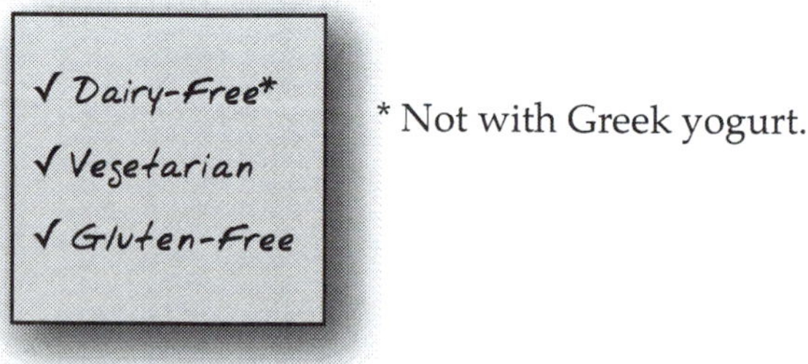

* Not with Greek yogurt.

Watermelon Refresher

1 to 2 cups watermelon
½ cucumber, peeled and chopped (frozen for 3 hours)
4 sprigs of mint
5 to 6 ice cubes

Optional:
1 soaked Medjool date or 4 drops of stevia
1 banana for creamy consistency

Place ingredients into blender and blend until smooth. Garnish with mint.

Makes 1 to 2 servings.

Nutrition per serving: calories 150, fat 2.15 g, cholesterol 0 mg, sodium 9 mg, carbohydrates 32 g, fiber 2.75 g, sugar 10.5 g, protein 3 g.

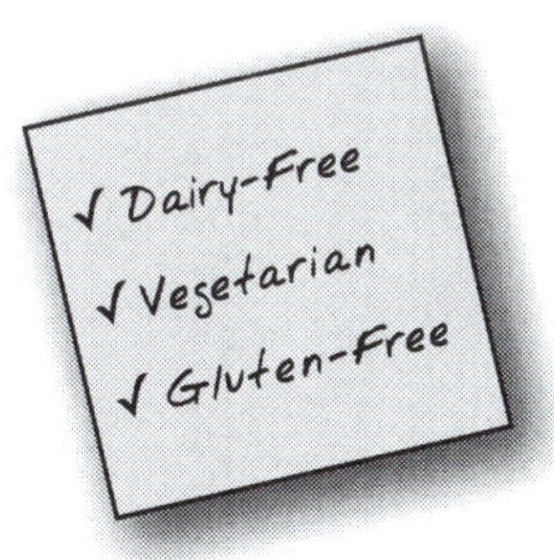

Recipes: Lunch and Dinner

"You don't have to cook fancy or complicated masterpieces—just good food from fresh ingredients."
— Julia Child

Asian Beef Stir-Fry

4 portions lean, grass-fed steak (about 1 pound)
⅛ teaspoon crushed red pepper flakes
3 cloves garlic, minced
1 onion, cut up
4 celery stalks, cut up
1 head napa cabbage, shredded
2 tablespoons reduced sodium soy sauce

Slice steak lengthwise into 2-inch strips. Cut crosswise into ⅛-inch slices. Lightly coat a large skillet or wok with cooking spray. Over medium to high heat, stir-fry red pepper flakes and garlic for 1 minute. Add the steak strips to the skillet, then stir-fry only until no longer pink (approximately 2 minutes). Remove the steak from skillet and set aside. Lightly re-coat the skillet with cooking spray. Stir-fry onion and celery until tender (approximately 5 minutes). Add cabbage and cook until crisp-tender, (approximately 2 more minutes). Return steak to the skillet. Add reduced sodium soy sauce, then mix and heat thoroughly.

Makes 4 servings.

Nutrition per serving: calories 240, total fat 9.9 g, saturated fat 3.5 g, sodium 532 mg, carbohydrates 10.3 g, fiber 3.8 g, protein 27.6 g.

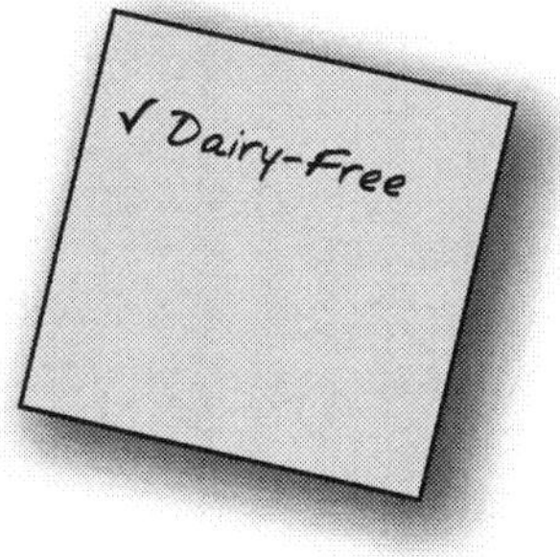

Asian Cabbage[1]

2½ cups finely shredded cabbage
1 cup grated carrots
1 cup fresh spinach
2 tablespoons extra-virgin olive oil
1 teaspoon grated ginger root
Lemon juice
1 tablespoon toasted sesame seeds

Optional: dash of Tabasco® or hot sauce

Stir-fry the cabbage, carrots and spinach in olive oil in a skillet or wok. Once the vegetables are tender, stir in the grated ginger root and hot sauce. Before serving, sprinkle with lemon juice. Put on a plate and top with toasted sesame seeds.

Makes 6 servings.

Nutrition per serving: calories 60, total fat 5 g, saturated fat .5 g, sodium 20 mg, carbohydrates 4 g, fiber 1 g, sugar 2 g, protein 1 g.

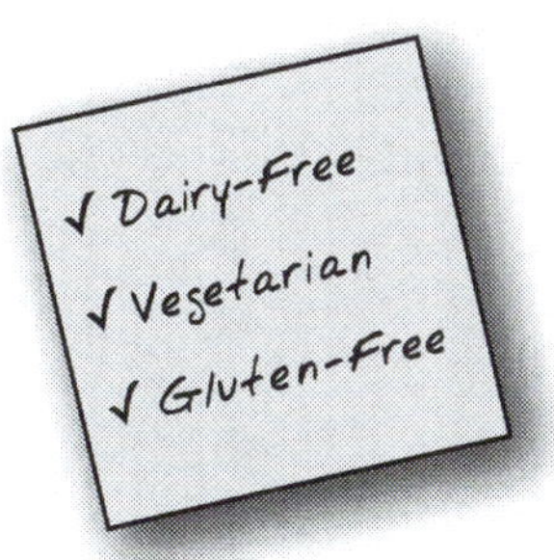

Baked Fish with Basil[2]

Organic nonstick cooking spray
6 (6 ounce) fish filets
1 cup chopped fresh basil
¼ cup extra-virgin olive oil
2 tablespoons minced garlic
1 tablespoon lemon juice
1 lemon, sliced

Optional: salt and pepper to taste

Preheat oven to 350°F. Place fish filets in baking dish sprayed with organic nonstick cooking spray (or use a spray pump mister filled with olive oil). Combine basil, olive oil, garlic and lemon juice in small bowl. Mix well and spoon evenly over fish. Bake for 20 to 25 minutes, until the fish flakes easily with a fork. Garnish with lemon slices and serve. Add salt and pepper if desired.

Makes 6 servings.

Nutrition per serving: calories 250, total fat 12 g, saturated fat 2.5 g, sodium 90 mg, carbohydrates 1 g, protein 35 g.

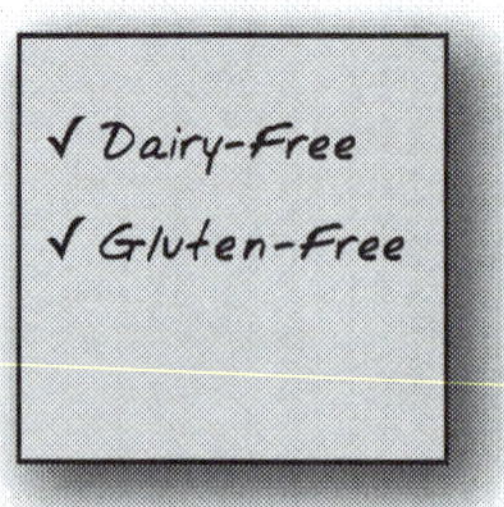

Baked Zucchini Fries

3 zucchinis (about 4 cups total)
Vegetable oil spray
2 teaspoons chili powder
1 teaspoon no salt seasoning
½ teaspoon garlic powder
¼ teaspoon black pepper

Optional: ⅛ teaspoon cayenne pepper (if you like spicy)

Preheat the oven to 500°F. Trim the ends off the zucchini and cut lengthwise into ¼-inch-thick slices. Then cut those slices into 3-inch-long fries, place flat on a nonstick sheet pan, and spray them and the pan liberally with vegetable oil spray. Place all the seasonings in a small bowl and mix well, then sprinkle evenly over all the fries. Bake for about 15 minutes or until well browned. Serve immediately.

Makes 4 servings.

Nutrition per serving: calories 29, total fat 0.4 g, saturated fat 0.1 g, sodium 16 mg, carbohydrates 4.6 g, fiber 2 g, protein 1.7 g.

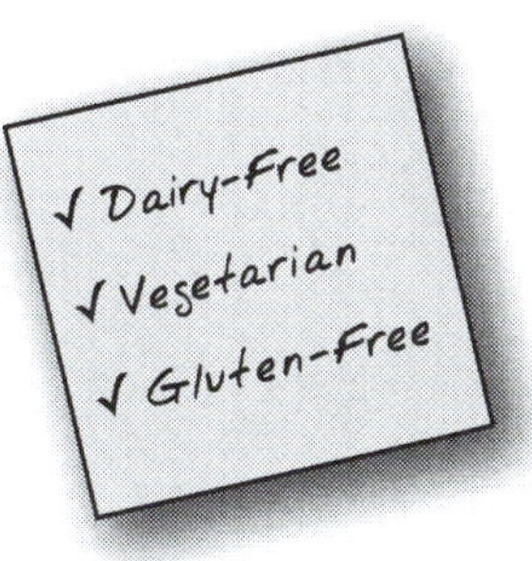

Balsamic-Marinated Flank Steak

½ cup balsamic vinegar
1 tablespoon packed light brown sugar
1 teaspoon dried rosemary
Salt and pepper
1½ pound flank steak

Combine vinegar, sugar, rosemary and 1½ teaspoon salt in a ziplock bag. Add steak to bag, then seal and turn bag several times to coat meat with marinade. Refrigerate 20 minutes, turning once or twice to redistribute marinade. Preheat gas grill to high. Remove steak from marinade and sprinkle both sides with salt and pepper. Discard leftover marinade. Grill steak for 4 to 6 minutes. Carefully turn over, then continue to grill until meat reaches desired doneness—3 to 4 minutes more for medium-rare, depending on thickness of meat and heat of grill. (Or, grill steak on a lightly oiled, ridged grill pan over medium to high heat on a stove for same amount of time.) Transfer steak to a cutting board, tent loosely with foil and let stand 5 minutes. Slice steak thinly against grain and serve.

Makes 6 servings.

Nutrition per serving: calories 199, fat 8 g, cholesterol 57 mg, sodium 471 mg, carbohydrates 5 g, fiber 0 g, protein 23 g.

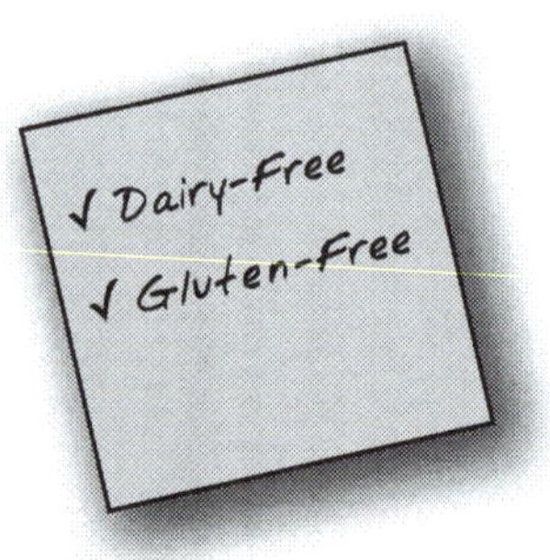

Balsamic Roasted Apple Butternut Squash[3]

2 large butternut squash, halved, and seeds and membrane removed
1-inch ginger peeled and finely chopped
1 cup balsamic vinegar
2 tablespoons brown sugar or 1 tablespoon agave
Olive oil cooking spray
2 Gala apples, cored and thinly sliced
¼ cup dried cherries, chopped

Heat oven to 400°F. Slice a small piece off the skin side of each squash half, so halves sit flat. Microwave on high in a covered bowl until flesh begins to soften, 2 minutes. Gently simmer ginger, vinegar, and sugar in a small saucepan over medium low heat until liquid decreases by ⅓, 8-10 minutes. Remove from heat and set aside. Line 2 large baking sheets with foil and coat with cooking spray. Place squash halves skin side down on baking sheets. Arrange apple slices in cavity of each half. Bake until apples soften, 25 minutes. Remove squash from oven, drizzle with balsamic sauce, return to oven and bake until apples brown, 5-6 minutes. Cut each squash half into quarters and transfer to a serving platter with any extra juices. Sprinkle with cherries. Serve as a side with rotisserie or simple baked chicken.

Makes 8 servings.

Nutrition per serving: calories 166, fat 0 g, cholesterol 0 mg, sodium 250 mg, carbohydrates 42 g, fiber 8 g, sugar 21 g, protein 3 g.

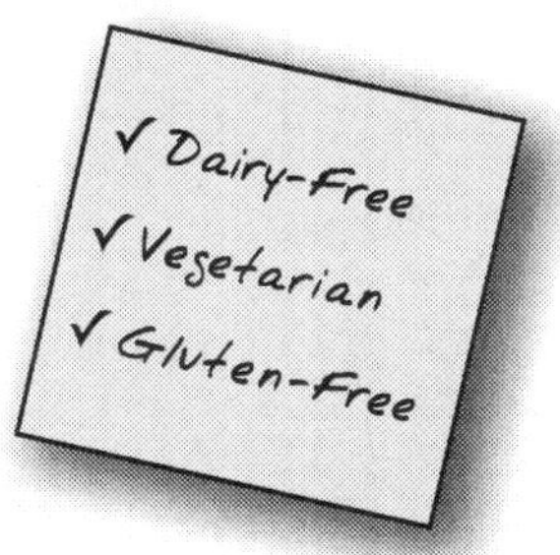

Beef & Quinoa Meatballs[4]

1 pound grass-fed ground beef, turkey or chicken
¾ cup cooked quinoa
¼ cup finely chopped onions
¼ cup grated zucchini
2 tablespoons natural ketchup
1 tablespoon chopped garlic
1 tablespoon soy sauce
½ teaspoon pepper
½ teaspoon salt
¼ teaspoon dried oregano
¼ teaspoon dried thyme
1 egg

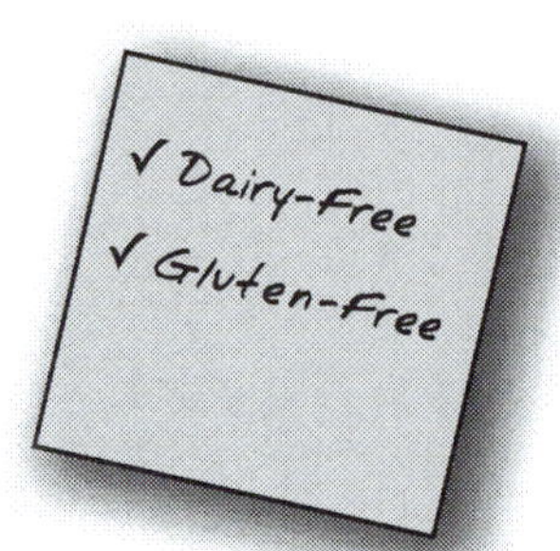

Optional: add chopped spinach, kale and carrots

Preheat oven to 500°F. Line a large baking sheet with foil then grease with cooking spray; set aside. To cook quinoa, bring 1 cup water to boil and pour ½ cup quinoa, cover, simmer until water is absorbed about 10-12 minutes, then fluff with fork. In a large bowl, mix together beef, quinoa, onions, carrots, zucchini, ketchup, garlic, soy sauce, pepper, salt, oregano, thyme, and egg until well combined. Shape beef mixture into 18 balls and transfer to prepared baking sheet. Roast until cooked through and golden brown, 12-15 minutes. Serve hot.

Makes 6 servings.

Nutrition per serving: calories 50, fat 5 g, cholesterol 75 mg, sodium 470 mg, carbohydrates 8 g, fiber 1 g, sugar 2 g, protein 17 g.

Black Bean Sweet Potato Burger

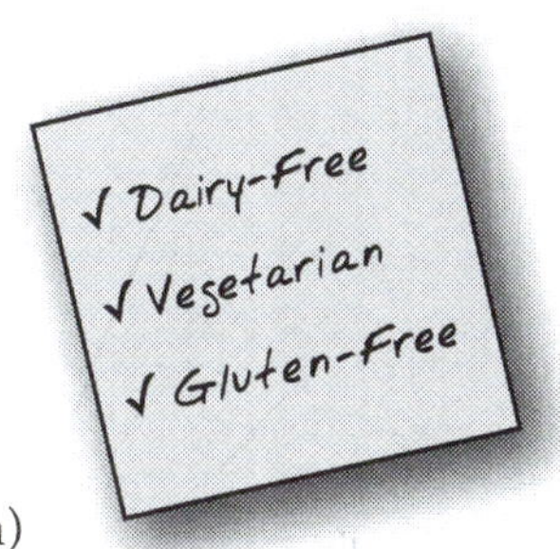

2 cups cooked black beans, mashed
2 cups sweet potatoes peeled and cut into small cubes
2 teaspoons olive oil
Salt and pepper
3 ounces yellow onion, diced
2 teaspoons garlic
3 tablespoons tamari
2 teaspoons ground cumin
7 cups cooked rice (brown rice or quinoa)
1½ teaspoons Worcestershire sauce
2 ounces cornmeal (substitute tapioca or rice flour)

Preheat oven to 350°F. Place mashed black beans in bowl. Peel and cut sweet potatoes, dropping them in cold water as you cut them. Drain well and toss with olive oil and salt. Spread them out evenly on lightly oiled baking sheet. Roast in oven for 25 to 30 minutes or until tender. Toss occasionally. Heat olive oil in large sauté pan over medium heat. Add onion and garlic and cook until lightly browned. Add onions to bowl of beans. Stir in tamari, cumin and salt and pepper to taste. Add cooked rice, sweet potatoes, Worcestershire sauce, and 1 ounce of cornmeal. Mix well and adjust the seasonings. Form 4½ ounce patties and dredge in remaining 1 ounce of cornmeal. Heat a cast iron skillet over medium heat and add more olive oil. Add burgers and brown lightly on each side. Place on baking sheet and bake for 10 minutes. Serve with guacamole on bun, lettuce wrap or salad.

Makes 10 servings (serving size of 1 burger).

Nutrition per serving: calories 175, fat 3.6 g, cholesterol 0 mg, sodium 220 mg, carbohydrates 20 g, fiber 2.2 g, sugar 2.2 g, protein 4 g.

Black Beanofritos[5]

2 cups (16 ounce can) black beans
1 medium tomato, chopped
1 small onion, minced
1 avocado
⅓ cup plain low-fat yogurt
4 low-fat whole-wheat tortilla wraps
2 teaspoons chili powder
1 teaspoon garlic powder

In a medium skillet, sauté black beans with tomato and onion until vegetables are soft and beans are hot. Add chili and garlic powders while mixture is cooking. Peel the avocado, mash with a potato masher, and mix well with yogurt. Remove bean mixture from skillet and drain any liquid. Using the potato masher, mash the bean mixture and then spoon it evenly onto the center of each tortilla, placed on a plate or platter. Fold the tortilla over. Top with a tablespoon of the avocado-yogurt mixture.

Makes 4 servings.

Nutrition per serving: calories 340, total fat 9 g, saturated fat 1 g, sodium 190 mg, carbohydrates 51 g, fiber 11 g, protein 14 g.

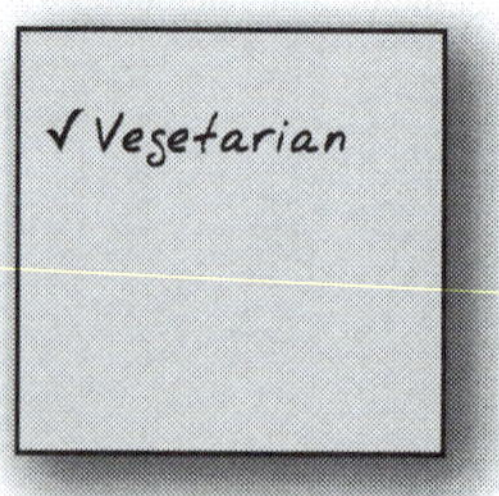

Blackened Rub for Fish

2 tablespoons paprika
1 tablespoon dried oregano
½ teaspoon salt
½ teaspoon freshly ground black pepper
¼ teaspoon ground red pepper

Combine all 5 ingredients in a small bowl. Sprinkle both sides of fish with the spice mixture.

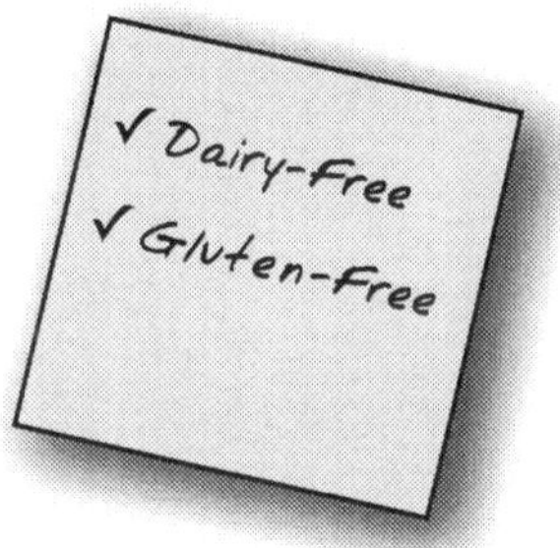

Blackened Cajun Salmon

6 filets salmon (or ahi tuna), 8 ounces each
Cajun seasoning
1 tablespoon cilantro
½ tablespoon coconut oil

Place ½ tablespoon coconut oil in skillet and heat for 2 minutes on medium heat. Rub salmon filet with Cajun rub on both sides. Place one side down for 4 to 5 minutes. Turn and sprinkle a little more Cajun seasoning, and heat for another 4 to 5 minutes, until salmon is cooked through.

Makes 6 servings.

Nutrition per serving: calories 450, fat 13.2 g, cholesterol 120 mg, sodium 200 mg, carbohydrates 10 g, fiber 3 g, sugar 3.2 g, protein 65 g.

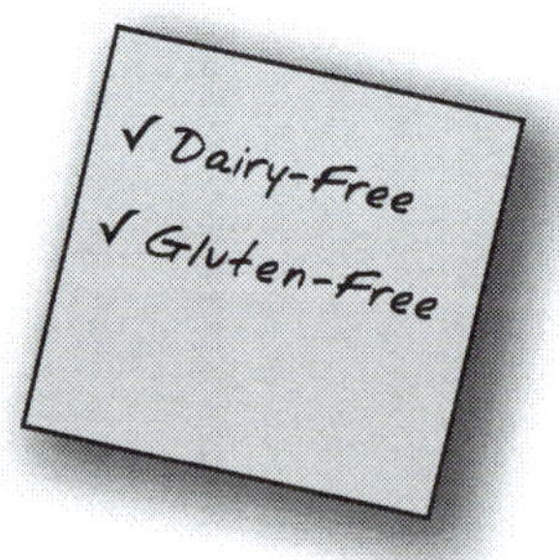

Blueberry Chicken

1 cup blueberries

1 small red onion

1 red bell pepper

1 jalapeño pepper

½ cup basil leaves

1 lime

1 teaspoon raw honey

¼ teaspoon salt

3 cooked chicken breasts, 6 ounces each

In a bowl, combine 1 cup blueberries, 1 diced small red onion, 1 diced red bell pepper, 1 seeded and diced jalapeño pepper, ½ cup torn basil leaves, juice of 1 lime, 1 teaspoon honey, ¼ teaspoon salt. Serve over seared chicken (or white fish).

Makes 3 to 4 servings.

Nutrition per serving: calories 238, fat 4.6 g, cholesterol 108 mg, sodium 346 mg, carbohydrates 11 g, sugar 6.2 g, fiber 2.7 g, protein 36.9 g.

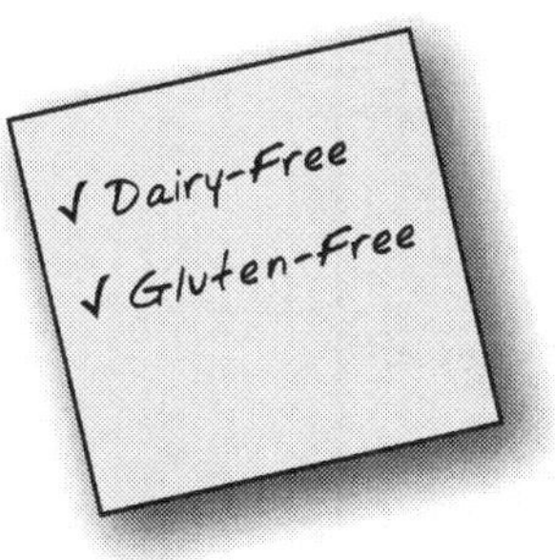

Broccoli with Almonds

1 pound broccoli flowerets
1 teaspoon olive oil
½ cup slivered almonds
Juice of 1 lemon

Optional: 2 tablespoons broccoli sprouts

Steam the broccoli flowerets for 5 to 10 minutes, or until they are just tender. Meanwhile, heat the olive oil in a pan over low heat, then fry the almonds until brown. Mix together the broccoli and almonds in a serving dish and sprinkle the lemon juice over.

Optional: top the dish with broccoli sprouts.

Makes 4 servings.

Nutrition per serving: calories 129, total fat 7.7 g, saturated fat 0.8 g, sodium 32 mg, carbohydrates 9 g, fiber 4.7 g, protein 5.8 g.

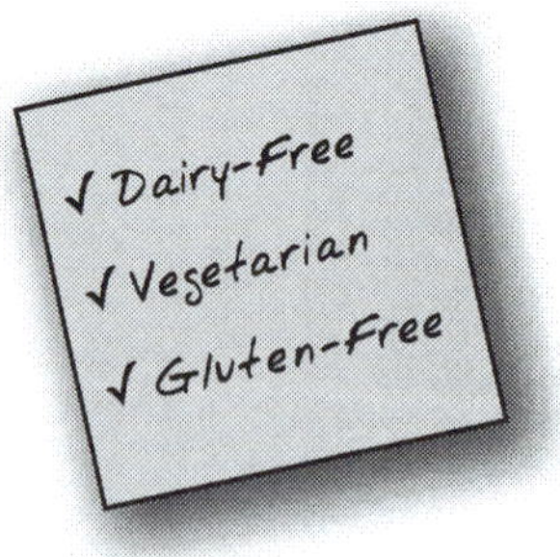

Broccoli with Turmeric and Tomatoes

2 tablespoons cooking oil

2 onions, cut into thin slices

¾ teaspoon turmeric

1½ pounds broccoli (about 2 large stalks), stems peeled and cut crosswise into ¼-inch slices, tops cut into florets (about 7 cups in all)

1 cup drained canned diced tomatoes (from a 15 ounce can)

⅓ cup water

¾ teaspoon salt

In a large, deep frying pan, heat the oil over moderate heat. Add the onions and cook while covered, stirring occasionally, for 5 minutes. Uncover and cook, stirring occasionally, until the onions are very soft—about 5 minutes longer. Stir in the turmeric to coat the onions. Stir in the broccoli, tomatoes, water and salt, then bring to a simmer. Reduce the heat and simmer, covered, until the broccoli is tender—about 10 minutes.

Makes 4 servings.

Nutrition per serving: calories 154, total fat 7.6 g, saturated fat 1 g, sodium 136 mg, carbohydrates 15.3 g, fiber 6.5 g, protein 6.2 g.

√ Dairy-Free
√ Vegetarian
√ Gluten-Free

Buckwheat Soba Noodles with Chicken

4 skinless chicken breast cut into 1-inch cubes
½ cup tamari (wheat free soy sauce) or Nama® Shoyu
½ teaspoon sesame oil
1 tablespoon grapeseed oil
2 cloves garlic
8 ounces soba noodles (buckwheat noodles), cooked and drained

Optional:
- ½ cup zucchini or carrots, chopped
- ½ head of cabbage, chopped

In a large skillet combine sesame oil, grapeseed oil and garlic. Cooke for 1 minute. Add chicken and ¼ cup of soy sauce and cook chicken. Remove mixture from pan and set aside. Place zucchini, cabbage, and carrot in pan and cook until cabbage wilts. Stir in remaining soy sauce, cooked noodles, and chicken mixture in pan and mix to blend.

Makes 4 servings.

Nutrition per serving: calories 220, fat 7 g, cholesterol 65 mg, sodium 500 mg, carbohydrates 10.75 g, fiber 1 g, sugar 3 g, protein 28.25 g.

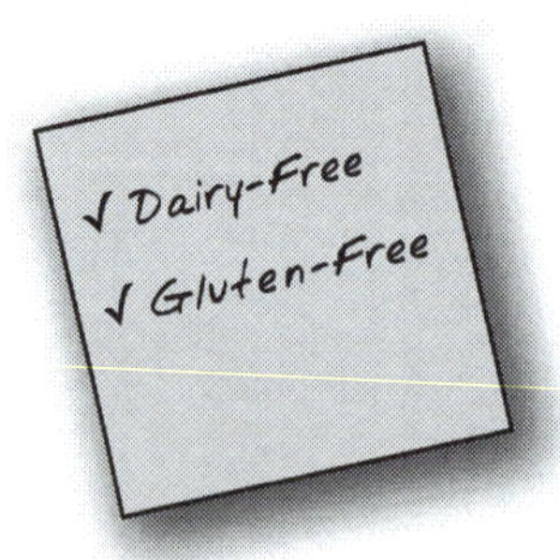

Caribbean Kale

2 bunches of kale
½ yellow onion
1 can red kidney beans
3 garlic cloves
1 to 2 tablespoons olive oil, avocado oil, or coconut oil
½ teaspoon salt or more to taste

Optional: add diced chicken

Boil chopped kale in a pot with water. Cook until tender, then drain water. Heat 1 tablespoon oil in large pot over medium heat. Add garlic cloves and cook for 2 minutes. Add onions and sauté until transparent. Add kidney beans and cook, stirring occasionally. Add kale, salt and pepper to pot, and cook. Drizzle with avocado oil.

Makes 2 servings.

Nutrition per serving: calories 168, fat 7.5 g, cholesterol 0 mg, sodium 44.5 mg, carbohydrates 2.05 g, fiber 6.4 g, sugar 0 g, protein 7.7 g.

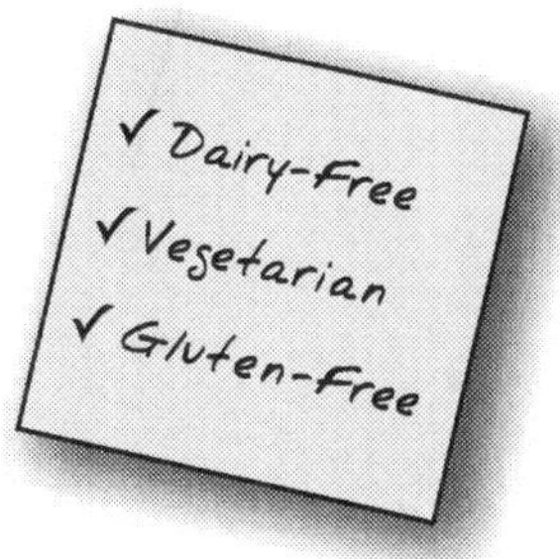

Caribbean Rice & Beans[6]

2 tablespoons grapeseed or olive oil
½ yellow onion, chopped
4 garlic cloves, chopped
2 cups long-grain rice
1 teaspoon salt
1 teaspoon grated fresh ginger
1 cup water
1 cup chicken or vegetable stock
1 cup light coconut milk
1 can red kidney beans (15 ounces), rinsed and drained
2 teaspoons thyme
1 whole scotch bonnet chili or habanero

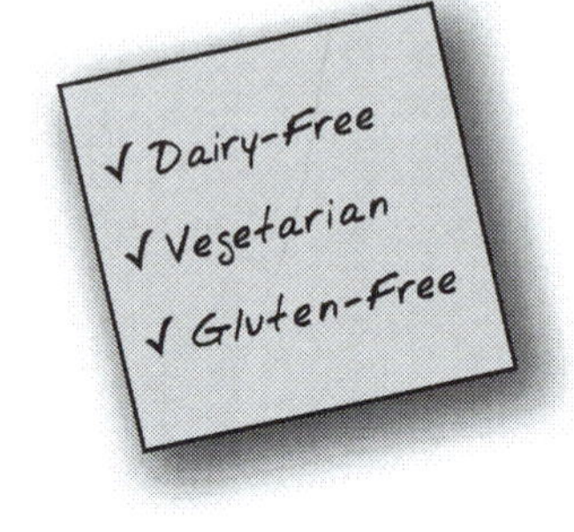

Heat the oil in a medium pot over medium high heat. Add onions and sauté for 4-5 minutes, until they begin to brown. Add the garlic and rice, stir well and cook for another 2 to 3 minutes, stirring often. Add the grated ginger, salt, water, stock and coconut milk and stir well. Add the kidney beans and sprinkle the thyme. Add the whole scotch bonnet chili or habanero. Bring to a simmer, then turn the heat to low and cover. The rice should be done in about 15 to 20 minutes. Check after 15 minutes. Once done, remove from heat and cover for about 10 minutes. Discard the habanero and sprinkle with lime juice if you want.

Makes 6 to 8 servings.

Nutrition per serving: calories 171, fat 7.16 g, cholesterol 0 mg, sodium 192.8 mg, carbohydrates 22.81 g, fiber 2 g, sugar 1.58 g, protein 3.84 g.

Cauliflower Rice

4 tablespoons olive oil or butter
1 medium onion, diced
1 head cauliflower, trimmed and coarsely chopped
¼ teaspoon Celtic Sea Salt®
Onion powder to taste

Optional:
Sun-dried tomato or celery, chopped
Garlic powder
2 cloves garlic

In a large skillet, heat olive oil over medium heat. Sauté onion and garlic over medium heat for 10 minutes, until soft and browned. Meanwhile, place cauliflower in a food processor and process until texture of rice (use S blade). Add cauliflower to skillet, cover and cook 5 to 10 minutes until soft, then uncover to add salt, garlic powder and onion powder to taste. Cook a little longer. If cooked longer it will become crispy like garlic-fried rice. Use as side dish, on top of salad or add to collard greens wraps.

Makes 3 servings.

Nutrition per serving: calories 113, fat 9.3 g, cholesterol 0 mg, sodium 20 mg, carbohydrates 7.3 g, fiber 3.1 g, sugar 0 g, protein 2.3 g.

✓ Dairy-Free
✓ Vegetarian
✓ Gluten-Free

Chicken Salad Collard Greens Wrap

3 boneless, skinless organic chicken breasts
4 tablespoons mayonnaise (preferably olive oil mayonnaise)
2 stalks celery, diced (¾ cup)
¼ cup pecan pieces
⅓ cup golden raisins, chopped
3 tablespoons lemon juice
2 teaspoons Dijon-style mustard
1 pear
½ teaspoon sea salt
½ teaspoon ground black pepper
7 to 10 collard greens leaves, cabbage leaves, or romaine lettuce leaves

√ Dairy-Free
√ Gluten-Free

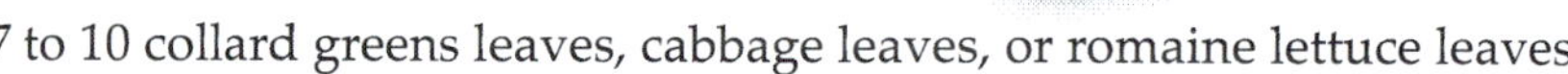

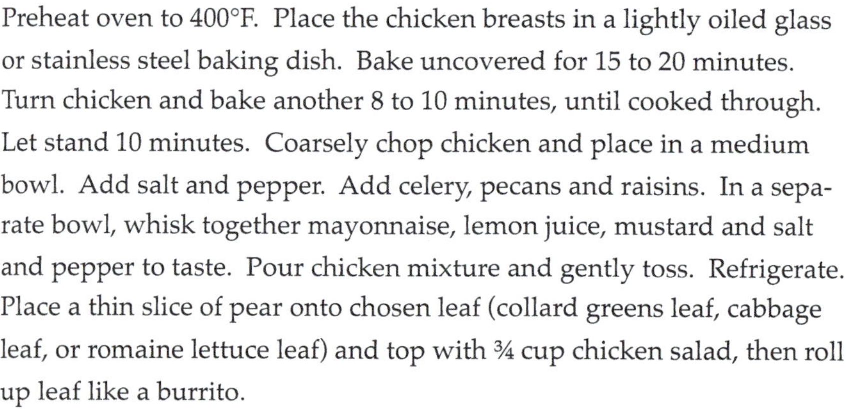

Preheat oven to 400°F. Place the chicken breasts in a lightly oiled glass or stainless steel baking dish. Bake uncovered for 15 to 20 minutes. Turn chicken and bake another 8 to 10 minutes, until cooked through. Let stand 10 minutes. Coarsely chop chicken and place in a medium bowl. Add salt and pepper. Add celery, pecans and raisins. In a separate bowl, whisk together mayonnaise, lemon juice, mustard and salt and pepper to taste. Pour chicken mixture and gently toss. Refrigerate. Place a thin slice of pear onto chosen leaf (collard greens leaf, cabbage leaf, or romaine lettuce leaf) and top with ¾ cup chicken salad, then roll up leaf like a burrito.

Makes 7 servings.

Nutrition per serving: calories 158, fat 10.47 g, cholesterol 30.7 mg, sodium 134.4 mg, carbohydrates 5.86 g, fiber 1 g, sugar 4.85 g, protein 10.6 g.

Chive Mashed Cauliflower

4 garlic cloves
1 pound cauliflower florets
1 tablespoon butter
2 tablespoons chopped chives
Olive oil for drizzling

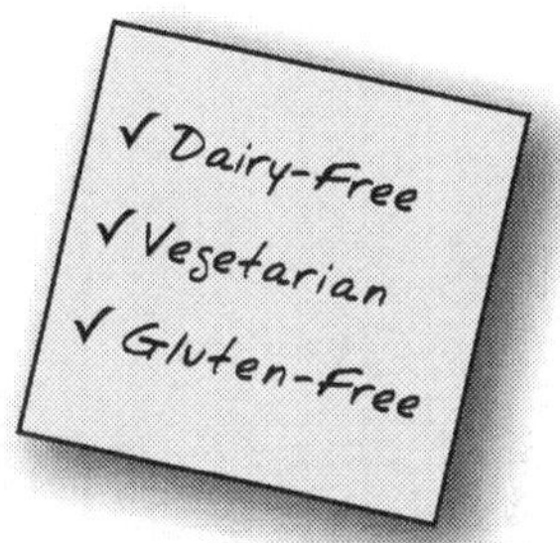

Optional:
1 cup diced celery
½ medium onion

Preheat oven to 400°F. Cut off top of garlic head to expose cloves. Place on a piece of foil big enough to form an envelope around the garlic. Drizzle with olive oil and enclose in foil. Roast until very tender and lightly browned—about 30 minutes. Cool slightly before squeezing out cloves and smashing them. Bring a large pot of water with a steamer basket to boil over medium-high heat. Steam cauliflower until it is very tender—for about 5 to 7 minutes. Remove cauliflower to a large mixing bowl and mash with a fork to reach desired consistency. (For a smoother consistency, add half or all the cauliflower to the bowl of a food processor and process until smooth, then return to mixing bowl before continuing.) Add peeled and smashed roasted garlic cloves, butter and 1 tablespoon of the chives to cauliflower and stir to combine. Garnish with remaining 1 tablespoon of chives.

Makes 4 servings.

Nutrition per serving: calories 82, fat 2.95 g, cholesterol 7.5 mg, sodium 200 mg, carbohydrates 11.2 g, fiber 5.25 g, sugar 5.05 g, protein 4.14 g.

Coconut Curry Chicken

1 can light organic coconut milk
8 ounces chicken breast, cooked and chopped
2 cups broccoli and zucchini
½ yellow onion, chopped
1 to 2 tablespoons curry powder
½ tablespoon ground cumin
1 teaspoon turmeric or curcumin
½ teaspoon ground coriander
¼ teaspoon paprika
Salt to taste

Optional: add 1 medium sweet potato, chopped

Sauté onions until browned. Place coconut milk in a sauce pan add broccoli, curry powder, cumin, coriander, paprika, chopped chicken and cook until warm. Add salt and pepper to taste. Let sit for 45 minutes. Adjust seasonings to taste.

Makes 2 servings.

Nutrition per serving: calories 233, fat 11.06 g, cholesterol 42.5 g, sodium 64.6 g, carbohydrates 9.74 g, fiber 1.68 g, sugar 2.76 g, protein 18.82 g.

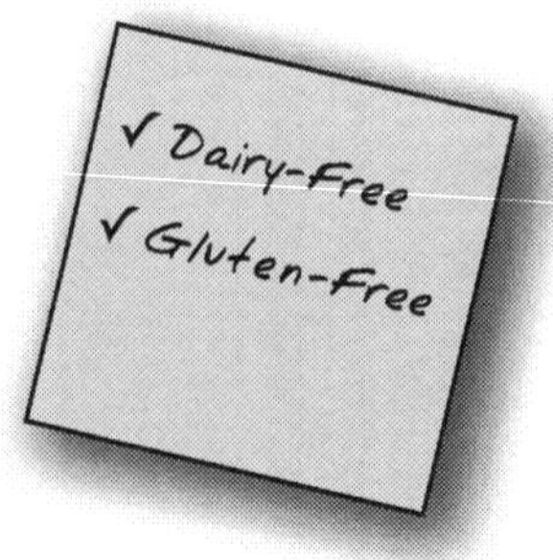

Coconut Rice

2 cups basmati rice
1 cup light coconut milk

Optional: add turmeric, curry, or garam masala

Cook rice directed on the box with 2 cups of water and 1 can of coconut milk.

Makes 6 to 8 servings.

Nutrition per serving: calories 142, fat 4.22 g, cholesterol 0 mg, sodium 5 mg, carbohydrates 24.35 g, fiber 0 g, sugar 2 g, protein 2.1 g.

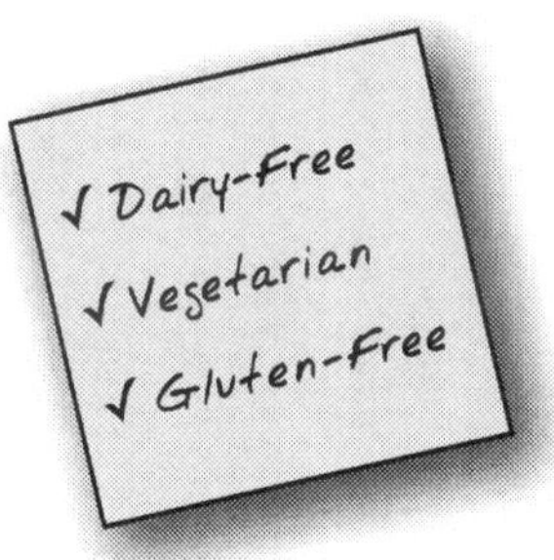

Crispy Kale

1 large bunch kale
Sea salt

Preheat the oven to 400°F. Coat two large baking sheets with oil spray. (The kale will be crispiest if baked directly on the baking sheet. Trim the kale and cut it into 2-inch pieces. Divide the kale pieces between the two baking sheets and spread them out into a single even layer. Liberally mist the kale with cooking spray, then lightly sprinkle with salt. Bake for 10 minutes, or until the kale is crispy to the touch and the edges are beginning to brown.

Makes 4 servings.

Nutrition per serving: calories: 35, total fat 0.5 g, saturated fat 0 g, sodium 150 mg, carbohydrates 7 g, fiber 1 g, protein 2 g.

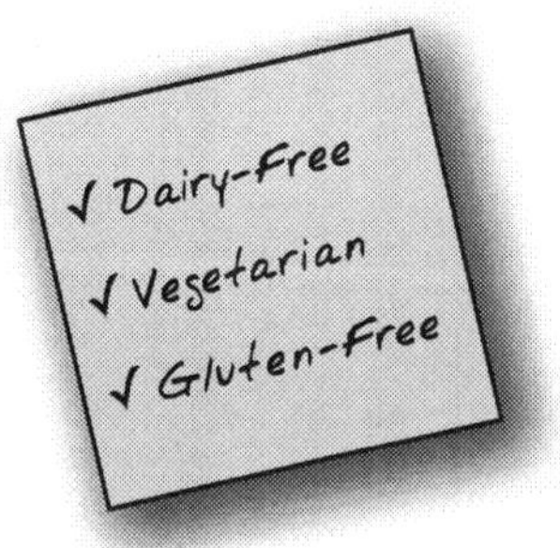

Cruciferous Couscous[7]

1 cup minced broccoli
1 cup fresh spinach
1 cup minced cauliflower
2 tomatoes, cubed
2 tablespoons minced garlic
2 tablespoons extra-virgin olive oil
3 cups water
2 cups quick-cook couscous
2 tablespoons balsamic vinegar
Salt and pepper to taste

Preheat oven to 350°F. Mix broccoli, spinach, cauliflower and tomatoes with garlic and 1 tablespoon of olive oil, then place on a baking sheet. Bake for 15 to 20 minutes, until tender. In a pot, bring water and remaining tablespoon of olive oil to a boil. Add couscous, return to a boil, then remove from heat and let stand for 5 minutes. Fluff with a fork and let cool. Place couscous on a plate and top with roasted vegetables. Drizzle with balsamic vinegar before serving.

Makes 8 servings.

Nutrition per serving: calories 220, total fat 4 g, saturated fat 0.5 g, sodium 20 mg, carbohydrates 38 g, fiber 3 g, protein 6 g.

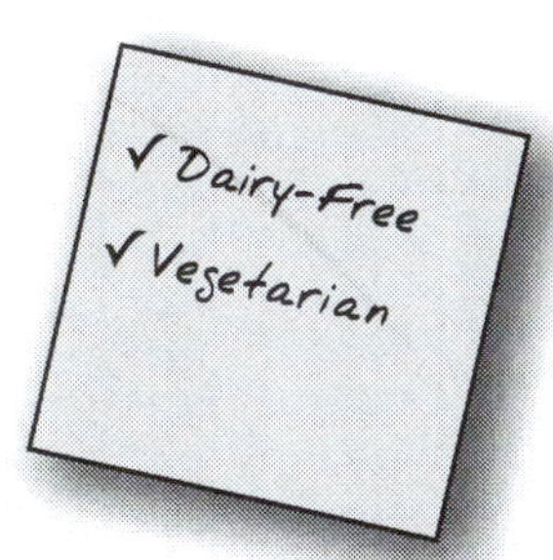

Cumin Carrots

1 tablespoon cumin seeds
3½ cups carrots, cut into thin sticks
1 tablespoon olive oil
2 garlic cloves, crushed
2 tablespoons white wine

Dry-fry the seeds briefly in a pan, then grind the seeds. Boil the carrots 5 minutes, or until nearly tender, then drain. Heat the oil in a skillet and sauté the garlic 1 minute. Add the wine and carrots, then cook until the wine evaporates. Stir in the cumin and serve immediately.

Makes 4 servings.

Nutrition per serving: calories 98, total fat 4.1 g, saturated fat 0.5 g, sodium 66 mg, carbohydrates 13.1 g, fiber 3.8 g, protein 2.3 g.

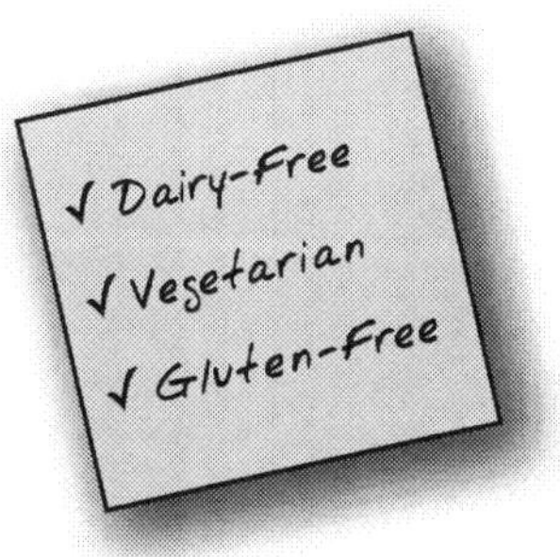

Curried Cauliflower

1 teaspoon curry powder
¼ teaspoon dried crushed red pepper
2 tablespoons vegetable oil
2 (10 ounces) packages fresh cauliflower florets
1 medium onion, chopped
¾ teaspoon salt

Cook curry powder and red pepper in hot oil in a large skillet over medium heat—stirring often—for 1 minute. Add cauliflower, onion and salt, then cook while stirring constantly—for 2 to 3 minutes, or until onion is crisp-tender. Reduce heat to low, then add 6 tablespoons water. Cover and cook—stirring occasionally—for 8 to 10 minutes, or just until cauliflower is tender.

Makes 4 servings.

Nutrition per serving: calories 54, fat 0.4 g, saturated fat 0.1 g, sodium 43 mg, carbohydrates 9.6 g, fiber 4.1 g, protein 3.2 g.

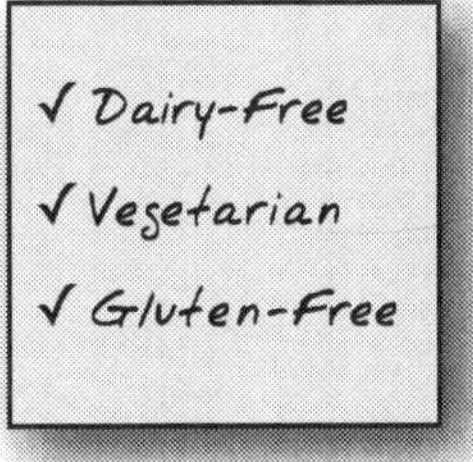

Curried Ginger Raisin Lentils

1 cup dry green lentils

½ cup raisins (golden raisins are the best)

1½ tablespoon garam masala seasoning

1 tablespoon ground ginger

1 teaspoon cumin

1 can tomato paste (6 ounces)

1 cup diced vegetables (carrots, broccoli, cauliflower or leftover cauliflower, rice, zucchini, etc.)

2 tablespoons coconut oil (or extra virgin olive oil)

1 tablespoon salt

Cook lentils with 2 cups of water on stovetop. Bring lentils and water to a boil, then cover and reduce heat. Simmer for 15 to 20 minutes. Add remaining ingredients. Stir, cover, and cook for another 10 minutes. Garnish with extra raisins, serve on top of a bed of spinach.

Makes 4 servings.

Nutrition per serving: calories 200, fat 21 g, cholesterol 0 mg, sodium 180 mg, carbohydrates 38 g, fiber 15 g, sugar 8 g, protein 13 g.

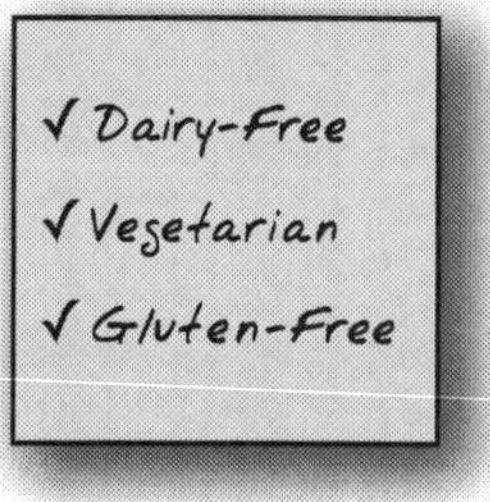

Dressed-Up Asparagus[8]

1 pound fresh asparagus

2 tablespoons extra-virgin olive oil

2 teaspoons lemon juice

1½ tablespoons finely chopped almonds

1 tablespoon toasted flaxseed

Optional: salt and pepper to taste

Wash asparagus and trim ends. Steam approximately 5 minutes until bright green and tender, but crisp. While asparagus is steaming, mix together olive oil, lemon juice, salt and pepper. In a separate bowl, mix the almonds and flaxseed. Drain the asparagus and arrange on a serving platter. Drizzle with olive oil-lemon juice mixture and then sprinkle with nut-seed mix.

Makes 4 servings.

Nutrition per serving: calories 120, total fat 9 g, saturated fat 1 g, carbohydrates 6 g, fiber 3 g, protein 3 g.

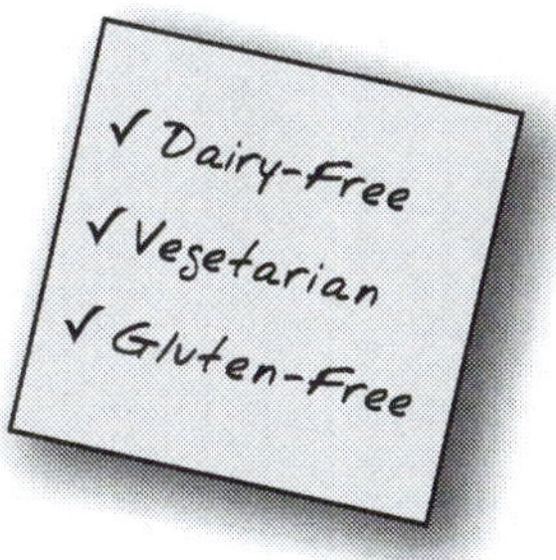

Garlic Butter Roasted Mushrooms

1 pound mushrooms (cremini or white) halved lengthwise
2 tablespoons capers, rinsed and chopped
3 large garlic cloves, minced
2 tablespoons olive oil
3 tablespoons organic butter, cut into pieces
2 teaspoons fresh lemon juice
¼ cup chopped parsley

Preheat oven to 450°F. Toss mushrooms with capers, garlic, oil, ⅛ teaspoon salt and several grinds of pepper in a 1½ to 2 qt shallow, baking dish. Top with butter and roast, stirring occasionally until mushrooms are tender and golden and a bubbly garlic sauce forms below—15-20 minutes. Stir in lemon juice and parsley. Serve immediately.

Makes 8 to 10 servings.

Nutrition per serving: calories 84, fat 7.5 g, cholesterol 11.25 mg, sodium 35.62 mg, carbohydrates 4 g, fiber 0 g, sugar 0 g, protein 1.5 g.

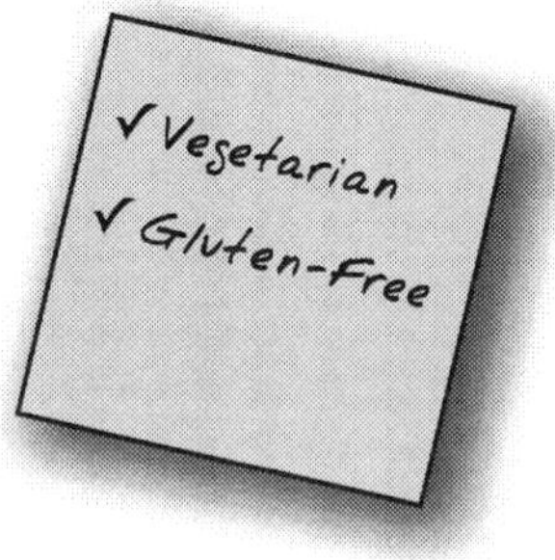

Garlic Chickpeas and Pasta

1 can (16 ounces) chickpeas (garbanzo beans) or 2 cups dried chickpeas, cooked
1 can (8 ounces) crushed tomatoes with basil
1 cup steam broccoli, chopped
3 tablespoons chopped garlic
1 cup water
½ teaspoon extra-virgin olive oil
Salt and pepper to taste
1 cup uncooked whole-grain pasta (to reduce calories, substitute with Miracle Noodle®—page 481)

In saucepan, mix chickpeas, tomatoes, broccoli and garlic. Cook on low heat until warmed. Add water, olive oil, salt and pepper to a large pot and bring to a boil. Add pasta and cook according to the time recommended on the package. Remove pasta, drain, then toss with chickpea mixture. Serve immediately.

Makes 6 servings.

Nutrition per serving: calories 210, total fat 2.5 g, saturated fat 0 g, sodium 135 mg, carbohydrates 39 g, fiber 9 g, protein 11 g.

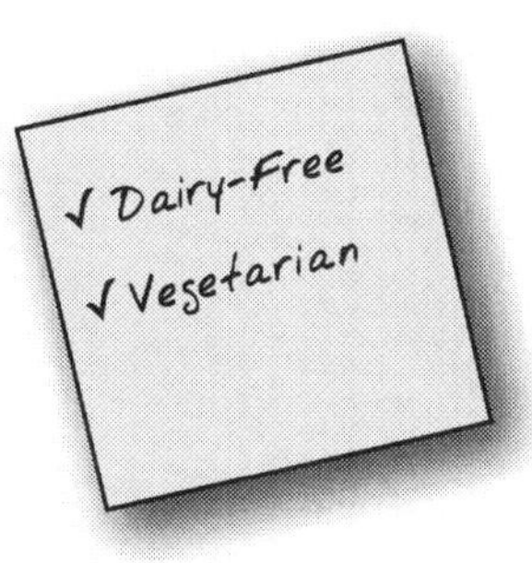

Goat Cheese Swiss Chard with Rice[9]

16 red Swiss chard leaves (choose smallish leaves around 10-inch long)
2 cups water
Salt to taste
1½ tablespoons ghee or regular butter, divided
1½ tablespoons olive oil, divided
1 small yellow onion, chopped
1 clove garlic, finely chopped
⅔ cup brown and wild rice mix, prepared according to package directions, cooled
¼ cup pine nuts
⅓ cup raisins
8 ounces soft goat cheese
Pepper to taste

In a saucepan or skillet large enough to submerge chard without folding, bring water and salt to a boil. Blanch leaves, one at a time for about 20 to 30 seconds, just to soften. They should remain bright green with limp stems. Drain in a single layer on a paper towel-covered cookie sheet. Set aside. Preheat oven to 400°F. Grease a baking pan with ½ tablespoon of the ghee, then set aside. Heat ½ tablespoon of the remaining ghee and ½ tablespoon of the oil in a large skillet over medium heat. Add onions and garlic and cook, stirring occasionally, until tender. Transfer to a large bowl with cooked and cooled rice and toss gently to combine.

In a separate small, heavy skillet, heat remaining ½ tablespoon of the ghee and ½ tablespoon of the oil. Add pine nuts and cook, stirring constantly, until golden brown. Add to rice mixture along with raisins and goat cheese. Season with salt and pepper.

To assemble, cut off thickest part of stem by cutting a "V" shape about 1-inch up from bottom of leaf. Turn leaf face side up and overlap bottom cut edges. Spoon a heaping tablespoon of filling near stem. Fold bottom sides in and roll to enclose the filling. Place open edge down in prepared baking pan. Repeat with remaining leaves and filling. Drizzle remaining ½ tablespoon oil over finished packets. Cover loosely with foil. Bake about 15 minutes, until heated through.

Makes 8 servings.

Nutrition per serving: calories 240, fat 14 g, cholesterol 20 mg, sodium 600 mg, carbohydrates 21 g, fiber 3 g, sugar 6 g, protein 9 g.

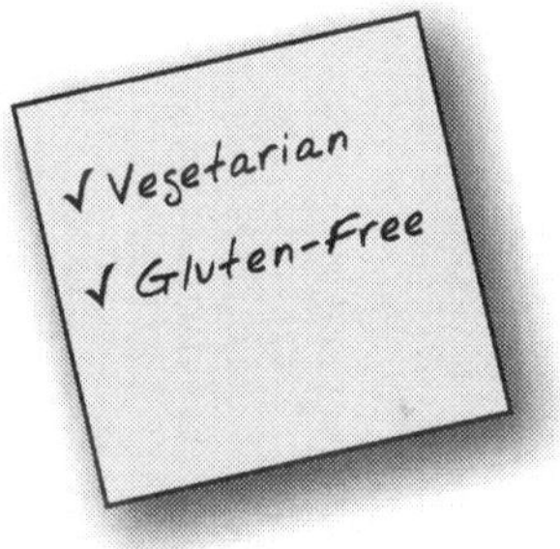

Grilled Asparagus with Sesame Seeds[10]

4 tablespoons extra-virgin olive oil

1 pound fresh asparagus, trimmed and peeled

1 teaspoon salt

1 tablespoon sesame seeds

Drizzle the olive oil over the asparagus and turn spears until they are coated. Sprinkle with salt. Grill asparagus for 5 minutes on a hot grill, turning each minute or so. Remove and toss with sesame seeds.

Makes 4 servings.

Nutrition per serving: calories 90, total fat 8 g, saturated fat 1 g, carbohydrates 5 g, fiber 3 g, protein 3 g.

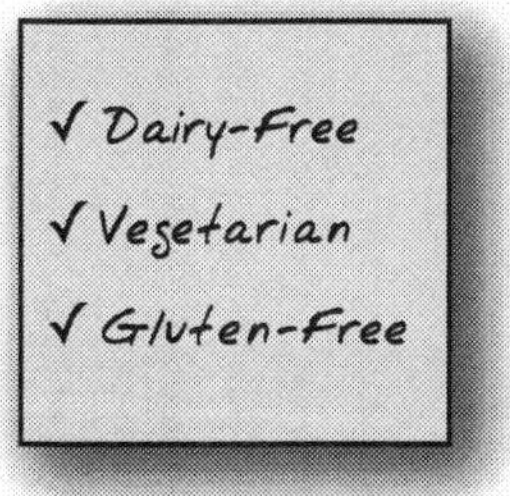

Grilled Basil-Marinade Chicken

1 tablespoon olive oil
1 tablespoon red wine vinegar
1 tablespoon chopped basil leaves
1 tablespoon finely chopped red onion
1 garlic clove chopped
4 boneless, skinless chicken breast halves (about 1½ pounds)

Whisk together the oil, vinegar, basil, onion and garlic in a bowl. Transfer the marinade to a plastic bag with the chicken and shake to combine. Refrigerate for at least 3 hours and up to overnight. When ready to cook, preheat a gas grill. Remove the chicken from the marinade. Grill the chicken, turning once, until browned and just cooked through, about 4 minutes per side.

Makes 4 servings.

Nutrition per serving: calories 301, total fat 9.5 g, saturated fat 2.1 g, sodium 126 mg, carbohydrates 1.3 g, fiber 0 g, protein 52.8 g.

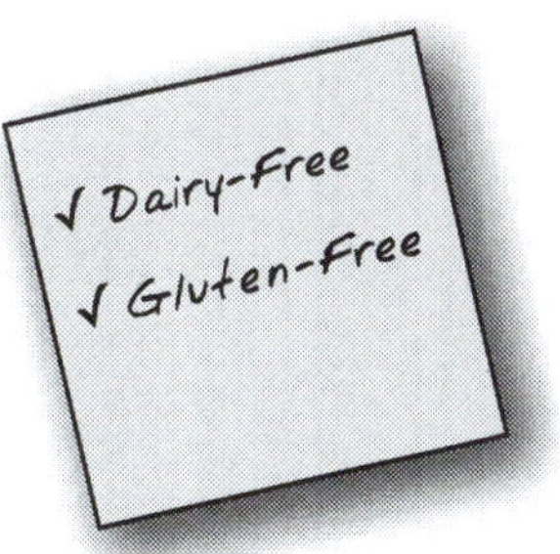

Grilled Caribbean Chicken

4 (4-ounce) skinned, boned chicken breast halves
2 teaspoons lime juice
1 teaspoon vegetable oil
2 teaspoons jerk seasoning or Mrs. Dash® Caribbean Citrus Seasoning
Cooking Spray

Place chicken between 2 sheets of heavy-duty plastic wrap and flatten to ¼-inch thickness by using a meat mallet or rolling pin. Combine lime juice and oil; brush over both sides of chicken. Rub both sides of chicken with jerk seasoning. Coat grill rack with cooking spray; place rack on grill over medium to hot coals (350°F to 400°F). Place chicken on rack and grill—covered—for 5 to 6 minutes on each side, or until done.

Makes 4 servings.

Nutrition per serving: calories 199, total fat 11.6 g, saturated fat 3.1 g, sodium 71 mg, carbohydrates 0.2 g, fiber 0 g, protein 23.6 g.

Grilled Fish with Citrus Marinade[11]

¼ cup extra-virgin olive oil
2 tablespoons grapefruit juice
3 tablespoons lime juice
4 (6 ounce) fish fillets

Optional: salt and pepper to taste

Combine olive oil, grapefruit juice, lime juice, salt and pepper (if desired. Pour over fish and marinate in the refrigerator for 2 or more hours. Grill and serve.

Makes 4 servings

Nutrition per serving: calories 200, total fat 6 g, saturated fat 1.5 g, sodium 90 mg, carbohydrates 0 g, protein 34 g.

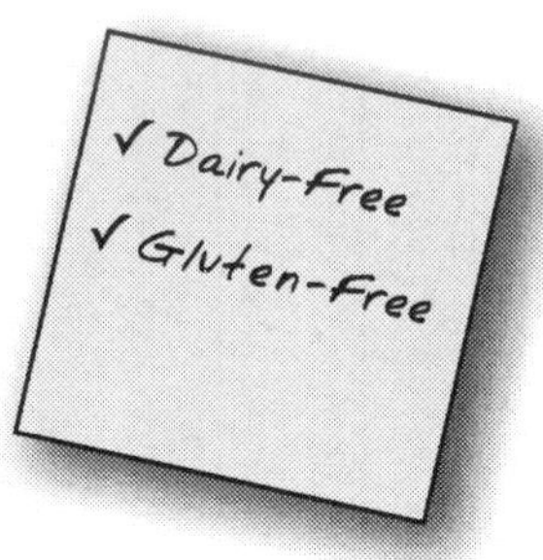

Grilled Glazed Dijon Chicken

1 tablespoon olive oil
2 tablespoons Dijon-style mustard
2 tablespoons honey
1 tablespoon Mrs. Dash® Original Blend
4 boneless, skinless chicken breast halves (4 ounces each)

Prepare grill for medium to high heat. Spread olive oil over chicken breasts. Sprinkle Mrs. Dash® over chicken. Combine mustard and honey, then mix well. Place chicken on grill. Brush half of mustard mixture over chicken. Grill covered for 4 minutes. Turn chicken and brush remaining mustard mixture over chicken. Continue grilling covered for 4 to 5 minutes, or until juices run clear.

Makes 4 servings.

Nutrition per serving: calories 122, total fat 5.3 g, saturated fat 0.6 g, sodium 19 mg, carbohydrates 10.4 g, fiber 0.8 g, protein 8.1 g.

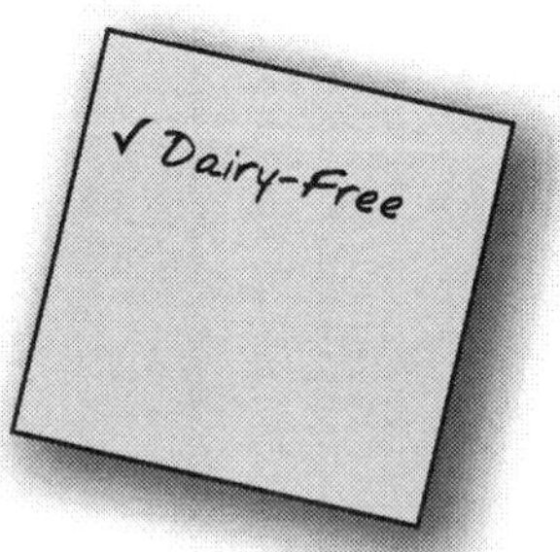

Grilled Portobello Mushrooms

3 portobello mushroom caps
3 tablespoons olive oil
1 tablespoon lemon juice
3 tablespoons balsamic vinegar
Black and red pepper

Brush the mushrooms with olive oil, balsamic vinegar, and plenty of black and red pepper.

Grill for 5 minutes on each side, or until tender. Or, broil mushrooms in the oven (on a rack 4 inches from preheated broiler) for 5 minutes. Drizzle with lemon juice.

Makes 6 servings.

Nutrition per serving: calories 43, total fat 1.5 g, saturated fat 0.2 g, carbohydrates 4.4 g, fiber 2 g, protein 3 g.

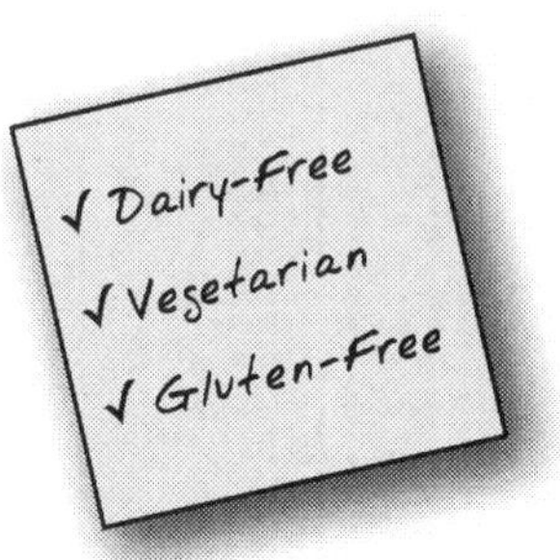

Grilled Portobellos, Peppers and Squash

2 portobello mushroom caps, stemmed
1 red bell pepper, cored, seeded, and quartered
1 medium yellow squash, halved lengthwise
1 medium zucchini, halved lengthwise
2 tablespoons olive oil
2 garlic cloves, minced

Optional: ½ teaspoon sea salt

Preheat gas grill Place all the vegetables on a baking sheet, season with salt and pepper, and toss with the olive oil and garlic. Place the vegetables, cut side down, on the grill. Cook for 4 to 5 minutes on each side, or until tender and nicely marked by the grill.

Makes 4 servings.

Nutrition per serving: calories 98, total fat 7.1 g, saturated fat 0.9 g, sodium 4 mg, carbohydrates 6.6 g, fiber 2 g, protein 1.8 g.

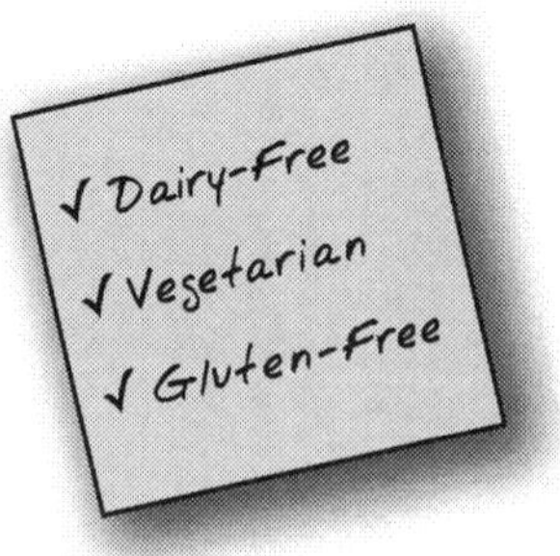

Grilled Rosemary Steak

1 tablespoon finely chopped fresh rosemary
1 teaspoon grated lemon rind
1 teaspoon freshly ground black pepper
1 teaspoon olive oil
¼ teaspoon sea salt
2 garlic cloves, minced
4 (4 ounce) grass-fed beef tenderloin steaks, trimmed (1-inch thick)
Cooking spray

Combine rosemary, lemon rind, pepper, olive oil, salt and garlic in a small bowl. Rub rosemary mixture evenly over steaks, then cover. Refrigerate 1 hour. Prepare grill. Place steaks on a grill rack coated with cooking spray. Grill 5 minutes on each side, or until desired degree of doneness.

Makes 4 servings (serving size of 1 steak).

Nutrition per serving: calories 179, total fat 7.9 g, saturated fat 2.7 g, sodium 168 mg, carbohydrates 1 g, protein 24.4 g.

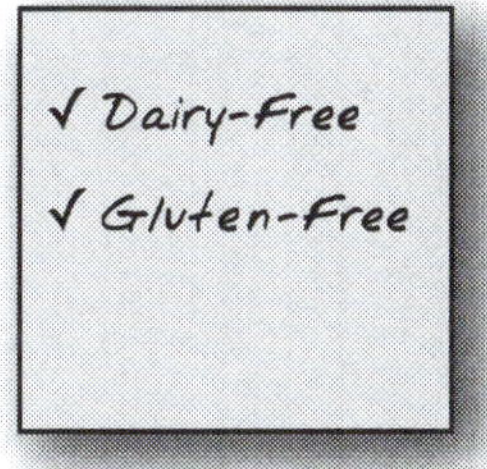

Grilled Vegetables

If any of these vegetables aren't in season, you may substitute other vegetables.

2 tomatoes
2 zucchini
1 summer squash
1 onion
1 teaspoon dried basil
1 teaspoon dried oregano

Slice the vegetables and place on aluminum foil leaving room at the sides to fold up. Drizzle with olive oil. Add basil and oregano. Stir to mix in olive oil and herbs. Fold up the foil around the vegetables, so that all ingredients are sealed inside. Place on upper rack of grill and cook for approximately 30 minutes on medium heat.

Makes 4 servings.

Nutrition per serving: calories 96, total fat 3.8 g, saturated fat 0.6 g, sodium 23 mg, carbohydrates 12.2 g, fiber 4.2 g, protein 3.2 g.

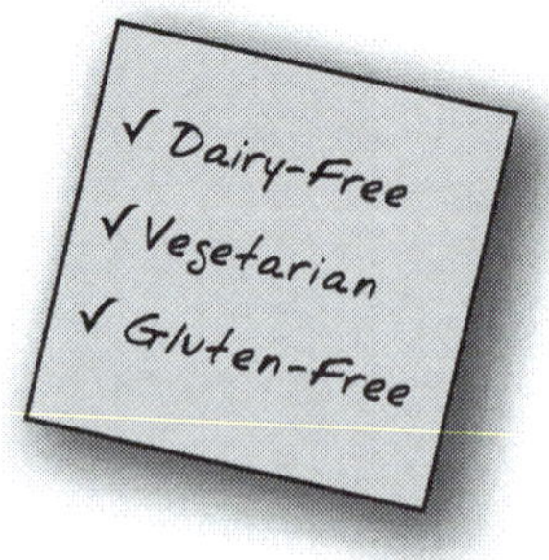

Indian-Spiced Salmon

½ teaspoon ground ginger
½ teaspoon garam masala
½ teaspoon ground coriander
¼ teaspoon ground turmeric
Freshly ground pepper
4 (6 ounce) skinless salmon fillets
Cooking spray

Preheat broiler. Combine ginger and the next 5 ingredients (through pepper). Rub spice mixture evenly over salmon. Place fillets on a broiler pan or baking sheet coated with cooking spray. Cover with foil; broil 7 minutes. Remove foil; broil an additional 4 minutes or until desired degree of doneness.

Makes 4 servings (serving size of 1 fillet).

Nutrition per serving: calories 250, total fat 11.3 g, saturated fat 2.4 g, sodium 79 mg, carbohydrates 0.4 g, fiber 0.1 g, protein 36.9 g.

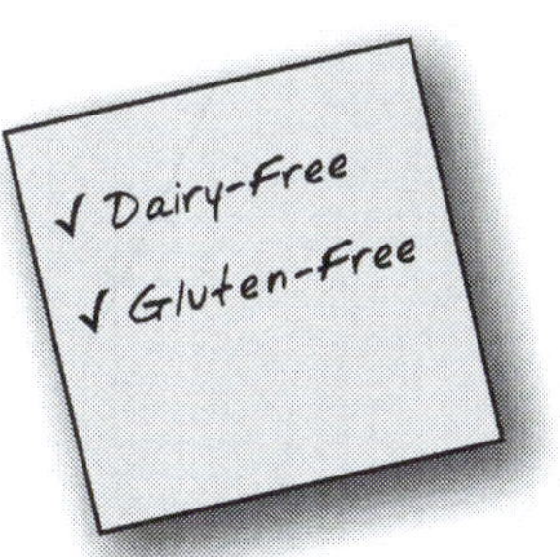

Italian Green Beans[12]

1½ pounds fresh green beans, trimmed
1 tablespoon olive oil
2 to 3 large tomatoes, chopped
2 large garlic cloves, minced
1 tablespoon chopped fresh basil, or 1 teaspoon dried
Salt and fresh ground black pepper to taste

Trim beans and break them into bite-size pieces. Steam until just tender—5 to 10 minutes—then chill in cold water. Drain and set aside. Heat oil in a large skillet, then add tomatoes and garlic. Simmer over medium heat for 10 minutes. Add the beans and basil, then cook 10 minutes longer, stirring occasionally. Add salt and pepper to taste and serve.

Makes 6 to 8 servings.

Nutrition per serving: calories 113, total fat 7.8 g, saturated fat 1.3 g, sodium 79 mg, carbohydrates 8.3 g, fiber 2.6 g, protein 2.8 g.

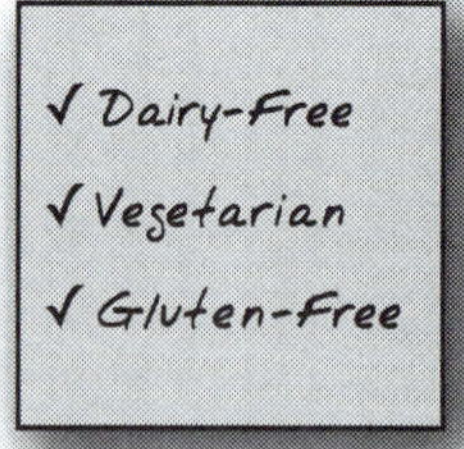

Japanese Raw Rice

1 cup chopped parsnips
¼ cup raw pine nuts
1 to 2 tablespoons raw honey (omit to make vegan)
1 tablespoon rice vinegar
3 tablespoons raw teriyaki sauce*

Pulse parsnips, pine nuts, honey and vinegar until mixture starts to look like brown rice. Add sauce and mix well.

*To make raw teriyaki sauce: combine 1 cup Nama® Shoyu, 1 cup pure maple syrup, 1 teaspoon ginger, 1 clove garlic, 1 drizzle toasted sesame oil.

Makes 2 servings.

Nutrition per serving: calories 188, fat 6.7 g, cholesterol 0 mg, sodium 921.5 mg, carbohydrates 25.45 g, fiber 3.75 g, sugar 14.7 g, fiber 5.8 g.

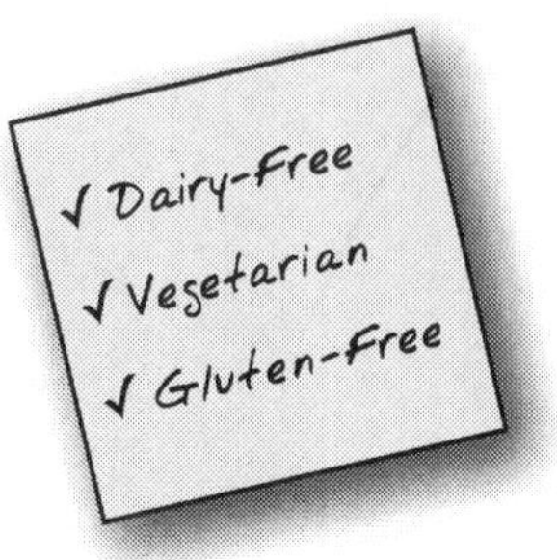

Jamaican Jerk Chicken

1 teaspoon salt
1 teaspoon ground allspice
1 teaspoon packed brown sugar
1 teaspoon onion powder
½ teaspoon dried minced garlic
½ teaspoon ground nutmeg
½ teaspoon black pepper
½ teaspoon ground ginger
¼ teaspoon cayenne pepper
pinch or ¼ teaspoon ground cinnamon
¼ teaspoon dried thyme leaves
2 chicken breasts (4 to 6 ounces each)
¼ cup oil (extra virgin olive oil or coconut oil)
1 lime

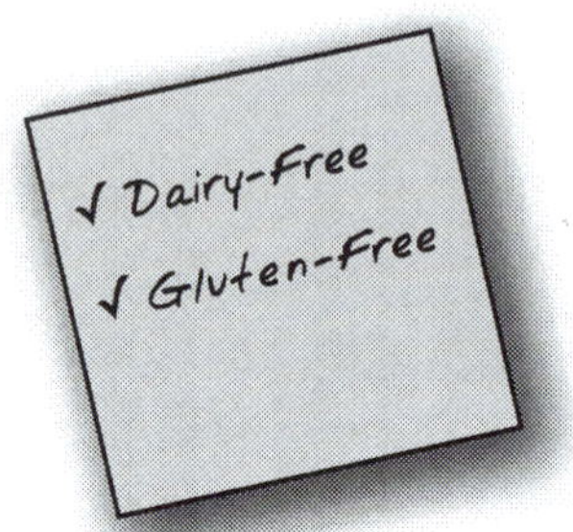

Mix all the herbs together in a bowl to make jerk mix. Squeeze the lime onto the chicken, then rub jerk mix on the chicken. Marinade in refrigerator for 2 to 4 hours. Preheat oven to 350°F. Pour oil into baking dish and place chicken pieces skin-side up into the baking dish. Bake in oven for 45 minutes, or until cooked. Then turn oven on to broil for 2 to 5 minutes.

Makes 2 servings.

Nutrition per serving: calories 180, fat 1.25 g, cholesterol 85 g, sodium 98.75 mg, carbohydrates 4.5 g, fiber 0 g, sugar 0.13 g, protein 33.75 g.

Kale Chips

1 large bunch of Tuscan kale (~10-12 leaves)
1 tablespoon olive oil
Sea salt and ground pepper to taste

Preheat oven to 275°F. Remove stalks and ribs from kale, rinse and then dry leaves. Toss in large bowl with olive oil. Add salt and pepper to taste. Bake for 25 minutes, or until crisp.

Makes 2 servings.

Nutrition per serving: calories 117, fat 7.5 g, cholesterol 0 mg, sodium 166 mg, carbohydrates 11.4 g, fiber 2.3 g, protein 3.8 g.

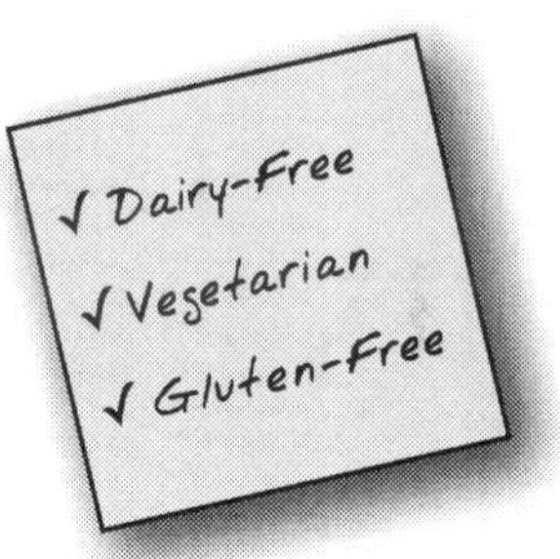

Lemon-Asparagus Packets

½ pound asparagus
2 teaspoons olive oil
½ teaspoon Mrs. Dash® seasoning

Snap off tough ends of asparagus. Place asparagus on a square of heavy-duty aluminum foil. Drizzle 2 teaspoons olive oil over asparagus, and sprinkle with ½ teaspoon Mrs. Dash® seasoning. Fold aluminum foil tightly to seal. Place on grill rack and grill over medium-hot coals for 10 minutes.

Makes 2 servings.

Nutrition per serving: calories 35, fat 2.6 g, saturated fat 0 g, protein 1.4 g, carbohydrates 2.9 g, fiber 1.3 g.

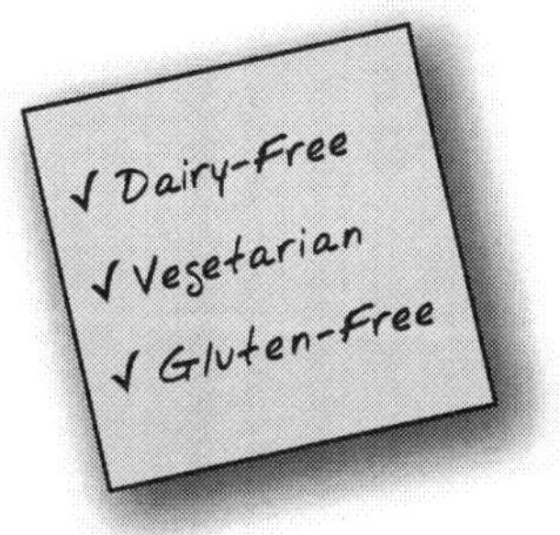

Lemon-Curry Cauliflower and Kale[13]

1 teaspoon curry powder
2 teaspoons lemon zest
3 tablespoons lemon juice
1 bunch kale
1 head cauliflower

Mix curry powder, lemon zest, and lemon juice. Set aside. Boil kale and cauliflower in a large pot of water with salt and pepper for 4 to 5 minutes, or until tender. Drain and toss with lemon juice mixture.

Makes 4 servings.

Nutrition per serving: calories 70, total fat 0.5 g, saturated fat 0 g, sodium 70 mg, carbohydrates 15 g, fiber 5 g, protein 5 g.

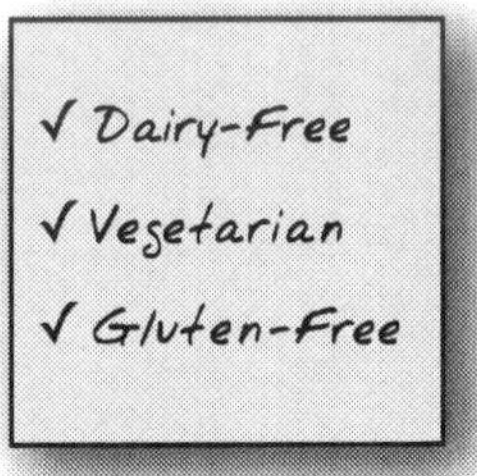

Mango Shrimp

1 pound shrimp, peeled

1 mango

1 jalapeño

1 teaspoon cumin

Puree mango, cumin powder and jalapeño in food processor. Skewer shrimp and cover with only half of the marinade for 30 minutes in the refrigerator. Cook on grill or pan until pink, and then top with the remaining marinade. Serve with side of quinoa or brown rice and salad.

Makes 2 to 3 servings.

Nutrition per serving: calories 225, fat 2.5 g, cholesterol 330 mg, sodium 381.5 mg, carbohydrates 14.05 g, fiber 1.25 g, sugar 12.2 g, protein 36.24 g.

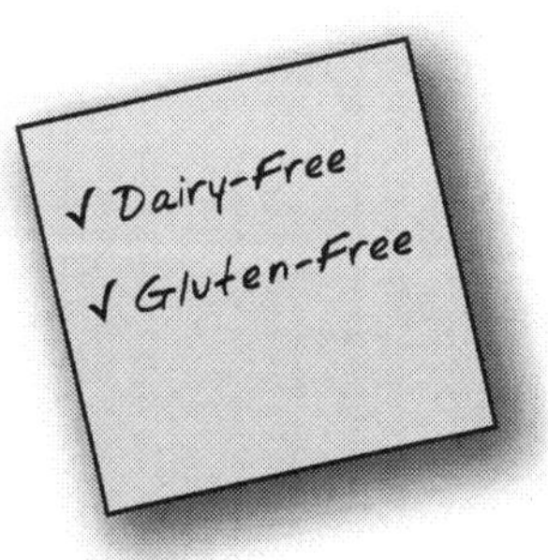

Maple Glazed Root Vegetables

3 large carrots, peeled
3 large parsnips, peeled
2 tablespoons olive oil
2 tablespoons maple syrup, preferably grade B
Dash unrefined sea salt

Julienne the peeled parsnips and carrots by cutting them into thin matchsticks—no thicker than ¼ inch. Heat the olive oil in a skillet over medium heat. Add the julienned carrots and parsnips and stir continuously over medium heat until the vegetables become slightly tender (about 5 to 6 minutes). Note that some of the parsnips and carrots may become slightly caramelized. Gently stir in maple syrup and season with a dash of salt. Continue to stir the carrots and parsnips for about 1 to 2 minutes, or until the vegetables are well-glazed by the maple syrup. Serve warm.

Makes 6 servings.

Nutrition per serving: calories 45.6, carbohydrates 3.1 g, cholesterol 10 mg, total fat 3.8 g, saturated fat 2.4 g, fiber 0 g, sodium 1.1 mg, protein 2.9 g.

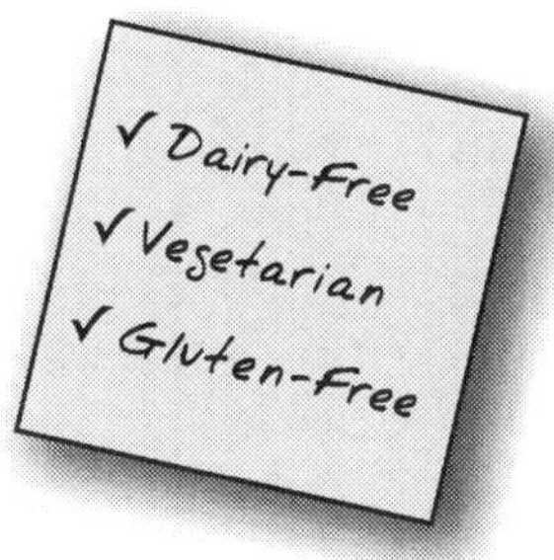

Marinara Sauce

1 tablespoon olive oil
1½ tablespoons minced garlic
6 pounds coarsely chopped and peeled tomato (about 6 cups)
¾ teaspoon salt
½ teaspoon black pepper
¼ cup chopped fresh basil
¼ cup chopped fresh parsley

Heat oil in a large saucepan over medium heat. Add garlic, then cook 2 minute while stirring frequently. Add tomato, salt, and pepper, then bring to a boil. Reduce heat and simmer 25 minutes, while stirring occasionally. Stir in basil and parsley, then cook 1 minute.

Makes 6 servings (serving size of 1 cup).

Nutrition per serving: calories 139, total fat 3.8 g, saturated fat 0.5 g, sodium 113 mg, carbohydrates 22.1 g, fiber 5.2 g, protein 4.1 g.

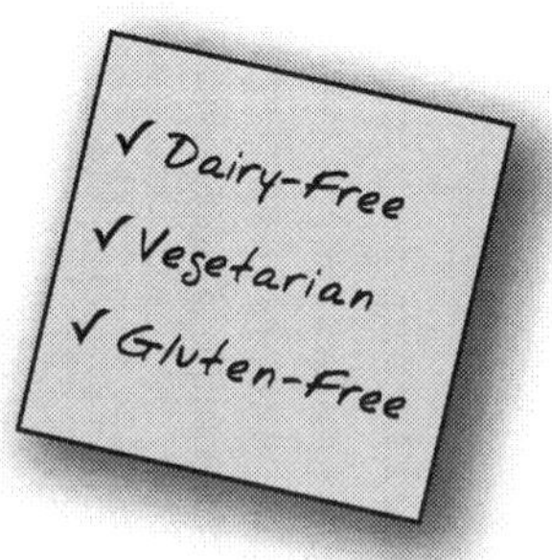

Marinated London Broil[14]

½ cup red wine

2 tablespoons red wine vinegar

4 teaspoons soy sauce

1 teaspoon black pepper

4 cloves garlic, minced

48 ounces London broil or sirloin steak

Put the wine, wine vinegar, soy sauce, black pepper and garlic in a resealable plastic bag or a covered bowl and mix well. Add meat and marinate in the refrigerator 6 hours. Heat broiler. Broil meat 6 inches from heating element, turning and basting once with marinade—20 minutes for medium rare. Slice very thin and serve.

Makes 12 servings (serving size of 4 ounces).

Nutrition per serving: calories 217, protein 28 g, carbohydrates 0 g, fat 8 g.

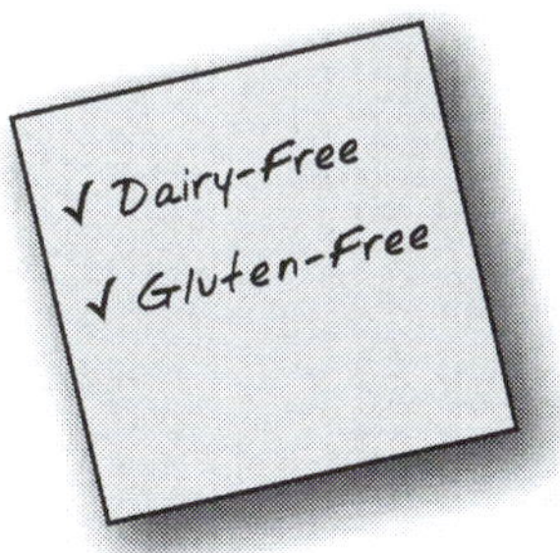

Mediterranean Beef Stew

2 medium zucchini, cut into bite-size chunks
¾ pound grass-fed beef stew meat, cut into ½-inch pieces
2 (14½ ounce) cans Italian-style diced tomatoes, undrained
½ teaspoon pepper
1 (2-inch) stick cinnamon or ¼ teaspoon ground cinnamon

Place zucchini in bottom of a 3½ quart electric slow cooker. Add beef and remaining ingredients. Cover and cook on high setting 5 hours, or until meat is tender. Or, cover and cook on high setting 1 hour, then reduce to low setting and cook 7 hours. Remove and discard cinnamon stick before serving.

Makes 4 servings.

Nutrition per serving: calories 193, fat 4.0 g, saturated fat 1.3 g, sodium 572 mg, carbohydrates 16.9 g, fiber 1.5 g, protein 22.8 g.

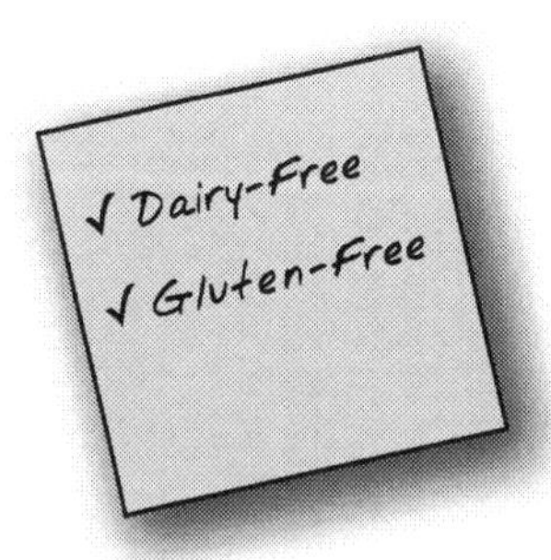

Mrs. Dash® Fish

1 teaspoon Mrs. Dash® Original Blend
1 tablespoon butter or olive oil
2 (4 ounce) haddock (or cod) fillets
1 tablespoon chopped parsley

Heat 1 tablespoon olive oil in skillet. Fry haddock (or cod) fillets in pan for 3 minutes. Turn over, sprinkle with 1 teaspoon Mrs. Dash® Original Blend. Cook for another 3 to 4 minutes, or until fish flakes easily. Sprinkle chopped parsley over fish, serve.

Makes 2 servings.

Nutrition per serving: calories 100, total fat 6.2 g, saturated fat 3.7 g, sodium 98 mg, carbohydrates 0 g, protein 11 g.

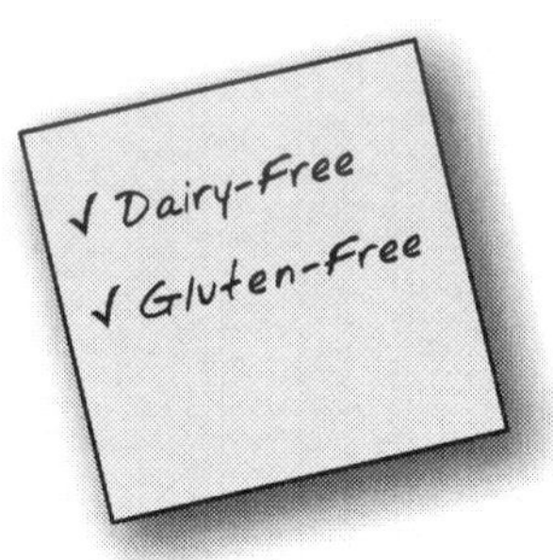

Orange-Ginger Salmon

¼ cup extra-virgin olive oil
½ cup orange juice
2 garlic cloves minced
4 (5 ounce/1-inch) salmon steaks
Fresh ginger slivers

Mix the olive oil, orange juice and garlic. Pour the mixture over the salmon and marinate at least 2 hours (or refrigerate overnight). Preheat the oven to broil. Broil the fish 2 to 3 inches from the heating element for 5 minutes, then turn and broil on the other side. You may also heat any saved marinate and spoon it over the fish just before serving.

Makes 4 servings.

Nutrition per serving: calories 310, total fat 18 g, saturated fat 2.5 g, sodium 75 mg, total carbohydrates 2 g, protein 34 g.

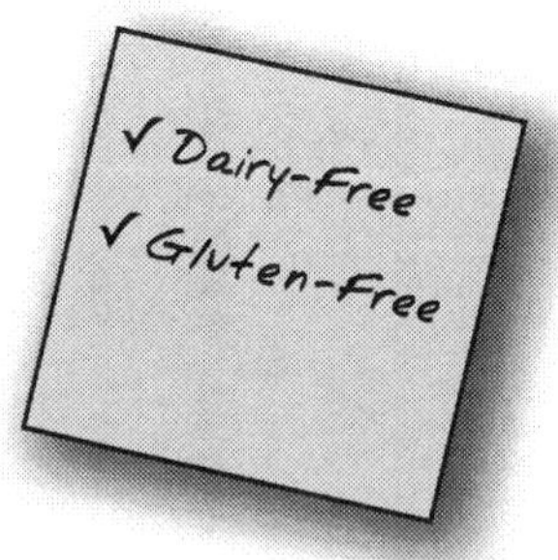

Orange Juice Scallops

10 ounces large scallops
1 pound broccoli florets
1 pound cauliflower florets
1 cup freshly squeezed orange juice
Cooking oil spray
1 teaspoon curry powder
Salt and pepper to taste

Coat nonstick skillet with cooking spray and heat skillet. Add scallops and season with curry powder, salt and pepper, then cook until scallops are golden brown. Add broccoli, cauliflower and orange juice. Cook until broccoli is tender. Drizzle with orange sauce.

Makes 1 to 2 servings.

Nutrition per serving: calories 307, fat 3 g, cholesterol 36 mg, sodium 184 mg, carbohydrates 40 g, fiber 13 g, sugar 24 g, protein 28 g.

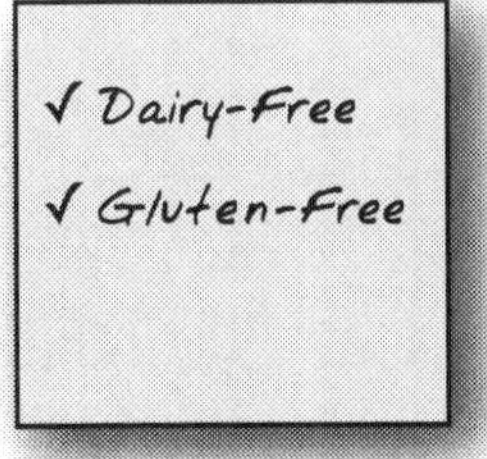

Pan-Browned Brussels Sprouts[15]

2 tablespoons olive oil
1 pound Brussels sprouts, trimmed and cut in half
¼ teaspoon freshly ground pepper
⅓ cup water
½ teaspoon lemon zest

Optional: ½ teaspoon kosher salt

Heat the olive oil in a medium skillet over medium-high heat. Add the Brussels sprouts, pepper, and salt if desired, and cook, stirring occasionally, for 2 to 3 minutes, until they begin to brown. Add the water, then cover the pan and cook for about 4 or 5 minutes, or until almost done. Remove the lid and turn the heat to high. Cook until brown and no liquid remains. Sprinkle with the lemon zest.

Makes 4 servings (serving size of ¾ cup).

Nutrition per serving: calories 107, fat 7 g, saturated fat 1 g, carbohydrates 9 g, fiber 4 g, protein 3 g.

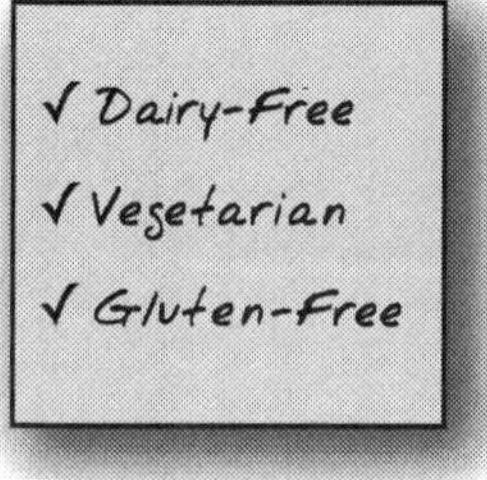

Pan-Seared Grass-Fed Beef

4 to 6 ounces grass-fed beef
Salt and black pepper, to taste
1 tablespoon extra virgin olive oil

Preheat oven to 425°F. Place steak in a oven-safe sauté pan and brown on one side for about 5 minutes, then turn over and place in oven for 4 to 5 minutes for medium-done.

Makes 1 serving.

Nutrition per serving: calories 216, fat 15.99 g, cholesterol 68 mg, sodium 76 mg, carbohydrates 0 g, fiber 0 g, sugar 0 g, protein 20 g.

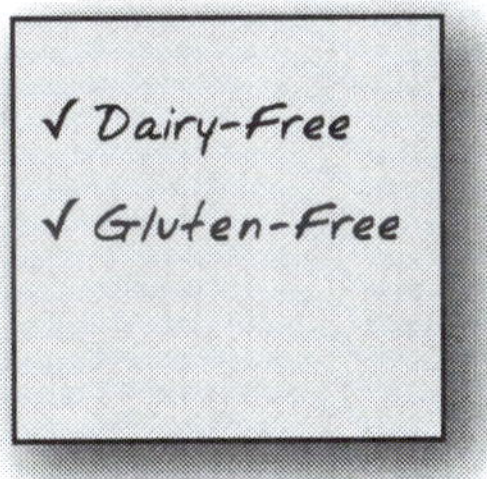

Pesto Filet

1 filet of halibut, salmon or sea bass (6 ounces)
1 to 2 tablespoons olive oil
½ cup pesto
Sprig of cilantro
Grated parmesan

Brush fish with olive oil, lemon and salt. Grill for 3 to 5 minutes on each side. Top with cilantro. Place fish onto bed of quinoa, brown rice pasta or Miracle Noodle® (page 481). Top with pesto sauce and grated parmesan.

Makes 1 serving.

Nutrition per serving: calories 227, fat 12.6 g, cholesterol 30 mg, sodium 86 mg, carbohydrates 1.8 g, fiber 1 g, sugar 0 g, protein 24.2 g.

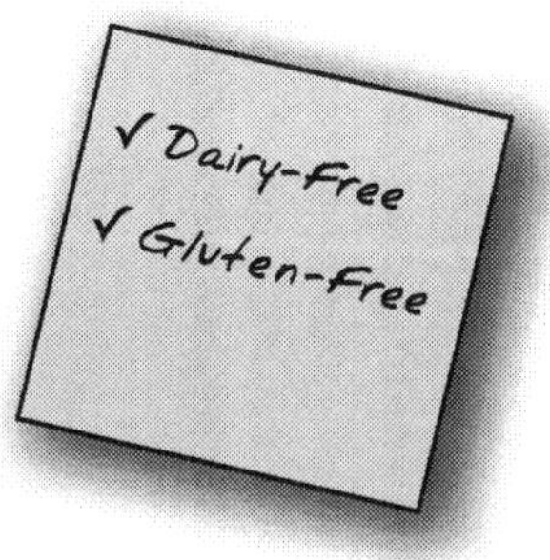

Pizza Roasted Vegetables

3 cups vegetables of choice (zucchini, broccoli, cauliflower)
½ cup marinara sauce (recommended: Paesana or Seeds of Change)
1 teaspoon Italian seasonings

Optional: ¼ cup shredded Alta Dena cheddar style goat cheese

Preheat oven to 350°F. Rinse and chop vegetables into bite size pieces. Transfer to mixing bowl and toss with marinara sauce to coat. Arrange on baking sheet and roast in oven for 15 minutes. Flip vegetables and roast another 10 to 15 minutes. Remove from oven. Shred raw goat cheese over vegetables and return to oven for 5 more minutes.

Makes 1 serving.

Nutrition per serving: calories 210, fat 3.5 g, cholesterol 0 mg, sodium 320 mg, carbohydrates 33 g, fiber 20 g, sugar 0 g, protein 10 g.

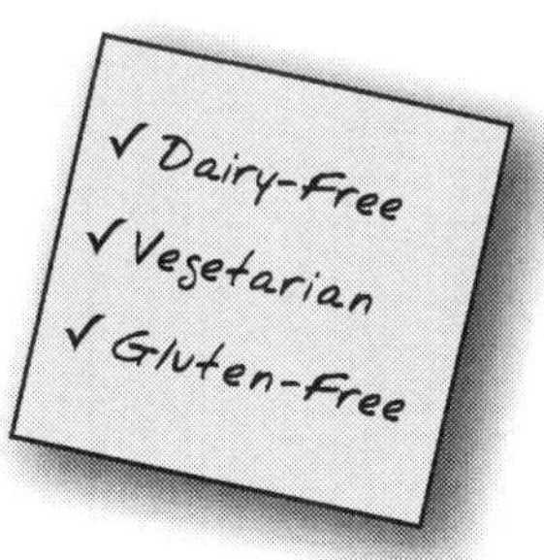

Plantain Encrusted Halibut

4 portions of halibut (7 ounces each)
½ pound banana chips
2 tablespoons olive or grapeseed oil
½ onion, thin-sliced
½ apple, sliced
1 yellow plantain, sliced
2 ounces curry powder
1 can organic light coconut milk
2 tablespoons butter
1 bunch scallions, sliced

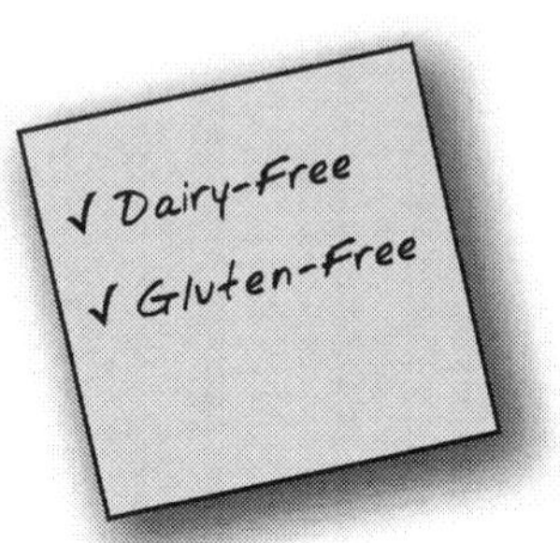

Heat oil in heavy bottom pot. Sauté onions, apple and plantains until soft, then add curry and sauté 1 minute longer. Add 1 can of coconut milk and 1 cup water—simmer 15 minutes. Puree all in blender with the butter. Puree banana chips in blender or coffee bean grinder until a course powder. Heat 2 sauté pans to medium. Season filets with salt and pepper. Coat one side of fish with ground banana chips and sauté for 2 minutes on each side. Serve on a bed of coconut rice—drizzle curry sauce around fish and garnish with sliced scallions.

Makes 1 to 2 servings.

Nutrition per serving: calories 374, fat 20.31 g, cholesterol 60 mg, sodium 226.5 mg, carbohydrates 21.05 g, fiber 1.72 g, sugar 4.84 g, protein 23.61 g.

Poppyseed Brussels Sprouts[16]

1½ pounds Brussels sprouts, ends trimmed
1 tablespoon lemon juice
1 tablespoon oil
1 tablespoon butter
1 garlic clove, minced
½ teaspoon salt
½ teaspoon lemon zest
2 teaspoons poppyseeds
¼ cup chicken or vegetable stock

Finely chop Brussels sprouts into small pieces. Place in a bowl with lemon juice and toss. Heat butter and oil over medium heat and sauté the Brussels sprouts for 3 minutes. Add salt, garlic, lemon zest and poppyseeds, then cook for 2 more minutes. Then add chicken stock and cook another minute.

Makes 6 servings.

Nutrition per serving: calories 76, fat 4.38 g, cholesterol 5 g, sodium 127 mg, carbohydrates 6.16 g, fiber 3.25 g, sugar 0 g, protein 2.98 g.

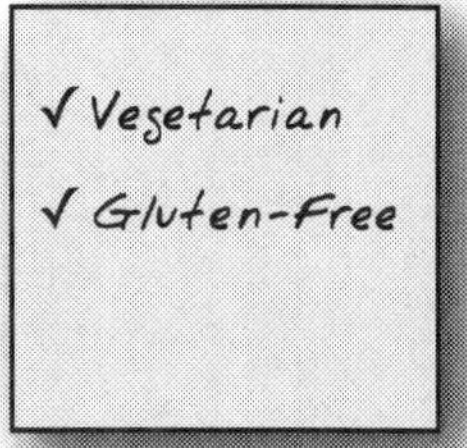

Quick Skillet Asparagus

4 teaspoons olive oil
1 pound medium asparagus spears, trimmed
½ teaspoon grated lemon rind
1 teaspoon fresh lemon juice

Optional: ¼ teaspoon salt

Heat a large skillet over medium-high heat. Add oil to pan; swirl to coat. Add asparagus to pan, then cook for 3 minutes, or until asparagus is crisp-tender and browned, stirring frequently. Transfer to a serving platter. Add rind, juice and salt—if desired—then toss to coat.

Makes 4 servings (serving size of 3 ounces).

Nutrition per serving: calories 71, fat 4.7 g, saturated fat 0.7 g, sodium 148 mg, carbohydrates 5 g, fiber 2.5 g, protein 2.5 g.

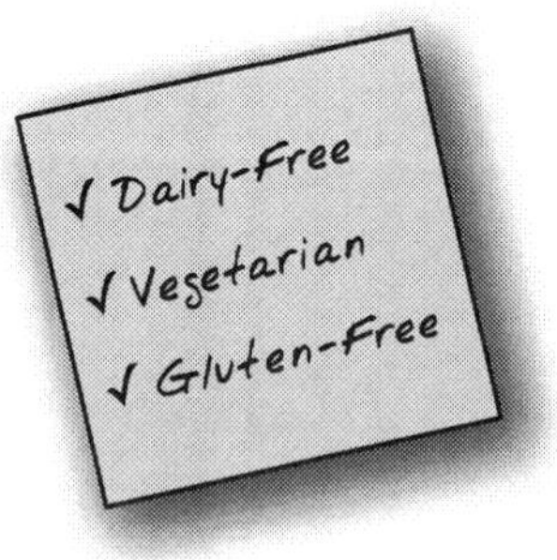

Quinoa Stuffed Bell Peppers[17]

1 tablespoon olive oil
1 red onion, chopped
½ pound sliced mushrooms
6 bell peppers (cored, seeded, tops removed)
½ cup chopped parsley
¼ pound baby spinach
1½ teaspoons ground cinnamon
¾ teaspoon ground cumin
1 cup quinoa, cooked
Salt and pepper to taste

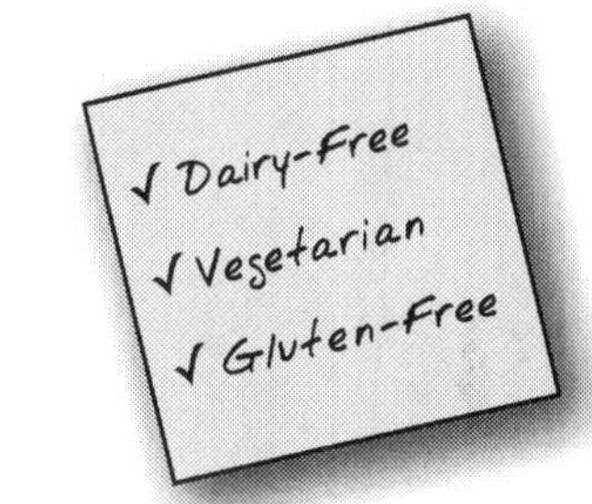

Optional: ½ cup roasted chopped cashews

Preheat oven to 350°F. Heat oil in a large skillet over medium high heat. Add onion and cook until transparent—8 to 10 minutes. Add mushrooms and cook until softened—4 to 5 minutes. Add parsley and spinach. Let spinach wilt, then stir in cinnamon, cumin and cooked quinoa, then toss gently to combine. Add salt, pepper and cashews, then cook 1 to 2 minutes. Divide quinoa mixture evenly among bell peppers, gently packing down to fill each pepper. Top each pepper with reserved top and arrange upright in pan. Cover with foil and bake for 1 hour.

Makes 6 servings.

Nutrition per serving: calories 250, fat 10 g, cholesterol 0 mg, sodium 280 mg, carbohydrates 36 g, fiber 7 g, sugar 6 g, protein 9 g.

Quinoa with Corn and Peppers

½ cup uncooked quinoa
1 cup water
1 cup diced bell pepper
1 cup frozen corn kernels, cooked
½ cup chopped onion
Juice and grated zest of one lime
½ teaspoon cumin
3 tablespoons extra virgin olive oil
Freshly ground pepper

Place the quinoa in a fine strainer and rinse thoroughly with cold water. In a small saucepan, bring 1 cup water and the quinoa to a boil. Reduce temperature to low, cover and cook for 15 minutes—or until the grains are translucent and the germ has spiraled out from each grain. Transfer to a large bowl and chill. Add the bell pepper, corn and onion to the chilled quinoa. Toss to combine. In a small bowl, whisk together the lime zest, juice, cumin and olive oil. Pour over the quinoa mixture and toss well. Season with pepper.

Makes 4 servings.

Nutrition per serving: calories 228, total fat 12 g, saturated fat 2 g, sodium 11 mg, carbohydrates 29 g, fiber 4 g, protein 5 g.

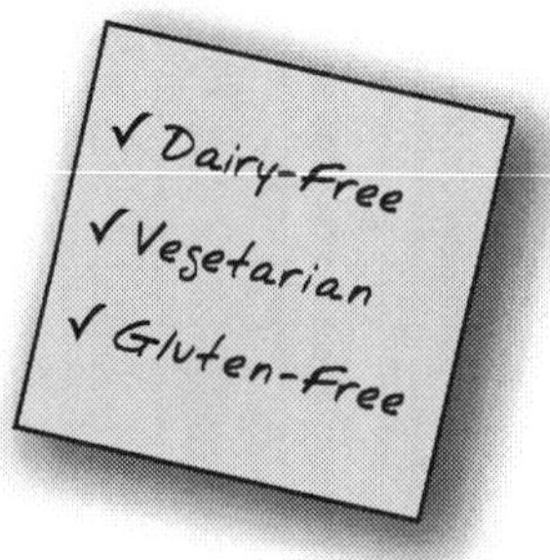

Quinoa with Roasted Garlic, Tomatoes and Spinach

2 to 3 garlic cloves, crushed
1 tablespoon olive oil
1 tablespoon finely chopped shallots
½ cup uncooked quinoa, rinsed and drained
1 tablespoon dry white wine
1 cup fat-free, less-sodium chicken broth
½ cup baby spinach leaves
⅓ cup chopped seeded tomato (1 small)
1 tablespoon shaved fresh Parmesan cheese
¼ teaspoon salt

Optional: ¼ teaspoon crushed red pepper—for spicy

Heat oil in a saucepan over medium heat. Add garlic, shallots and red pepper to pan, then cook 1 minute. Add quinoa to pan, cook 2 minutes while stirring constantly. Add wine, cook until liquid is absorbed, stirring constantly. Add broth and then bring to a boil. Cover, reduce heat and simmer for 15 minutes, or until liquid is absorbed. Remove from heat, stir in spinach, tomato, cheese and salt. Serve immediately.

Makes 4 servings (serving size of ½ cup).

Nutrition per serving: calories 130; total fat 5 g, saturated fat 0.7 g, sodium 305 mg, carbohydrates 16.6 g, fiber 1.8 g, protein 4.1 g.

Ratatouille

2 eggplants, peeled and cut in chunks
2 tablespoons olive oil
2 onions, chopped
3 cloves garlic, crushed
4 zucchinis, chopped
2 cans (15 ounces each) organic tomatoes

Sprinkle the eggplants with salt and leave for 30 minutes, then rinse and dry. Heat the oil in a pan and fry the onions and eggplants for 5 minutes. Add the remaining ingredients, then bring to a boil and simmer for 10 minutes until the zucchini are tender. Serve.

Makes 6 servings.

Nutrition per serving: calories 137, total fat 5.1 g, saturated fat 0.7 g, sodium 216 mg, carbohydrates 19.1 g, fiber 5.9 g, protein 3.6 g.

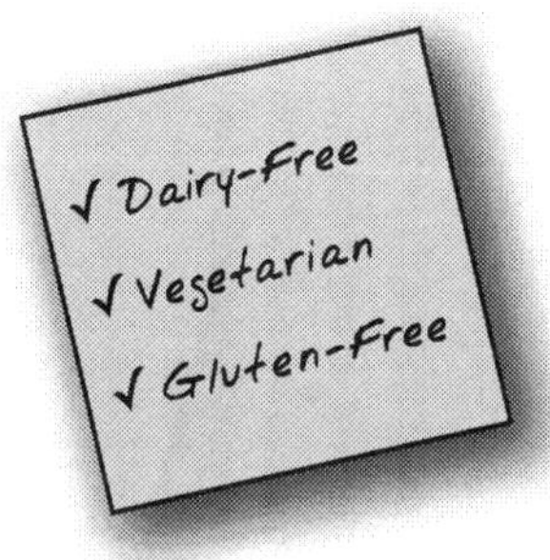

Roast Turkey Breast

1 fresh (or frozen and thawed) turkey breast (5 to 7 pounds)
Ground pepper
Dried herbs and spices of choice: sage, thyme, garlic or onion powder
Vegetable oil

Optional: sea salt

Preheat the oven to 325°F. Brush the turkey breast with vegetable oil. Sprinkle liberally with salt (if using), pepper, herbs, and spices. Insert meat thermometer to the center of the breast. Wrap and seal the breast in extra-heavy aluminum foil, with the face of the meat thermometer on the outside of the foil for viewing. Place on a wire rack in a shallow roasting pan. Roast the turkey breast until the meat thermometer reaches 170°F. (about 2 to 2¾ hours). Open the aluminum foil about 30 minutes before the breast is done and baste 2 times with the drippings.

Makes 8 servings.

Nutrition per serving: calories 277, total fat 5.4 g, saturated fat 1.3 g, sodium 2130 mg, carbohydrates 10.5 g, protein 46.8 g.

✓ Dairy-Free
✓ Gluten-Free*

* Basting solutions injected in turkey during processing may contain gluten. Be sure to read label.

Roasted Brussels Sprouts

1½ pounds Brussels sprouts
2 tablespoons olive oil
Cooking spray
Salt or Herbamare®

Preheat oven to 400°F. Wash Brussels sprouts and trim ends. Cut in half. Coat with butter or olive oil. Sprinkle with salt or Herbamare®. Place on baking sheet and roast for 20 minutes. Take out of oven and serve.

Makes 2 to 3 servings.

Nutrition per serving: calories 113, fat 9.3 g, cholesterol 0 mg, sodium 16 mg, carbohydrates 6.45 g, fiber 3.2 g, sugar 0 g, protein 2.82 g.

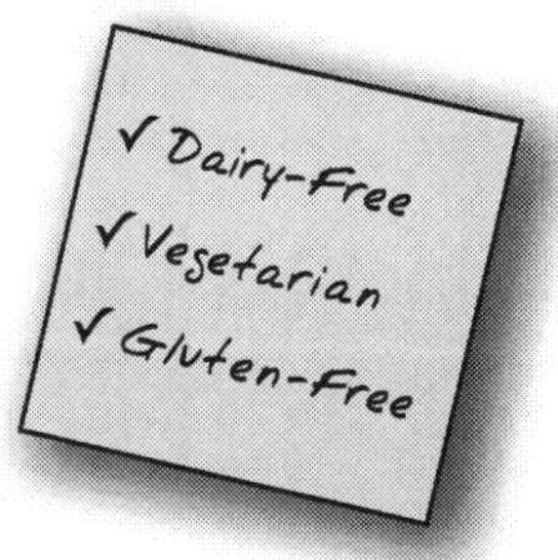

Roasted Red Pepper Hummus[18]

⅓ cup tahini

⅛ cup water

2 tablespoons olive oil

¼ cup chopped bottled roasted red pepper, rinsed and drained

2 tablespoons fresh lemon juice

1 garlic clove, minced (if omitting salt, increase up to 3 garlic cloves)

1 (15½ ounce) can chickpeas, rinsed and drained

Optional:

¼ teaspoon salt

¼ teaspoon crushed red pepper

Place all ingredients in a food processor. Process until smooth.

Makes 8 servings (serving size of ¼ cup).

Nutrition per serving: calories 178, fat 6.7 g, saturated fat 1 g, sodium 258 mg, carbohydrates 21.3 g, fiber 7.3 g, protein 8.3 g.

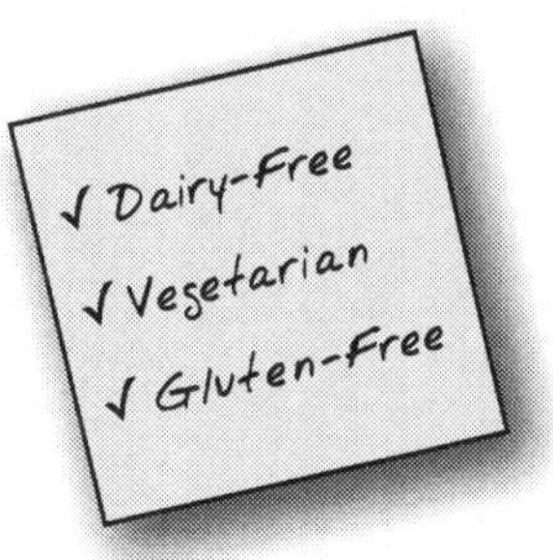

Roasted Sweet Potatoes[19]

4 large (about 2¼ pounds) sweet potatoes, peeled and each cut into 8 pieces
3 tablespoons extra-virgin olive oil
½ teaspoon kosher or sea salt
½ teaspoon freshly ground black pepper
⅛ teaspoon ground red pepper
½ teaspoon ground cinnamon

Preheat oven to 425°F. Place the potatoes on baking sheet. Drizzle with olive oil, salt, black pepper, red pepper and cinnamon. Toss to combine the ingredients. Bake for about 40 minutes (until brown and soft) while turning twice during cooking.

Makes 4 servings (serving size of ¾ cup).

Nutrition per serving: calories 217, fat 11 g, saturated fat 1.5 g, sodium 294 mg, carbohydrates 36 g, fiber 5 g, protein 3 g.

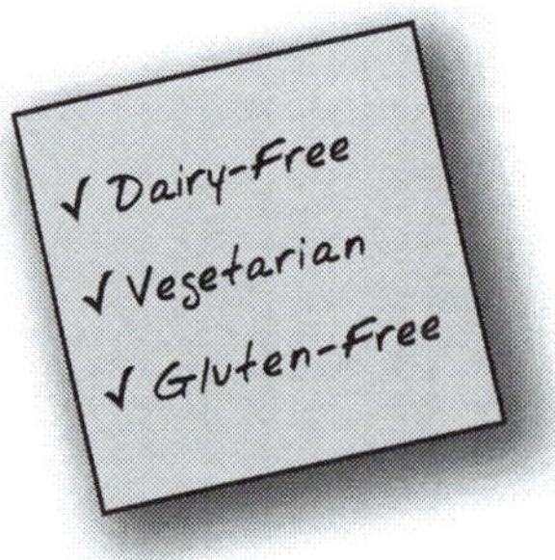

Rosemary Baked Chicken Breast[20]

4 skinless, boneless chicken breasts
2 tablespoons minced garlic
3 tablespoons fresh rosemary or 4 tablespoons dried
2 tablespoons lemon juice

Optional: salt and pepper to taste

Preheat oven to 375°F. Put the chicken breasts in a baking dish and cover them with garlic. Sprinkle with rosemary, lemon juice, salt, and pepper. Bake uncovered for 25 minutes.

Makes 4 servings.

Nutrition per serving: calories 140, total fat 1.5 g, saturated fat 0 g, sodium 80 mg, protein 28 g.

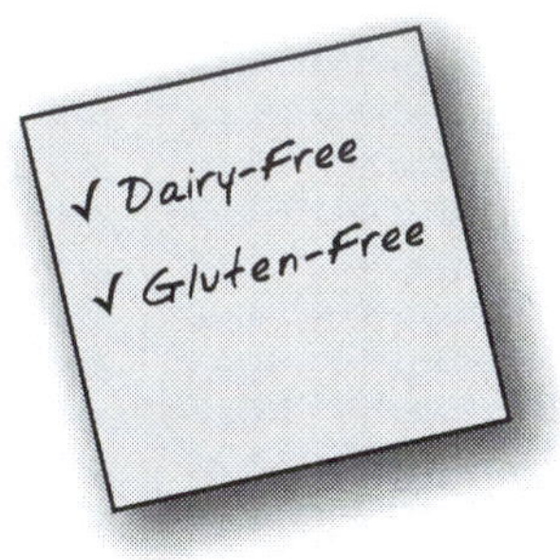

Sage-Crusted Chicken Tenders[21]

1 egg white
1 tablespoon sesame seeds
1 tablespoon shelled roasted sunflower seeds, chopped
¾ teaspoon chopped sage
⅛ teaspoon fresh ground black pepper
2 boneless chicken tenders (2 ounces each)
1 tablespoon spicy brown mustard
1 teaspoon honey

Preheat the oven to 400°F. Coat baking sheet with cooking spray. Place egg white into shallow bowl. Combine sesame seeds, sunflower seeds, sage and black pepper in another small bowl. Using a fork, dip the tenders in the egg white to coat both sides, then dip in the sesame seed mixture, coating both sides. Transfer to one half of the baking sheet and mist surface of chicken with spray. Flip tenders with fork and mist the other side. Bake 15 to 17 minutes, or until chicken is cooked through. Combine mustard and honey in a small bowl and serve as dipping sauce for tenders or top salad.

Makes 1 serving.

Nutrition per serving: calories 312, fat 8.14 g, cholesterol 0 mg, sodium 225.2 mg, carbohydrates 8.13 g, fiber 0.6 g, sugar 4.8 g, protein 52.48 g.

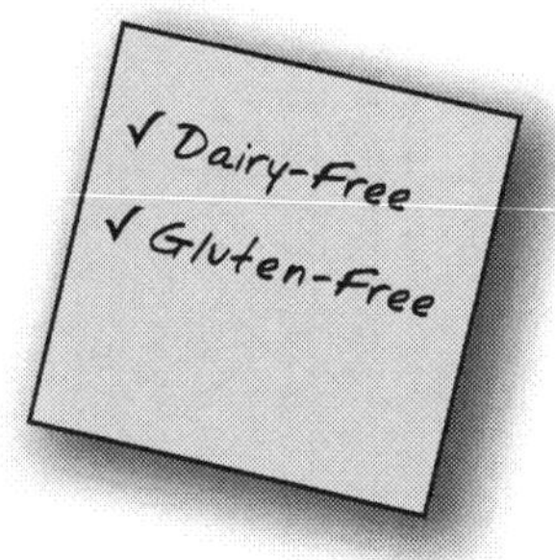

Sage Cranberries & Butternut Squash with Caramelized Onions[22]

1 medium butternut squash

4 tablespoons extra virgin olive oil

2 medium onions

2 tablespoons chopped sage

4 tablespoons dried cranberries or cherries

Sea salt and ground pepper

Preheat oven to 375°F. Peel squash and cut in half lengthwise. Scoop out seeds from the center and discard. Cut squash into large chunks. Coat with 2 tablespoons of the olive oil. Season with salt and pepper to taste and arrange on a parchment-lined baking sheet. Bake for about 30 minutes, or until well caramelized. Peel onions and cut into large chunks. Coat with remaining 2 tablespoons olive oil. Season to taste with salt and pepper and spread on a second lined baking sheet. Bake for about 20 minutes, or until well caramelized. When squash and onions are done, toss with sage and cranberries. Serve immediately.

Makes 4 to 6 servings.

Nutrition per serving: calories 210, fat 11 g, cholesterol 0 mg, sodium 240 mg, carbohydrates 29 g, fiber 6 g, sugar 9 g, protein 2 g.

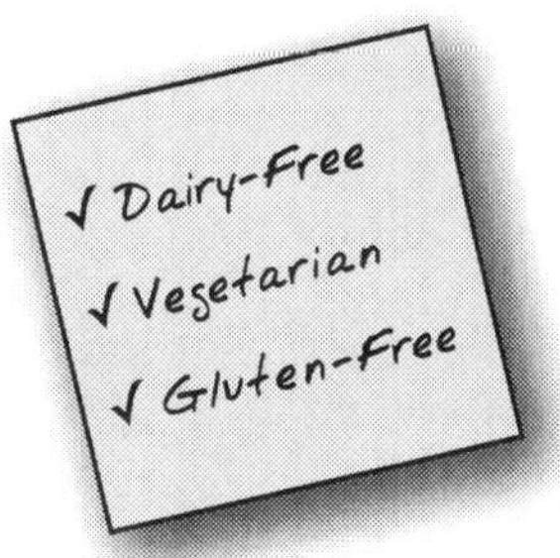

Salmon Florentine

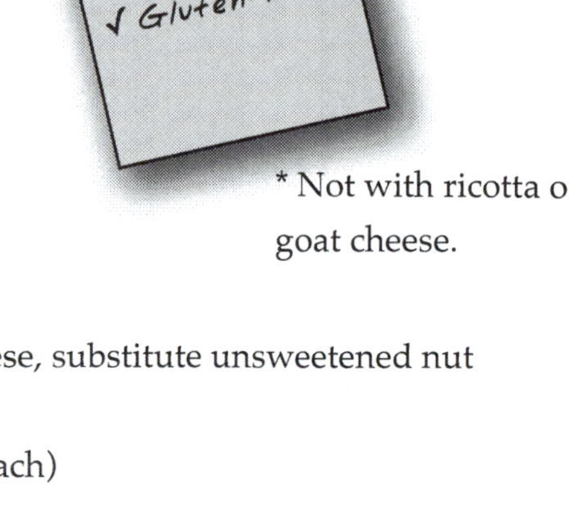

* Not with ricotta or goat cheese.

10 ounces spinach
1 tablespoon olive oil
¼ cup minced shallots
2 teaspoons minced garlic
5 sun-dried tomatoes, chopped
½ teaspoon salt
¼ teaspoon red pepper flakes
¼ teaspoon fresh ground pepper
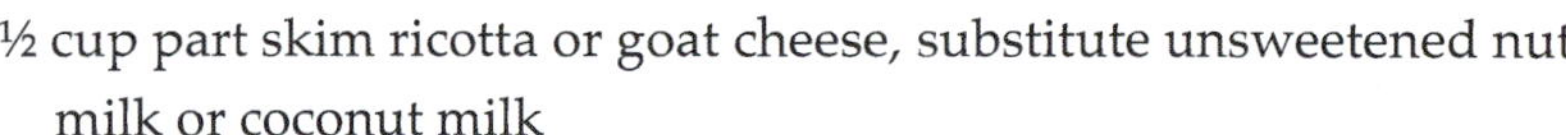
½ cup part skim ricotta or goat cheese, substitute unsweetened nut milk or coconut milk
4 skinless salmon fillets (6 ounces each)

Heat oven to 350°F. Heat oil in a large skillet over medium heat. Add shallots; cook, stirring until soft, which should take about 3 minutes. Add garlic, then cook 1 minutes more. Add spinach, tomatoes, salt, pepper flakes and pepper, then stir and cook 2 minutes more. Remove from heat and let cool about 15 minutes. Add ricotta, then stir to combine. Season with salt and pepper. Pack ½ cup spinach mixture on top of each fillet, matching the shape of the fillet. Place fillets on a rimmed baking sheet or in a glass baking dish, then bake until cooked through—about 15 minutes. Serve with a side of quinoa.

Makes 4 servings.

Nutrition per serving: calories 334, fat 14 g, cholesterol 50 mg, sodium 300 mg, carbohydrates 11 g, fiber 8 g, sugar 0 g, protein 43 g.

Salmon with Buckwheat Noodles[23]

1¼ pounds fresh skinless salmon fillet, about 1-inch thick
¼ cup olive oil
¼ cup balsamic vinegar
1 tablespoon cracked black pepper
½ pound buckwheat (or whole wheat) noodles
⅓ cup orange juice
1 oranges, peeled, sectioned, and chopped
1 clove garlic, minced
½ of a red onion, chopped or 2 green onions, thinly sliced
2 teaspoons anise seed, crushed

√ Dairy-Free
√ Gluten-Free

Combine 1 tablespoon of olive oil and 1 tablespoon balsamic vinegar and cracked pepper in a baking dish. Place fish in the mixture, turning to coat both sides. Marinate at room temperature for 10 minutes. Place salmon on rack of a broiler pan. Broil 4-inches from the heat for 4 to 5 minutes per ½-inch thickness of fish. Meanwhile, cook buckwheat noodles in boiling water in a large saucepan for 4 minutes until just slightly chewy. Drain and place in a large bowl. Add remaining oil and vinegar, the orange juice and orange sections, garlic, onion and anise seed, then toss to coat. To serve, divide noodle mixture among 4 dinner bowls and top each with a piece of salmon.

Makes 4 servings.

Nutrition per serving: calories 372, fat 6 g, cholesterol 25 mg, sodium 538 mg, carbohydrates 55 g, fiber 2 g, sugar 15 g, protein 29 g.

Savory Meatballs

1 pound lean ground turkey breast
½ cup part-skim ricotta cheese
1 egg
½ cup dry breadcrumbs
¼ cup chopped fresh basil
¼ teaspoon pepper
¼ teaspoon salt

Preheat oven to 375°F. Combine one pound ground turkey breast with above ingredients in a bowl, then shape mixture into about 18 meatballs. Heat a large nonstick skillet over medium-high heat. Coat pan with cooking spray. Add meatballs, then brown on all sides. Remove from skillet and transfer to broiler pan coated with cooking spray, then bake for 15 minutes or until done.

Makes 4 servings.

Nutrition per serving: calories 237, total fat 6.2 g, saturated fat 2.7 g, sodium 388 mg, carbohydrates 11.7 g, fiber 0.3 g, protein 33.5 g.

Sesame Noodles

1 package (8 ounces) of brown rice or quinoa spaghetti (to reduce calories, substitute with Miracle Noodle®—page 481)
¼ cup, reduced sodium tamari
2 tablespoons sesame tahini
2 tablespoons smooth almond butter
1 tablespoon brown rice vinegar
1 tablespoon lemon juice
1 tablespoon sesame oil
1 cup shredded cabbage
1 cup sliced green onions
½ tablespoon toasted sesame seeds

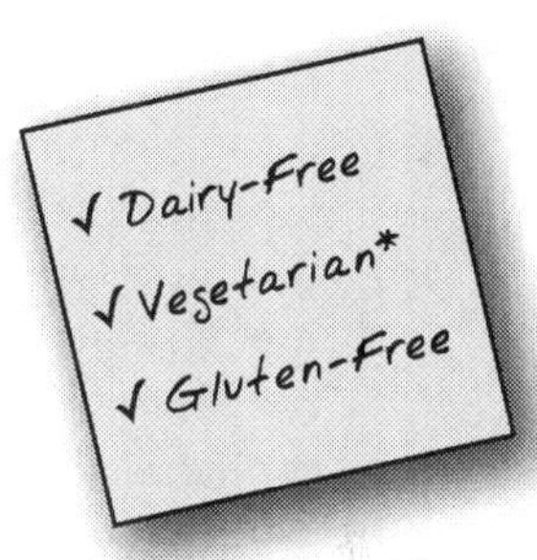

* Not with optional chicken or shrimp.

Optional:
Hot sauce to taste
Cooked or grilled chicken or shrimp

Cook pasta until al dente. Drain pasta thoroughly. In a large bowl, whisk together tamari tahini, almond butter, vinegar, lemon juice and toasted sesame oil. Add pasta, cabbage and green onions. Toss to coat noodles thoroughly with sauce. Sprinkle with sesame seeds. Add optional hot sauce and/or cooked or grilled chicken or shrimp.

Makes 4 servings.

Nutrition per serving: calories 390, fat 14 g, cholesterol 0 mg, sodium 970 mg, carbohydrates 55 g, fiber 4 g, sugar 4 g, protein 10 g.

Simple Grilled Chicken Breast[24]

4 (about 1½ pounds total) boneless, skinless chicken breast halves
2 tablespoons olive oil
½ teaspoon tarragon
½ teaspoon freshly ground black pepper

Rub the chicken breasts with the olive oil and spices. Preheat an outdoor grill, or a grill pan that has been brushed with olive oil to medium-high. Grill or sauté the chicken for about 4 to 5 minutes on each side, or until the juices run clear. Cooking time will vary with the thickness of the chicken.

Makes 4 servings (serving size of 4 ounces).

Nutrition per serving: calories 245, total fat 11 g, saturated fat 2.1 g, carbohydrates 0 g, protein 34 g.

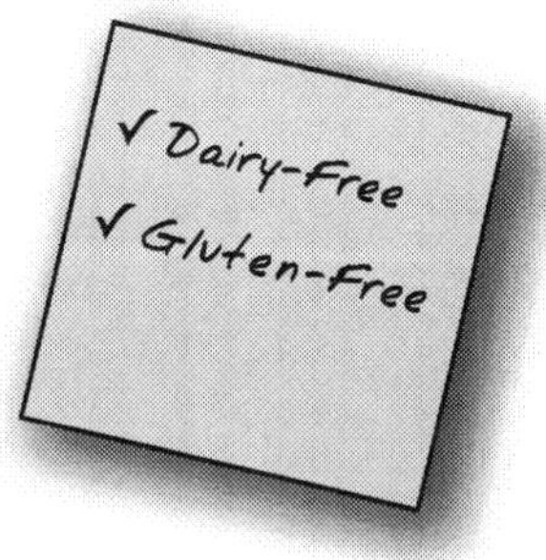

Simple Steamed Artichokes[25]

4 large artichokes
1 fresh lemon
½ teaspoon kosher salt

Trim the artichoke leaves and stems. Rub the cut surfaces with fresh lemon. Place the artichokes upside down on a steaming rack over boiling water. Cook for 25 to 30 minutes, or until a leaf pulls out easily from the artichoke and the bottom is tender when pierced with a small knife or fork. Place the cooked artichokes in a bowl of ice water or rinse under cold water to stop the cooking. Transfer to a plate and place upside down to drain. Serve cold or at room temperature.

Alternate method: If you don't have a steaming rack you may place the artichokes in a pot or deep sauté pan large enough to hold them in a single layer. Put 1-inch of boiling water in the pot with ½ teaspoon salt. Bring to a simmer and cook the artichokes, covered, for 25 to 30 minutes. Then, continue as above with the steaming method.

Makes 4 servings.

Nutrition per serving: calories 85, fat 0 g, carbohydrates 20 g, fiber 10 g, protein 7 g.

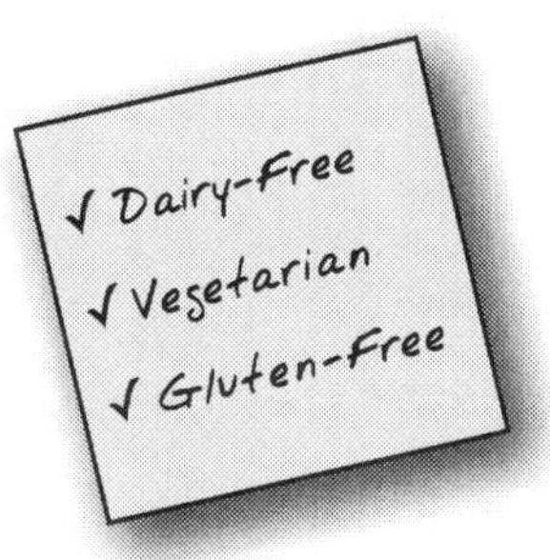

Simple Sweet Potato

1 medium sweet potato
1 teaspoon ground cinnamon

Optional: ½ tablespoon butter

Wash sweet potato with water and rub off dirt. Do not dry. Pierce potato lightly with a fork about 8 to 10 times. Wrap potato in a paper towel—potato should still be wet. Place potato on a dish, then microwave for 8 minutes, rotate and cook for another 1 to 2 minutes. When potato is cool, cut down the middle and sprinkle with cinnamon and butter.

Makes 1 serving.

Nutrition per serving: calories 205, fat 2.75 g, cholesterol 7.5 mg, sodium 95.75 mg, carbohydrates 41 g, fiber 7 g, sugar 13 g, protein 4 g.

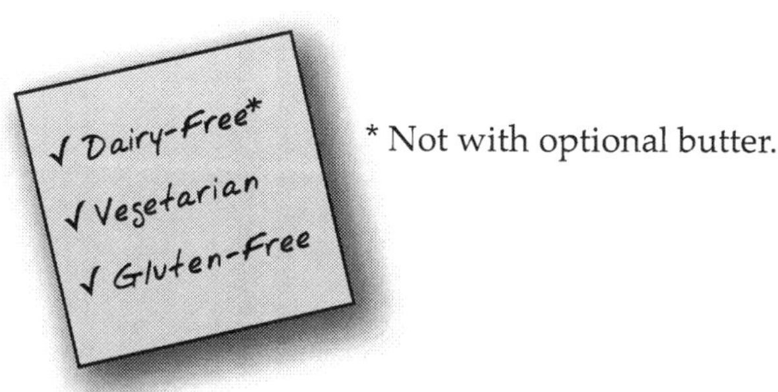

* Not with optional butter.

Skillet Broccoli (or Asparagus) with Sesame Seeds

2 large stalks fresh broccoli (or 12 to 14 asparagus spears)
2 tablespoons olive oil
2 tablespoons sesame seeds
2 or 3 cloves garlic, peeled and sliced

Optional: salt and pepper to taste

Wash broccoli and cut the florets into medium to large pieces. Peel the outer layer from the stems and slice the inner tender, juicy portion in half. (If using asparagus, wash the spears and trim off the ends.) In a large skillet with a lid, heat the oil over high heat. Add sesame seeds and sauté, stirring until lightly toasted (be careful not to overcook as they tend to burn quickly). Keep the lid handy because the sesame seeds may start to pop. Add the broccoli or asparagus and garlic, then stir for a few seconds. Add optional salt and pepper to taste, then stir. Cover the skillet and remove from heat, then let sit for about 15 minutes. The broccoli or asparagus will retain their color and be tender and crisp.

Makes 6 servings.

Nutrition per serving: calories 70, total fat 6 g, saturated fat 1 g, carbohydrates 3 g, fiber 1 g, protein 1 g.

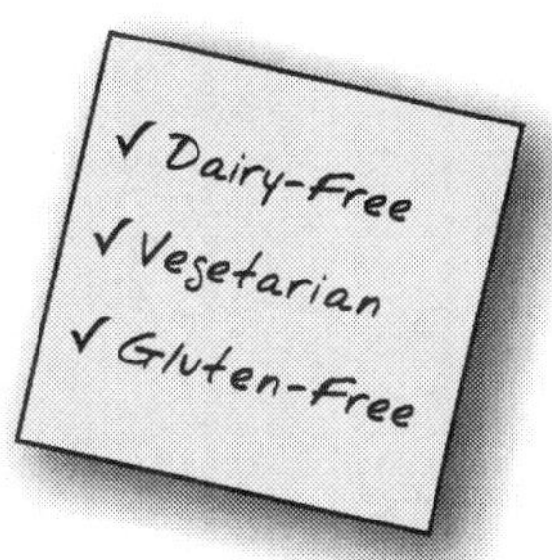

Skillet Zucchini

1 tablespoon olive oil
1 teaspoon minced garlic
2 medium zucchinis
½ teaspoon salt substitute
¼ teaspoon pepper

Optional: 1 tablespoon parmesan cheese

Coat a large nonstick skillet with 1 tablespoon olive oil and place over medium heat. Add 1 teaspoon minced garlic and sauté for 1 minute. Add 2 medium zucchinis (sliced and halved), then sprinkle with ½ teaspoon salt substitute and ¼ teaspoon pepper. Cook until zucchini is tender, stirring occasionally. Sprinkle with 1 tablespoon Parmesan cheese (optional).

Makes 4 servings.

Nutrition per serving: calories 16, total fat 0.5 g, saturated fat 0.3 g, carbohydrates 2.3 g, fiber 0.3 g, protein 1.3 g.

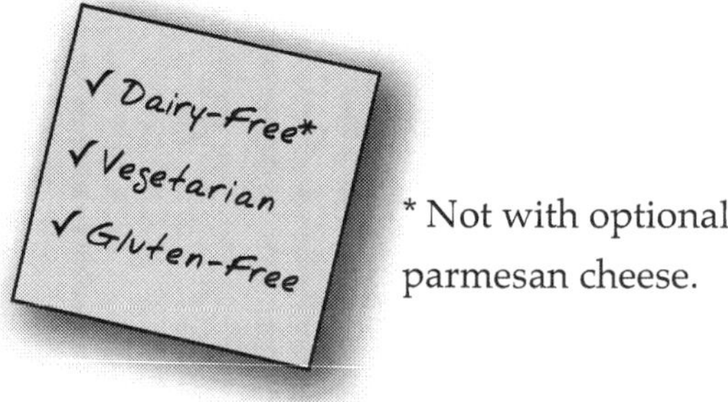

* Not with optional parmesan cheese.

Smothered Mushrooms and Kale

2 tablespoons olive oil
4 garlic cloves, chopped
24 small cremini mushrooms, wiped clean and halved
1¼ pounds kale (1 large bunch)
¼ cup sherry
Black pepper

Heat a medium skillet with the olive oil over medium to medium-high heat. Add the mushrooms and place a lid which is too small for the skillet down into the pan, thereby pressing and smothering the mushrooms. Cook them for 5 or 6 minutes, stirring once, then add the garlic. Cook another minute or two. While the mushrooms cook, strip the kale from its stems and coarsely chop. Add to the pan with the mushrooms, turning the kale with tongs to combine it with the mushrooms. Smother the greens for a minute or two, then add the sherry.

Makes 4 servings.

Nutrition per serving: calories 168, total fat 8.2 g, saturated fat 1.1 g, sodium 110 mg, carbohydrates 16.8 g, fiber 3.5 g, protein 6.8 g.

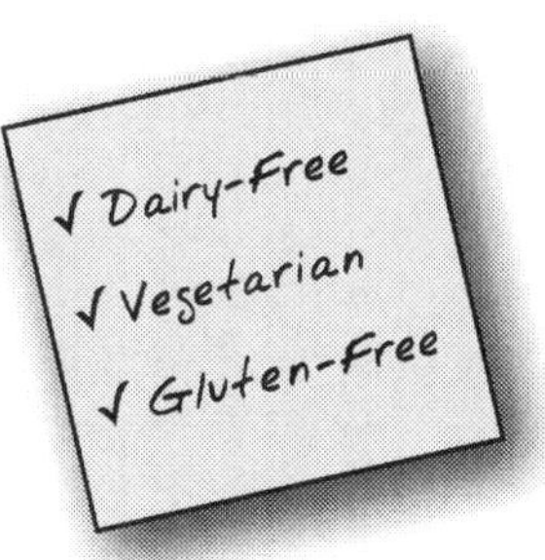

Southwestern Stuffed Sweet Potato

1 baked sweet potato
1 can of organic black beans
½ can organic fire-roasted tomatoes
1 lime
1 shallot
1 garlic clove
1 teaspoon chili powder
1 pinch of cayenne
½ teaspoon cumin
Sea salt and pepper to taste
1 tablespoon olive oil

Sauté shallot and garlic in olive oil. Add chili powder, cayenne, cumin, sea salt, pepper, and zest of one lime. Add black beans and ½ can organic fire-roasted tomatoes. Top baked sweet potato and serve.

Optional: top with scallions, goat cheese, or shredded cheese.

Makes 1 to 2 servings.

Nutrition per serving: calories 370, fat 2.3 g, cholesterol 0 mg, sodium 472 mg, carbohydrates 70.8 g, fiber 14 g, sugar 21.9 g, protein 9 g.

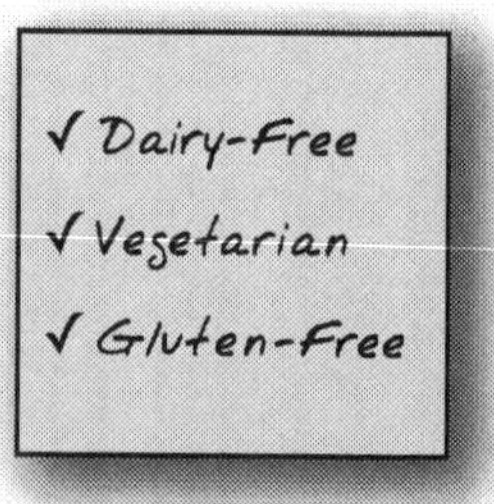

Spaghetti Squash

1 spaghetti squash (about 3½ pounds)

Preheat oven to 375°F and halve squash lengthwise. Use a spoon to scoop out and discard seeds from the middle of each half. Arrange squash in a 9x13 casserole dish, cut sides down. Pour ½ cup water into the dish and bake until just tender (30 to 35 minutes). Rake a fork back and forth across the squash to remove its flesh in strands like spaghetti.

Makes 6 servings (serving size of 9 ounces).

Nutrition per serving: calories 70, total fat 0.5 g, saturated fat 0 g, sodium 50 mg, carbohydrates 17 g, fiber 4 g, protein 2 g.

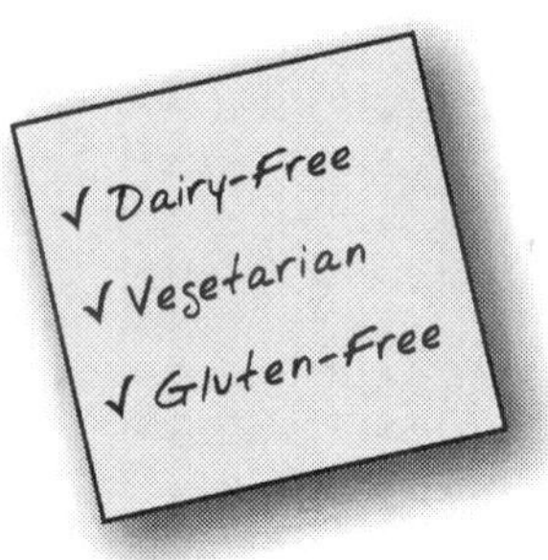

Spiced Cauliflower

1 large cauliflower, broken into flowerets
1 tablespoon olive oil
1 teaspoon ground coriander
1 teaspoon ground black pepper
1 large onion, chopped
1 tablespoon turmeric

Steam the cauliflower 10 minutes. Meanwhile, heat the oil in a pan over low heat and briefly fry the coriander and black pepper. Add the onion and stir-fry for 3 to 5 minutes until translucent. Add the turmeric. Stir in the cauliflower until well-coated and serve.

Makes 4 servings.

Nutrition per serving: calories 48, total fat 3.6 g, saturated fat 0.6 g, sodium 2 mg, carbohydrates 3.6 g, fiber 1 g, protein 0.5 g.

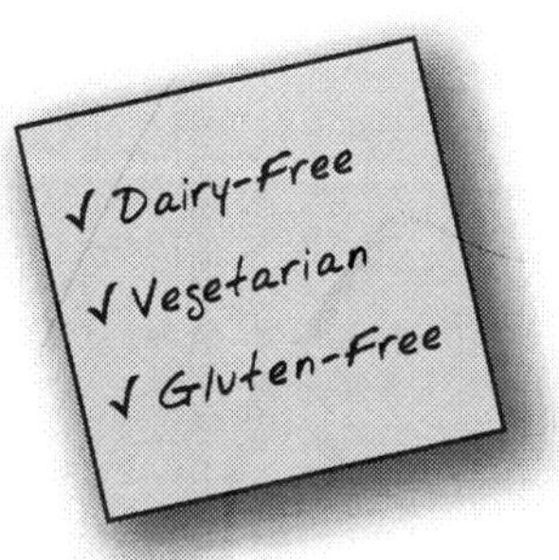

Spicy Grilled Tuna with Salsa[26]

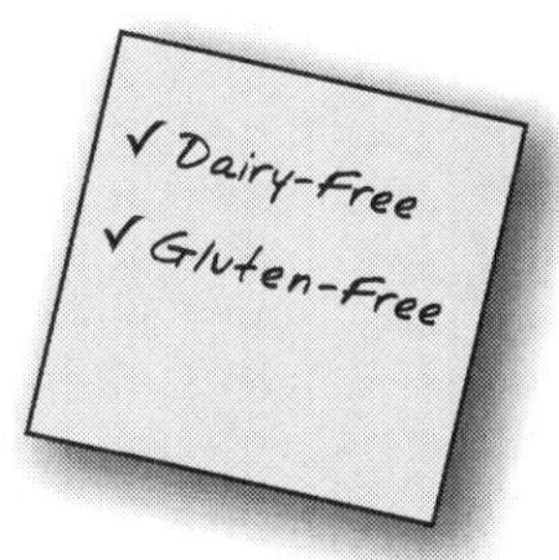

6 cloves garlic (large), peeled
3 jalapeño chilies, stemmed
¼ cup fresh lime juice
1 teaspoon salt
4 tuna steaks (5 ounces each)
2 cups diced heirloom tomatoes
¼ cup red onion, diced
1 tablespoon fresh cilantro, finely chopped
1 tablespoon fresh mint, finely chopped
1 tablespoon fresh basil, finely chopped
Olive oil cooking spray

Roast garlic and jalapeños in a small, dry skillet over medium heat, turning occasionally, until soft, both will blacken in spots: 5 to 10 minutes for jalapeños, 15 minutes for garlic. Cool, then peel garlic. Puree garlic, jalapeños, lime juice and ½ teaspoon salt in a blender until smooth. Scoop ½ cup puree into a glass baking dish. Place fish on puree, flipping once to coat both sides. Cover dish and refrigerate 10 to 20 minutes to marinate. Transfer remaining puree into another bowl for salsa. Mix in tomatoes. Rinse onion in a small strainer under cold water, then drain. Add to tomato mixture. Stir in cilantro, mint and basil. Season with ½ teaspoon salt. Coat grill with cooking spray, then heat to medium-high (about 375°F). Remove fish from marinade and place on grill. Cover grill and cook 3 minutes, then flip fish and cook until done—about 2 more minutes for medium rare. Place on plate, then spoon salsa on top. Serve with spring mix or side of steamed vegetables.

Makes 4 to 5 servings. Nutrition per serving: calories 237, fat 7.2 g, carbohydrates 7.8 g, fiber 1.6 g, protein 34.4 g.

Sweet Lentil Brussels Burger[27]

2 cups cooked lentils
1 sweet potato (small), steamed and mashed
1 cup Brussels sprouts (steamed)
¾ teaspoon ground ginger
½ teaspoon turmeric
½ teaspoon paprika
1 teaspoon cumin
1 teaspoon ground coriander
½ teaspoon dulse flakes or ½ teaspoon sea salt

Place ingredients into food processor and pulse until combined. If texture is wanted, do not pulse all the way. Form into patties. Place over medium heat on a lightly oiled skillet and cook 3 to 4 minutes on each side. Note: for crispy crust, coat burgers in garbanzo bean flour. Serve in romaine lettuce with ketchup or avocado cream (blend: 1 avocado, 1 tablespoon apple cider vinegar and 5 tablespoons water) or top with arugula and sliced tomatoes.

Makes 6 to 8 servings.

Nutrition per serving: calories 180, fat 5 g, cholesterol 0 mg, sodium 44 mg, carbohydrates 30 g, fiber 8 g, sugar 4 g, protein 10 g.

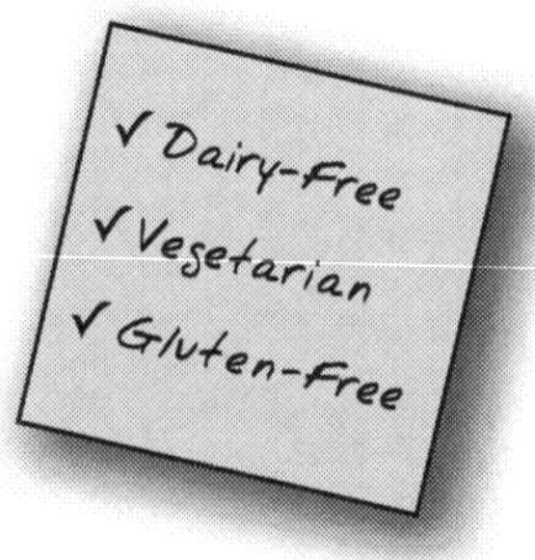

Sweet Potato Fries

2 sweet potatoes, peeled and sliced into thin strips
Cooking spray
Black pepper
Garlic powder
Paprika
Salt, to taste
1 tablespoon olive oil

Preheat oven to 450°F. Mix pepper, garlic powder, salt and olive oil. Line a sheet tray with parchment paper. In a large bowl, toss sweet potatoes in with mix to coat. Sprinkle with paprika and spread sweet potatoes in a single layer on baking sheet. Bake about 25 minutes or until sweet potatoes are golden brown, turning occasionally.

Makes 3 to 4 servings.

Nutrition per serving: calories 160, fat 4.5 g, cholesterol 0 mg, sodium 48 mg, carbohydrates 27.3 g, fiber 4.6 g, sugar 8.6 g, protein 2.67 g.

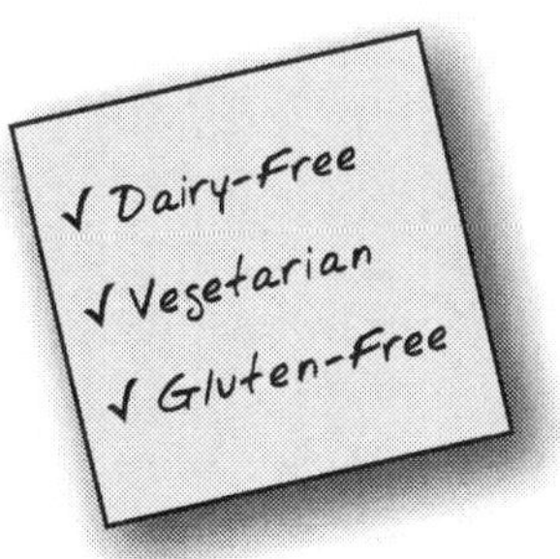

Swiss Chard with Shallots

1 tablespoon olive oil
1 shallot, finely chopped
⅛ teaspoon red pepper flakes
2 bunches Swiss chard, rinsed well
1 tablespoon apple cider vinegar
½ teaspoon salt

Cut off and discard chard stems and any tough center ribs. Thinly slice leaves. Heat oil in large skillet over medium high heat. Add shallot and pepper flakes, then cook, stirring often, until softened—about 2 minutes. Add chard, vinegar and salt, then continue cooking, while tossing often—until wilted and softened—for 3 to 4 minutes more.

Makes 4 servings.

Nutrition per serving: calories 90, fat 7 g, cholesterol 10 mg, sodium 680 mg, carbohydrates 7 g, sugar 2 g, fiber 3 g, protein 3 g.

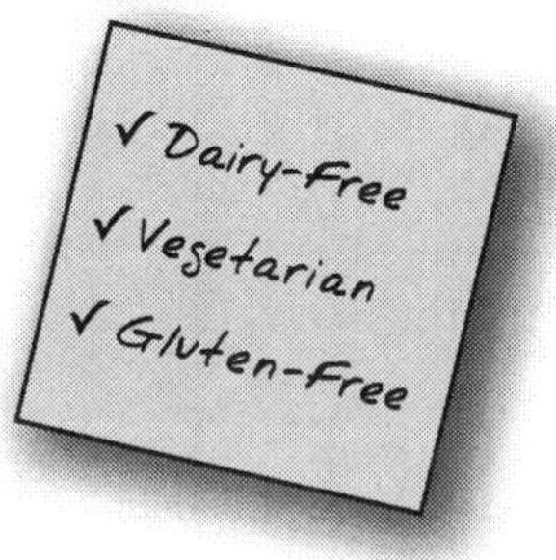

Thai Chicken Peanut Butter Pasta

Pasta of choice (quinoa, buckwheat, whole wheat or Miracle Noodle®—page 481)
3 chicken breasts, grilled or roasted
2 carrots, julienned
3 scallions, chopped
2 cups spinach, chopped
1 cup broccoli, chopped
1 cup mung bean sprouts
¼ cup fresh cilantro, chopped
1 cup dry roasted, chopped peanuts (¼ cup for sauce)

Sauce:
4 tablespoons creamy natural peanut butter
4 tablespoons low-sodium soy sauce or tamari
4 tablespoons hot water
2 teaspoons sesame oil
1 tablespoon ground ginger
1 dash of cayenne

Cook pasta until tender. While pasta is cooking, whisk together ingredients for peanut sauce. Add ¼ cup remaining peanuts into sauce. Toss pasta with chicken, carrots, scallions and bean sprouts, then pour peanut sauce over gently and toss to coat. Garnish with cilantro and remaining peanuts.

Makes 3 servings.

Nutrition per serving: calories 468, fat 21 g, cholesterol 68 mg, sodium 1679 g, carbohydrates 26 g, fiber 5.97 g, sugar 3.91 g, protein 7.53 g.

Vegetable Chips

2 parsnips, large
1 beet
1 zucchini
2 tablespoons pure, organic butter
1 tablespoon sea salt
1 tablespoon chopped parsley

Using a mandoline slicer, slice the vegetables into diagonal coin-size slices. Place on baking sheet. Melt butter and drizzle over vegetables. Top vegetables with a bit of sea salt and parsley. Bake at 400°F for 1 hour, or until crispy. Enjoy with salad or dip into guacamole or salsa.

Makes 4 servings.

Nutrition per serving: calories 130, fat 5.85 g, cholesterol 15 mg, sodium 95.25 mg, carbohydrates 15.5 g, fiber 5 g, sugar 8 g, protein 2.25 g.

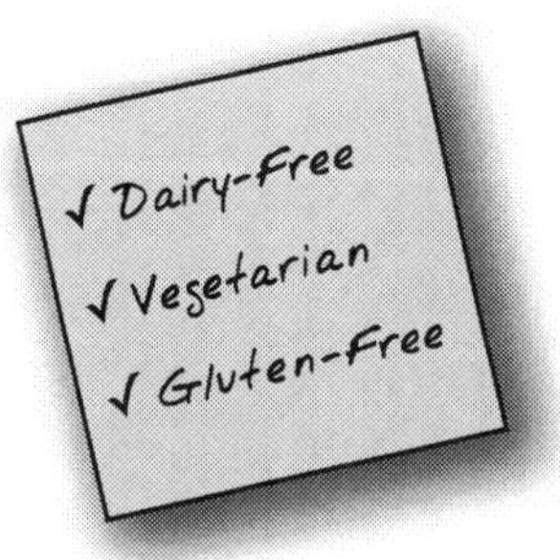

Vegetable Stir-Fry

Other vegetable combinations may also be used with this recipe.

1 tablespoon olive oil
1 medium zucchini, diced
Medium red pepper, diced
1 cup broccoli, sliced
1 cup cauliflower, sliced
Freshly ground pepper to taste

Optional: 2 tablespoons shredded fresh basil

Heat olive oil in skillet over medium high heat. Add vegetables and stir-fry until vegetables are crisp-cooked—2 to 3 minutes. Remove from the heat and stir in the basil and pepper.

Makes 4 servings.

Nutrition per serving: calories 67, total fat 3.7 g, saturated fat 0.5 g, sodium 16 mg, carbohydrates 6.3 g, fiber 2.6 g, protein 2 g.

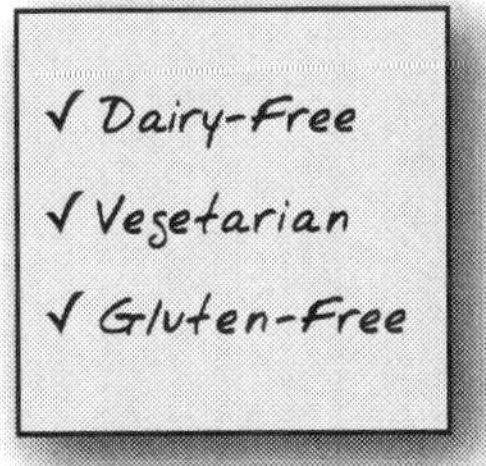

Wilted Spinach with Tomatoes

2 tablespoons olive oil
½ pint grape tomatoes
2 garlic cloves, chopped
Black pepper
1 pound spinach, triple washed, stemmed and coarsely chopped

Preheat a large skillet over medium-high heat with the olive oil. Add the grape tomatoes and cook until they start to burst, 4 to 5 minutes. Add the garlic, season the tomatoes with pepper, then cook for 2 more minutes. Add the spinach, turning it until partially wilted.

Makes 4 servings.

Nutrition per serving: calories 104, total fat 7.3 g, saturated fat 1 g, sodium 107 mg, carbohydrates 5.8 g, fiber 3.5 g, protein 3.8 g.

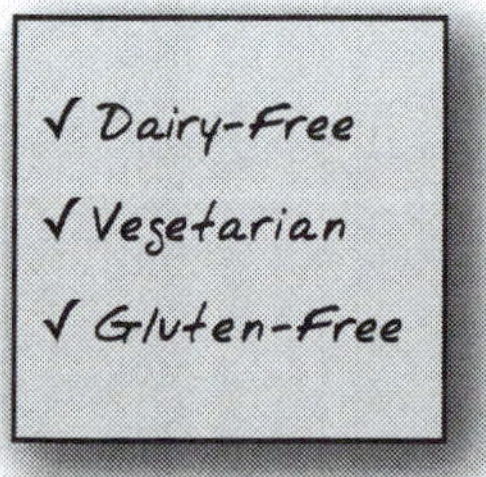

Zucchini Noodle Pasta

6 to 8 zucchinis, firm

2 garlic cloves, peeled

2 tablespoons extra virgin olive oil

Sea salt to taste

Optional:

Add tomato sauce

Add sun-dried tomato and basil

Add vegetables

Use a vegetable slicer to make thin, long noodles out of zucchini. If a slicer is not available, use a sharp knife to quarter the zucchini lengthwise, then cut into thinnest strips possible. Place ½ tablespoon olive oil in pan and roast the garlic. Add zucchini noodles and cook until warm. Turn off heat and drizzle olive oil.

Makes 4 servings.

Nutrition per serving: calories 142, fat 9.23 g, cholesterol 0 mg, sodium 33 mg, carbohydrates 15.92 g, fiber 5 g, protein 4 g, sugar 7.3 g.

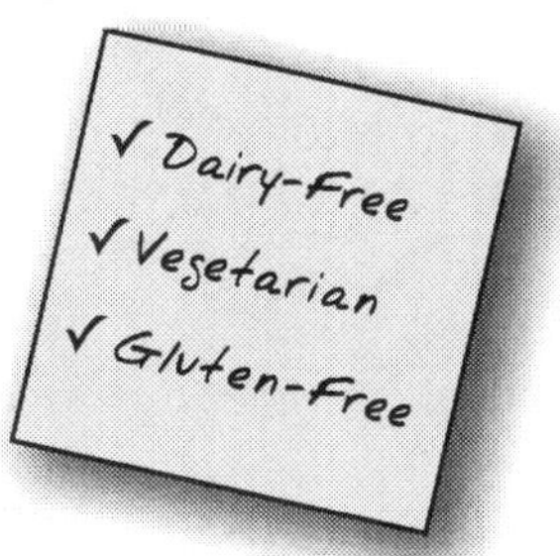

Recipes: Salads and Dressings

"If you have a complete set of salad bowls and they all say Cool Whip on the side, you might be a redneck."
— Jeff Foxworthy

Asian Chicken Salad[1]

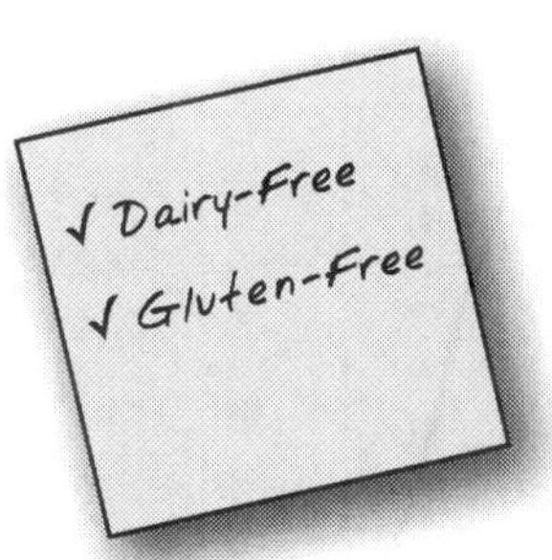

2 ounces snow peas, strings removed
3 cups cooked chicken breast, shredded
½ cup thinly sliced red bell pepper
½ cup julienne carrots
¼ cup onion
2 tablespoons toasted sesame seeds

Bring a large pan of salted water to a boil. Drop in the snow peas and cook for 30 seconds. Drain, and immediately place in a bowl of ice water to stop the cooking. Drain again, and cut the snow peas on the diagonal into thin slices. Place the snow peas in a large bowl. Add the chicken, red pepper, carrot and onions, then stir to combine. For salad dressing use *Lime-Rice Wine Vinaigrette* (page 409).

Makes 4 servings.

Nutrition per serving: calories 239, total fat 5.6 g, saturated fat 1 g, sodium 112 mg, carbohydrates 5.8 g, fiber 2.1 g, protein 41.3 g.

Apple, Almond, Spinach, Quinoa Salad [2]

√ Dairy-Free
√ Vegetarian
√ Gluten-Free

1 cup uncooked quinoa, washed well
3 tablespoons olive oil
1 cup chopped onion
2 to 3 cups chopped baby spinach
1 cup diced carrot
2 to 3 garlic cloves, minced
2 cups vegetable broth (low sodium, pacific brand is good)
½ teaspoon cinnamon
1½ cups diced granny smith apple, not peeled
15 to 20 almonds, toasted, can be sliced
½ cup dried cranberries
Sea salt (¼ to ½ teaspoon) and black pepper to taste
1 tablespoon maple syrup
1 teaspoon vanilla

Heat 1 tablespoon olive oil in pan over medium heat. Add chopped onion, carrots and garlic, then sauté until the onion is translucent. Add broth, quinoa, salt and cinnamon, then bring to a boil. Reduce heat to simmer, cover and let sit for 20 minutes or until liquid is gone. Be sure to keep an eye on it and stir often so it doesn't burn. Remove from heat, then stir to fluff. Meanwhile, heat oven to 350°F and toast almonds. Roughly chop toasted almonds, or use sliced almonds.
Heat 1 teaspoon olive oil in a nonstick pot or skillet. Add chopped apple and vanilla and sauté for about 5 minutes until apple starts to turn golden in color—but before it gets mushy. Add apple, spinach, almonds, cranberries and pepper to quinoa and mix thoroughly. Serve hot or cold, as a main dish or a side with a protein source.

Makes 4 to 5 servings. Nutrition per serving: calories 209, fat 6.2 g, cholesterol 0 mg, sodium 237 mg, carbohydrates 35.6 g, fiber 4.19 g, sugar 19.8 g, protein 3.43 g.

Apple Cabbage Salad

2 cups shredded green cabbage
2 cups shredded red cabbage
2 tablespoons Vegenaise® or olive oil
⅛ teaspoon sea salt
⅛ teaspoon black pepper
2 gala apples, very thinly sliced
½ cup walnuts, toasted and chopped
2 tablespoons chopped cilantro

Optional: add shredded turkey or chicken

Toss together cabbage, oil, salt and pepper. Add apples and walnuts and toss.

Makes 4 to 6 servings.

Nutrition per serving: calories 120, fat 8 g, cholesterol 0 mg, sodium 70 mg, carbohydrates 12 g, fiber 3 g, sugar 7 g, protein 4 g.

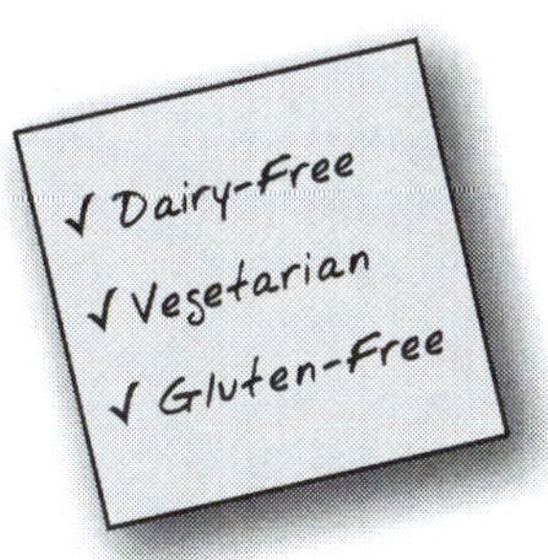

Baby Greens and Roasted Butternut Squash

4 cups baby greens
1 cup roasted butternut squash cubes
1 handful toasted pumpkin seeds

Preheat oven to 375°F. Peel and remove seeds from butternut squash. Cut flesh of butternut squash into small cubes and place on baking tray. Drizzle with extra virgin olive oil or coconut oil and a pinch of salt, then roast for 45 minutes until brown. In a large salad bowl, mix baby greens with roasted butternut squash. Sprinkle with pumpkin seeds and drizzle with balsamic or lemon vinaigrette.

Makes 1 serving.

Nutrition per serving: calories 181, fat 4.95 g, cholesterol 0 mg, sodium 360 mg, carbohydrates 29.5 g, fiber 4.4 g, sugar 8 g, protein 10 g.

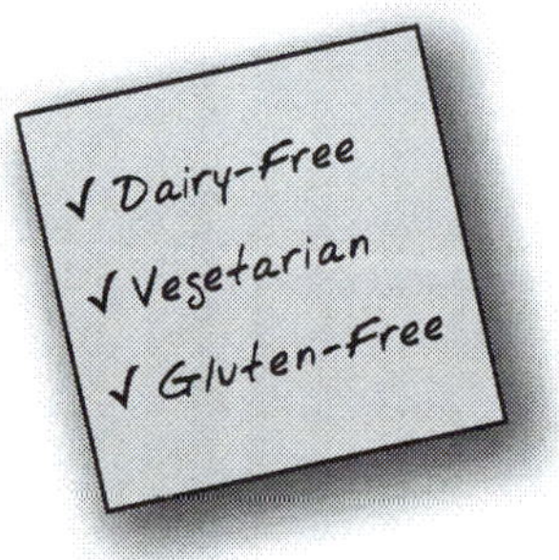

Basic Vinaigrette[3]

2 tablespoons fresh lemon juice
1 medium clove garlic, minced
½ teaspoon black pepper
1 teaspoon spices (basil, oregano, rosemary or thyme)
6 tablespoons extra-virgin olive oil

In a small bowl, combine the lemon juice, garlic, spices and pepper. Slowly whisk in the olive oil until the dressing is slightly thickened. Or, place all ingredients in a jar with a tight-fitting lid and shake until well combined.

Makes 8 servings (serving size of 2 tablespoons).

Nutrition per serving: calories 190, total fat 21 g, saturated fat 2.9 g, carbohydrates 0 g.

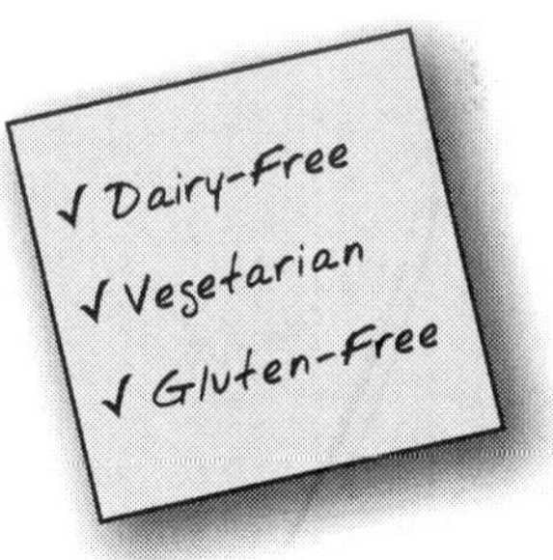

Broccoli Apple Chicken Salad with Poppyseed Dressing

6 cups broccoli florets, chopped
1 or 2 large Fuji apples, diced
½ cup dried cranberries
½ cup walnuts, chopped
Chopped parsley
8 ounces Brianna's Poppy Seed Dressing
2 chicken breasts, cooked and chopped

Optional: add romaine lettuce or spinach

Mix ingredients together. Toss with dressing.

Makes 4 servings.

Nutrition per serving: calories 314, fat 14.5 g, cholesterol 34 mg, sodium 304 g, carbohydrates 27.5 g, fiber 4.75 g, sugar 14.25 g, protein 18.125 g.

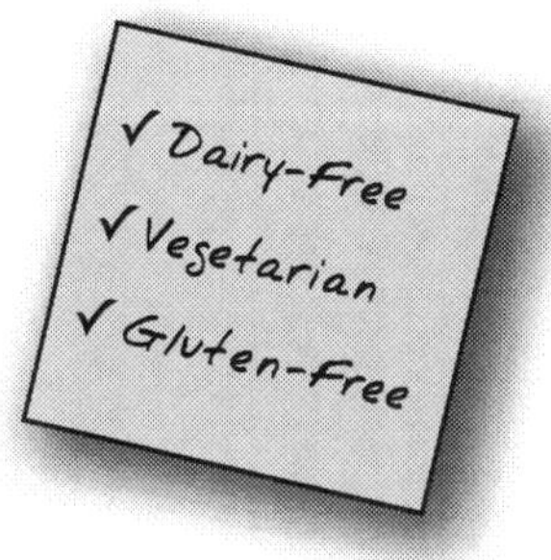

Butternut Squash and Kale Salad[4]

2 bunches kale, tough stems and ribs stripped out, leaves sliced

1 cup low sodium vegetable broth

1 butternut squash, peeled, seeded and cut into ½-inch cubes

1 red onion, sliced

4 pitted dates, finely chopped

2 tablespoons sherry vinegar

Put kale and ½ cup vegetable broth in a large pot and place over medium heat. Cook, covered, stirring frequently, until kale is wilted—about 3 minutes. Add squash and continue cooking, stirring occasionally, until kale and squash are tender but not mushy—10 to 12 minutes. Cool to room temperature. Meanwhile, combine the remaining ½ cup of broth, onion, dates and vinegar in a small saucepan. Bring to a boil, lower heat and simmer uncovered until onion is very tender and liquid is reduced by half—about 6 minutes. Cool, toss with kale and butternut squash. Serve at room temperature or chilled.

Makes 8 servings.

Nutrition per serving: calories 100, fat 0.5 g, cholesterol 0 mg, sodium 45 mg, carbohydrates 24 g, fiber 4 g, sugar 6 g, protein 3 g.

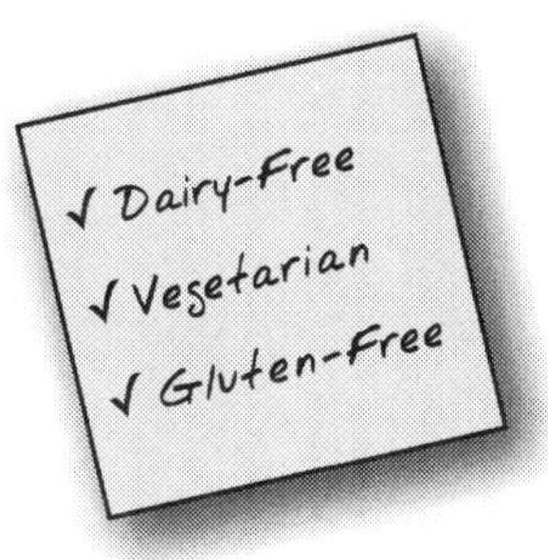

Cabbage-Apple Salad

1 cup shredded cabbage
1 cup diced apple
1 cup chopped celery
¼ cup plain low-fat yogurt
2 tablespoons flaxseed

Mix all ingredients in a large bowl. Toss, chill and serve.

Makes 6 servings.

Nutrition per serving: calories 45, total fat 2 g, saturated fat 0 g, sodium 25 mg, carbohydrates 7 g, fiber 2 g, protein 2 g.

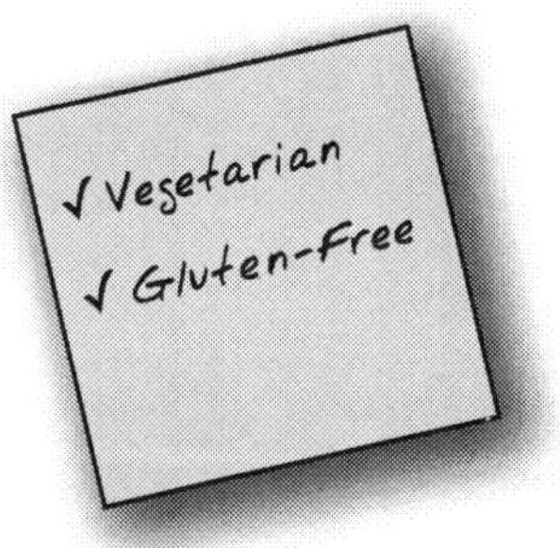

Carrot Ginger Dressing

1 large carrot, peeled and chopped
1 large shallot, peeled and chopped
2 tablespoons chopped fresh ginger
2 tablespoons rice wine vinegar
1 tablespoon sweet white miso
1 tablespoon sesame seed oil
¼ cup grapeseed oil
2 tablespoons water

Blend all ingredients in blender until smooth.

Makes 5 to 6 servings.

Nutrition per serving: calories 111, fat 11.25 g, cholesterol 0 mg, sodium 379.8 mg, carbohydrates 2.7 g, fiber 0.4 g, sugar 1.2 g, protein 0.4 g.

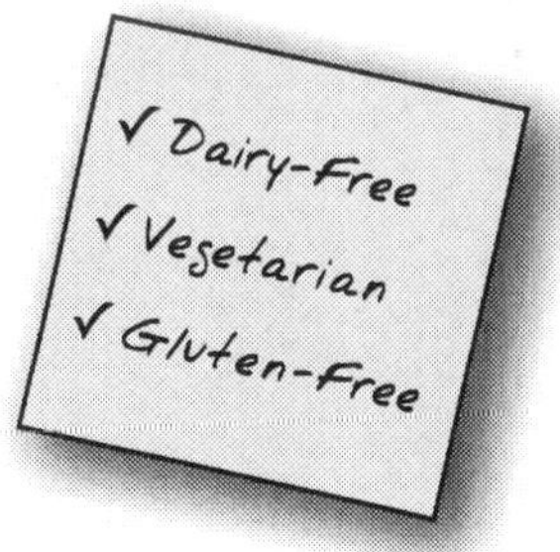

Citrus Salad Dressing

1 clementine orange (squeezed and scrape out pulp and use that)
1 tablespoon lime juice
1 tablespoon raw honey
1 teaspoon whole grain mustard
½ tablespoon Himalayan salt
½ tablespoon fresh ground black pepper
1 tablespoon extra virgin olive oil

Mix ingredients in a bowl and blend until smooth.

Makes 3 to 4 servings.

Nutrition per serving: calories 62, fat 3.75 g, cholesterol 0 mg, sodium 418.1 mg, carbohydrates 7 g, fiber 1 g, sugar 5 g.

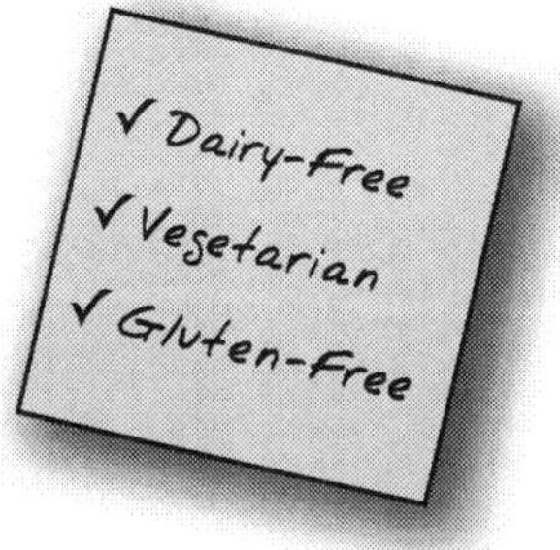

Creamy Coleslaw

4 cups shredded cabbage
1 cup grated carrots
1 cup plain low-fat yogurt
½ cup organic mayonnaise
1½ tablespoons finely chopped celery
1 teaspoon grated onion
3 tablespoons white vinegar
1 packet stevia
1 teaspoon Mrs. Dash® salt free seasoning
Dash of pepper

Mix all ingredients in a large bowl and toss well. Refrigerate at least 2 hours before serving.

Makes 10 servings.

Nutrition per serving: calories 119, total fat 9.5 g, saturated fat 1.6 g, sodium 105 mg, carbohydrates 6.1 g, fiber 1.2 g, protein 2.5 g.

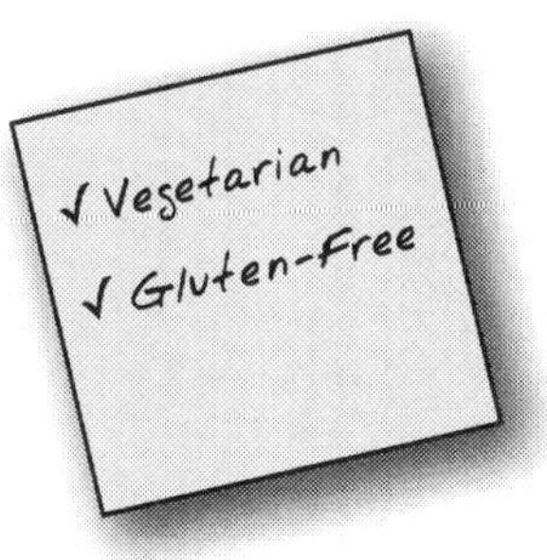

Everything But The Kitchen Sink Salad

Greens (Swiss chard, romaine, arugula, spinach, spring mix, kale)
Seeds or nuts (chopped almonds, walnuts, sunflower seeds, pumpkin seeds)
1 handful of sprouts (broccoli, mung bean, alfalfa, onion)
Vegetables (tomato, broccoli, carrots, zucchini, cauliflower, edamame, mushrooms, bell peppers, asparagus, red onion)
¼ avocado
Dressing of choice

Add anything you have on hand in the refrigerator to create a big flavorful salad!

Mix ingredients together.

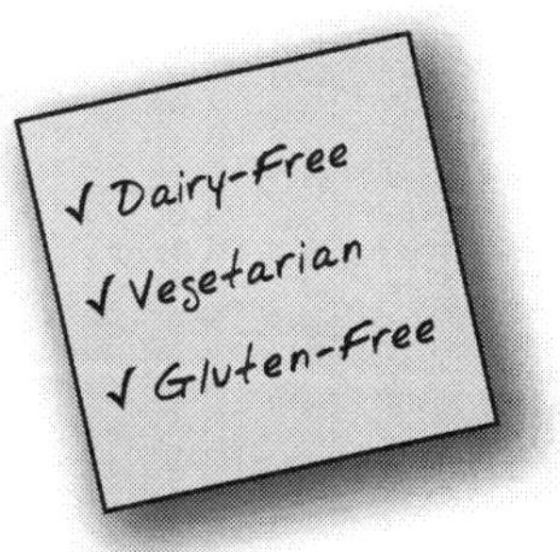

Fennel Avocado Salad [5]

3 to 4 cups romaine, mesclun greens, spinach, or red leaf lettuce
½ avocado
½ medium head of fennel, sliced thing
½ cup cherry tomatoes, chopped
5 sun-dried tomatoes, chopped
10 fresh basil leaves, chopped

Mix ingredient together and add choice of dressing.

Makes 1 serving.

Nutrition per serving: calories 195, fat 6.37 g, cholesterol 0 mg, sodium 597.06 g, carbohydrates 29.96 g, fiber 13.46 g, sugar 7.25 g, protein 7.86 g.

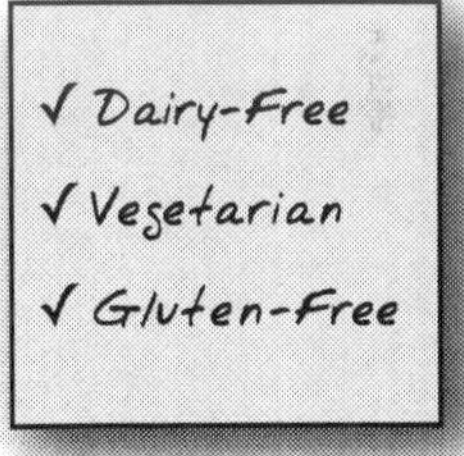

Garlic Avocado Dressing

½ cup water
¼ cup lime juice
¼ cup orange juice
1 avocado, pitted and peeled
2 cloves garlic
½ teaspoon sea salt

Blend all ingredients until smooth.

Makes 3 to 4 servings.

Nutrition per serving: calories 52, fat 3.76 g, cholesterol 0 mg, sodium 422.15 mg, carbohydrates 7.3 g, fiber 2.36 g, sugar 1.97 g, protein 0.69 g.

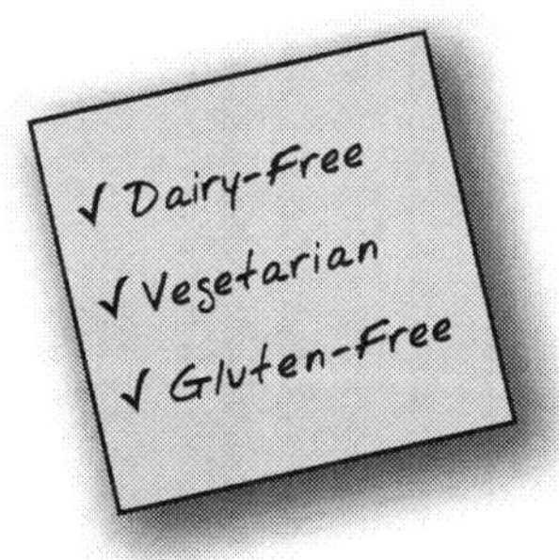

Ginger & Garlic Broccoli Salad

3 cups broccoli, cooked or raw

1 cup of cooked brown rice,

1 can of chickpeas (can be replaced with ground turkey or chicken)

1 inch grated ginger

2 minced garlic cloves

2 diced tomatoes

¼ cup olive oil

¼ cup lemon juice

1 teaspoon Herbamare® or sea salt

3 tablespoons chopped parsley

1 tablespoon fresh rosemary

Mix ingredient together.

Makes 3 servings.

Nutrition per serving: calories 346, fat 19.6 g, cholesterol 0 mg, sodium 34.6 g, carbohydrates 26 g, fiber 4 g, sugar 4.25 g, protein 5.33 g.

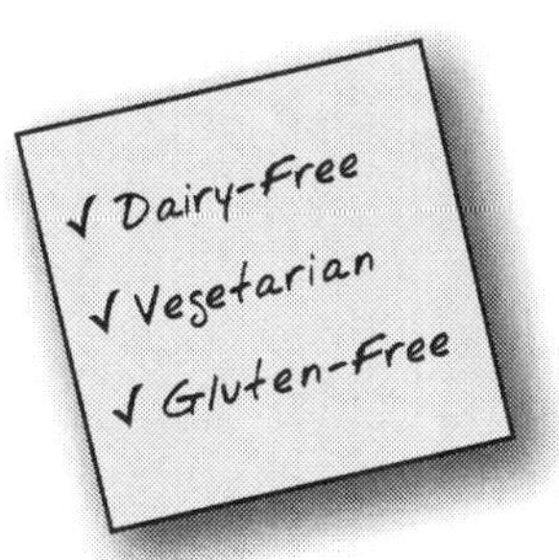

Green Salad with Strawberry Balsamic Vinaigrette

2 teaspoons strawberry jam (no sugar added)
1 tablespoon balsamic vinegar
3 tablespoons olive oil
Black pepper
6 strawberries, sliced
4 cups chopped romaine or mixed greens of any kind

Place the jam in a medium bowl and whisk in the vinegar and the olive oil. Season the dressing with pepper. Add the strawberries and greens to the bowl and toss to coat evenly with the dressing.

Makes 2 servings.

Nutrition per serving: calories 293, total fat 21.4 g, saturated fat 2.9 g, sodium 38 mg, carbohydrates 17.7 g, fiber 8.8 g, protein 7.6 g.

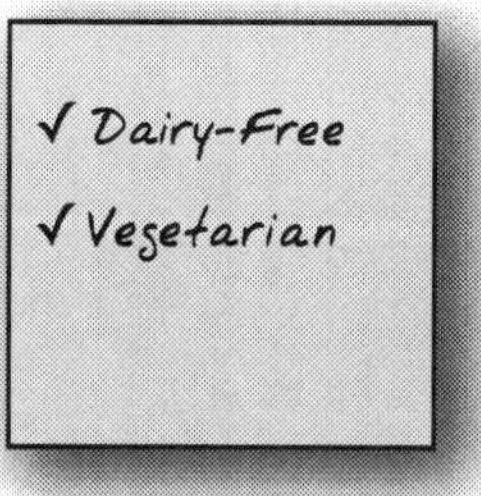

Italian-Style Green Bean Salad

2 cups green beans (fresh or frozen)
2 tablespoons freshly grated parmesan cheese
1 tablespoon fresh basil-finely chopped
2 tablespoons extra virgin olive oil
Balsamic vinegar
Fresh ground pepper

Place the green beans in a small pan with sufficient water to cover them and bring to boil. Remove from the heat when the beans are tender. Drain and leave to cool. In a large bowl, mix the chilled green beans with the basil. Season the salad with olive oil, balsamic vinegar and add fresh ground pepper to taste.

Makes 4 servings.

Nutrition per serving: calories 113, total fat 7.8 g, saturated fat 1.3 g, sodium 79 mg, carbohydrates 8.3 g, fiber 2.6 g, protein 2.8 g.

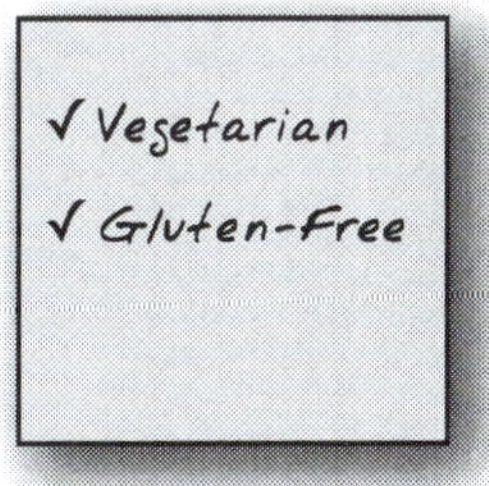

Lemon Oregano Vinaigrette

¼ cup fresh lemon juice (about 1½ lemons)
2 tablespoons apple cider vinegar
1 teaspoon Dijon-style mustard
½ teaspoon sea salt
½ teaspoon black pepper
¾ teaspoon garlic powder
1 teaspoon dried oregano
¼ cup extra virgin olive oil

Combine everything except oil in a food processor, or whisk, then add olive oil until blended.

Makes 5 to 6 servings.

Nutrition per serving: calories 100, fat 10.79 g, cholesterol 0 mg, sodium 358.7 mg, carbohydrates 0.77 g, fiber 0.05 g, sugar 0.29 g, protein 0.06 g.

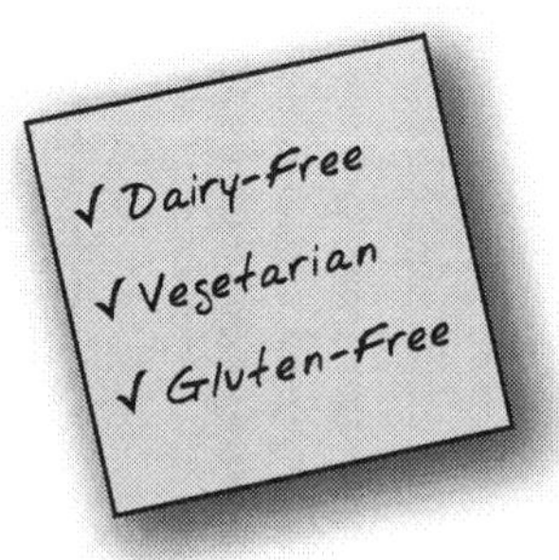

Lime-Rice Wine Vinaigrette[6]

2 teaspoons fresh lime juice
2 teaspoons unseasoned rice wine vinegar
¼ teaspoon pepper
¼ cup extra-virgin olive oil

Optional: ½ teaspoon sea salt

In a small bowl, combine the lime juice, vinegar, salt (if using) and pepper. Slowly whisk in the extra-virgin olive oil until the dressing is slightly thickened. Place all ingredients in a jar with a tight-fitting lid and shake until well combined.

Makes 4 servings (serving size of 2 tablespoons).

Nutrition per serving: calories 129, total fat 14 g, saturated fat 2 g, carbohydrates 1 g.

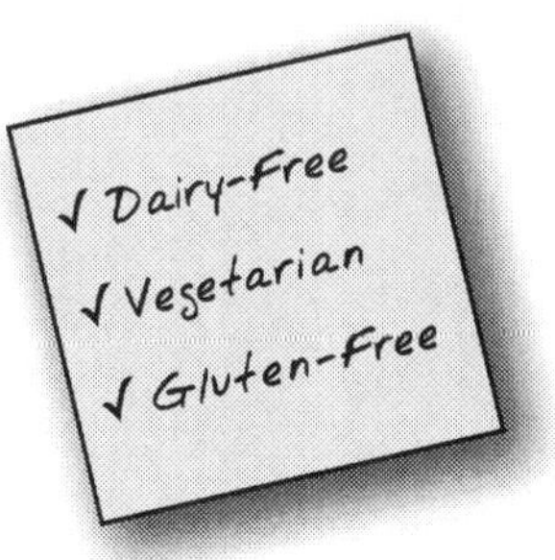

Mediterranean Quinoa Salad

1 cup quinoa
¼ red onion
¼ chopped tomato
1 ounce feta cheese
½ small garlic clove
1 tablespoon olive oil
Chopped parsley
Fresh black pepper to taste
Sea salt to taste

Mix ingredients together and squeeze some fresh lemon onto the salad. Add a little more olive oil as needed.

Makes 2 to 3 servings.

Nutrition per serving: calories 250, fat 10.27 g, cholesterol 67 mg, sodium 947 mg, carbohydrates 28.07 g, fiber 2.6 g, sugar 3.05 g, protein 15.7g.

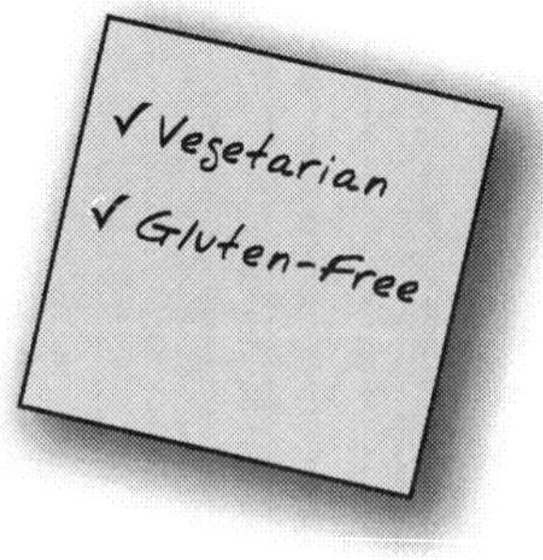

Oriental Chicken Salad

4 portions cooked chicken (about 1 pound total), cut into bite-size pieces
1 bag (16 ounces) coleslaw mix
4 green onions, chopped
2 tablespoons light sesame oil
⅓ cup rice vinegar
¼ cup lite soy sauce
½ teaspoon ground ginger
½ cup sliced almonds

In a large mixing bowl, combine cooked chicken, coleslaw mix and green onions. In a small mixing bowl, combine sesame oil, rice vinegar, soy sauce and ginger. Drizzle over chicken mixture and toss to coat. Divide the chicken salad into four portions. Top with sliced almonds.

Makes 4 servings.

Nutrition per serving: calories 390, total fat 17.4 g, sodium 667 mg, carbohydrates 17.2 g, fiber 5.7 g, protein 41 g.

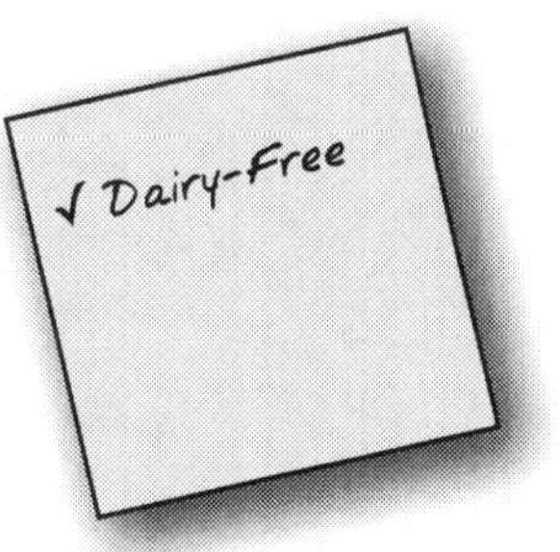

Papaya Salad

½ papaya, fresh
½ Avocado, sliced
½ tablespoon lime juice

Chop papaya and add avocado on top. Top with lime juice.

Makes 1 serving.

Nutrition per serving: calories 135, fat 7.59 g, cholesterol 0 mg, sodium 11 mg, carbohydrates 22.29 g, sugar 8.92 g, protein 1.84 g.

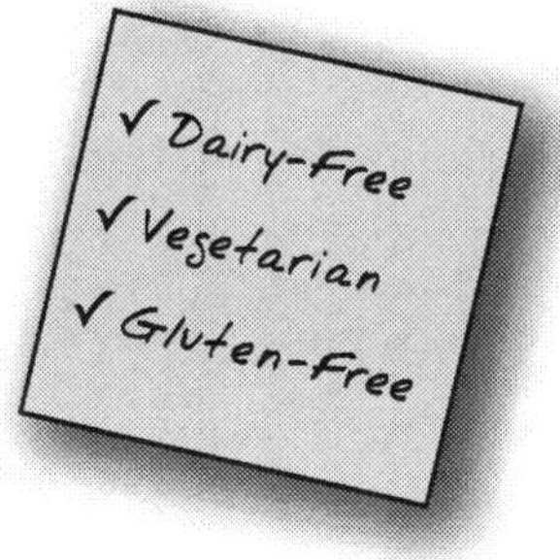

Pumpkin Caesar Salad Dressing[7]

2 tablespoons olive oil
Juice of one lemon
½ tablespoon cumin
1 to 1½ garlic cloves
¼ cup pumpkin seeds
Sea salt to taste

Optional: ½ tablespoon honey

Grind pumpkin seed in coffee grinder. Mix the remaining ingredients with the ground pumpkin seeds in a bowl.

Makes 3 to 4 servings.

Nutrition per serving: calories 102, fat 10.79 g, cholesterol 0 mg, sodium 1 mg, carbohydrates 1 g, fiber 0.03 g, sugar 0 g, protein 1.75 g.

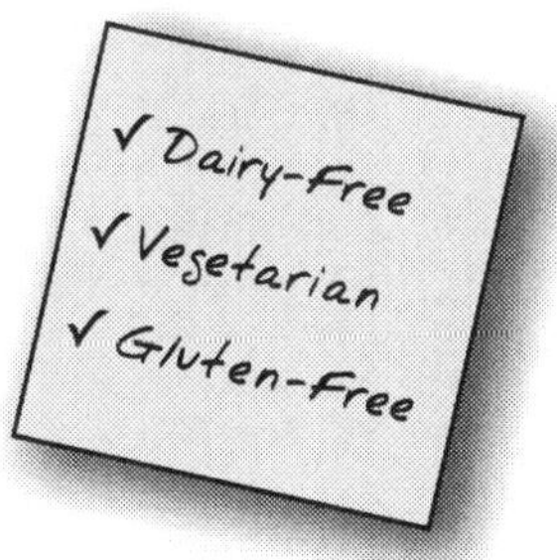

Radicchio and Spinach Salad with Walnuts

Vinaigrette:
2 tablespoons walnut oil
3 tablespoons balsamic vinegar
2 teaspoons honey

Salad:
2½ cups chopped radicchio
2½ cups baby spinach
¾ cup thinly sliced celery
3 tablespoons walnut pieces

In a small bowl, make the dressing by whisking the walnut oil, vinegar and honey to blend completely. In a large bowl, combine the radicchio, spinach, celery and walnuts. Toss the salad to combine. Add the vinaigrette and toss to coat.

Makes 2 servings.

Nutrition per serving: calories 276, total fat 20.8 g, saturated fat 2 g, sodium 84 mg, carbohydrates 18.2 g, fiber 2.8 g, protein 3.8 g.

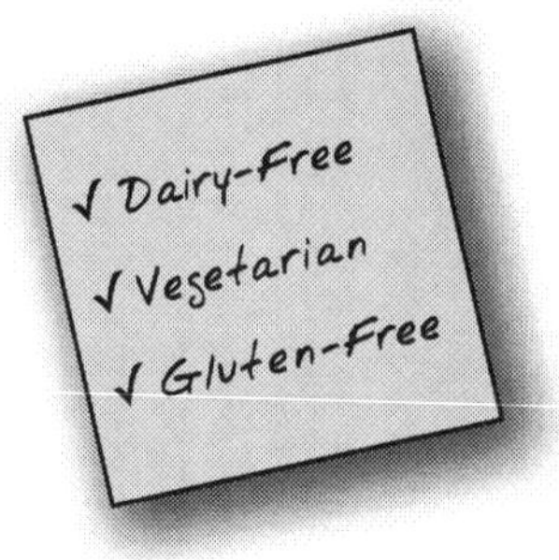

Red Vinaigrette

⅓ cup olive oil
1 teaspoon garlic powder
1 teaspoon dried oregano
1 teaspoon dried basil
¾ teaspoon pepper
¾ teaspoon sea salt
¾ teaspoon onion powder
¾ teaspoon Dijon-style mustard
½ cup red wine vinegar

Combine all ingredients and blend until smooth.

Makes 5 to 6 servings.

Nutrition per serving: calories 96, fat 10.79 g, cholesterol 0 mg, sodium 359 mg, carbohydrates 0 g, fiber 0 g, sugar 0 g, protein 0 g.

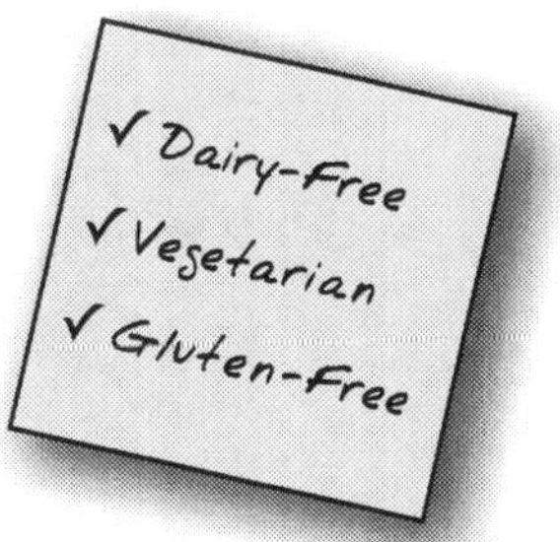

Refreshing Watermelon Salad[8]

2 to 3 cups watermelon, cut into 1-inch pieces
2 small ripe tomatoes, quartered
2 to 3 ounces fresh goat cheese, crumbled
2 tablespoons balsamic vinaigrette
2 to 3 tablespoons chopped fresh basil

In a bowl mix watermelon, tomatoes and goat cheese. Drizzle vinaigrette dressing, then top with fresh basil.

Makes 4 servings.

Nutrition per serving: calories 100, fat 6 g, cholesterol 5 mg, sodium 140 mg, carbohydrates 10 g, fiber 1 g, sugar 7 g, protein 3 g.

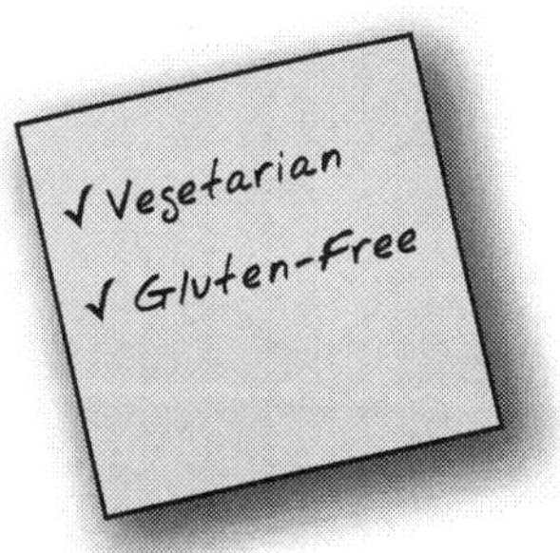

Seared Scallops with Farmers' Market Salad

2 cups chopped tomato
1 cup chopped fresh basil
1 tablespoon canola oil
1½ pounds sea scallops
2 cups corn kernels

Combine tomato, basil, ¼ teaspoon sea salt and ⅛ teaspoon freshly ground black pepper, Toss gently. Heat a large skillet over high heat. Add oil to pan, swirling to coat. Pat scallops dry with paper towels, then sprinkle with ½ teaspoon sea salt and ⅛ teaspoon ground black pepper. Add scallops to pan and cook 2 minutes, or until browned. Turn scallops and cook 2 more minutes, or until done. Remove scallops from pan and keep warm. Coat pan with cooking spray. Add corn to pan and sauté for 2 minutes, or until lightly browned. Add to tomato mixture and toss gently. Serve salad with scallops.

Makes 4 servings (serving size of 1 cup salad and 3 scallops).

Nutrition per serving: calories 251, total fat 5.7 g, saturated fat 0.5 g, sodium 641 mg, carbohydrates 19.4 g, protein 31.6 g.

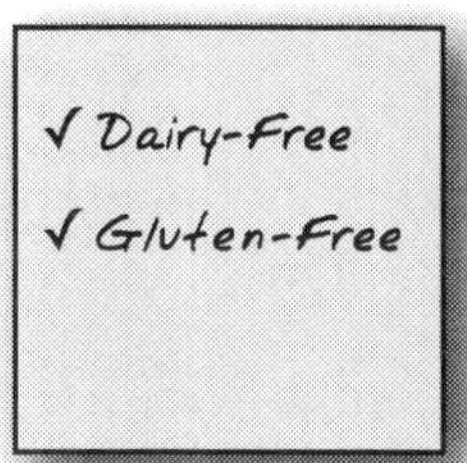

Shirazi Tomato Cucumber Salad

2 tomatoes, large, diced
2 cucumbers, medium, peeled and diced
1 onion, large, diced
1 tablespoon lemon juice
2 tablespoons olive oil
½ teaspoon salt

In a medium serving dish, toss the tomatoes, cucumbers and onion with lemon juice, olive oil and salt.

Makes 4 to 6 servings.

Nutrition per serving: calories 82, fat 4.7 g, cholesterol 0 mg, sodium 4.7 mg, carbohydrates 7 g, fiber 1.6 g, sugar 2.8 g, protein 1.5 g.

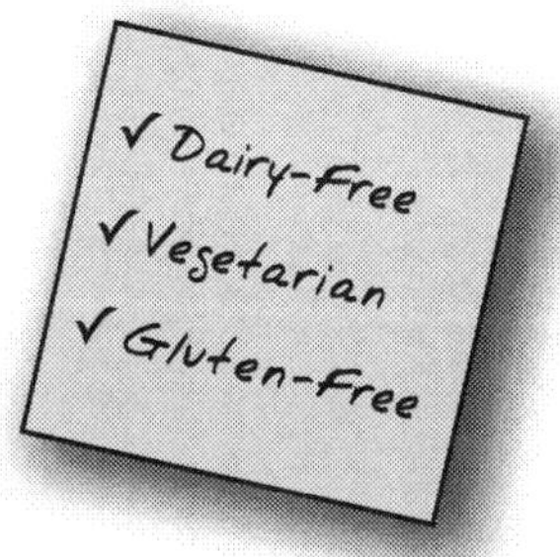

Sicilian Collard Greens[9]

1 bunch of collard greens
2 tablespoons pine nuts
3 garlic cloves, peeled and chopped
1 tablespoon olive oil
3 tablespoons raisins
2 tablespoons balsamic vinegar

Rinse collard greens, then cut out the central rib and stem from each collard leaf. Toast pine nuts over medium heat in a dry skillet for about 5 minutes, or until golden. Shake the pan often to keep pine nuts from burning. Transfer to a plate and set aside. Place garlic and oil in a large skillet, then sauté over medium heat for 1 minute, or until the garlic is fragrant. Add the damp collard greens and stir, then cover the pan and cook for 2 minutes longer. Add the raisins and pin nuts, then stir. Cover and cook for 2 minutes. Stir in balsamic vinegar, cover and cook for 1 to 2 minutes longer.

Makes 1 serving.

Nutrition per serving: calories 310, fat 24 g, cholesterol 0 mg, sodium 37 mg, carbohydrates 17.6 g, fiber 7.34 g, sugar 6.95 g, protein 7.24 g.

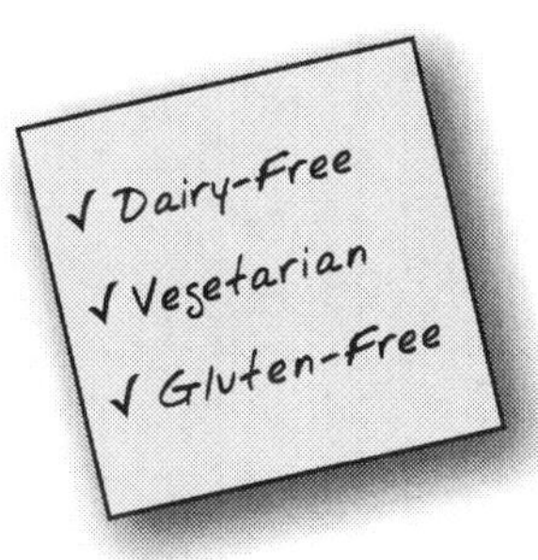

Simple Green Salad

½ Hass avocado, finely chopped
6 to 7 baby tomatoes, halved
1 bunch cilantro, chopped
1 pound baby romaine, mesclun, regular romaine lettuce
1 handful broccoli or onion sprouts
Dressing choice of: *Carrot Ginger Dressing* (page 399) or *Lemon Oregano Vinaigrette* (page 408)
Celtic Sea Salt® to taste
Ground black pepper to taste

Optional: add hard boiled eggs, turkey or chicken for protein salad

Mix all ingredients together and enjoy.

Makes 1 serving.

Nutrition per serving: calories 126, fat 7.5 g, cholesterol 0 mg, sodium 157 mg, carbohydrates 14.57 g, fiber 4.6 g, sugar 0.67 g, protein 7 g.

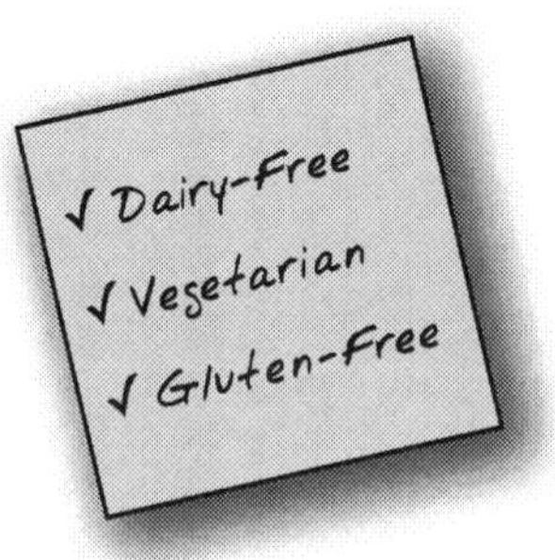

Simple Greens and Garlic[10]

This recipe works well for kale, spinach, turnip greens, collard greens or arugula

3 tablespoons extra-virgin olive oil
1 onion, chopped
3 cloves garlic, minced
2 pounds greens, washed, dried, and shredded
Salt and pepper

Heat olive oil over medium-high heat in a large frying pan. Add onion and garlic, then cook and stir until soft. Stir in greens and cook until wilted. Salt and pepper to taste. Serve hot or cold.

Makes 4 servings.

Nutrition per serving: calories 180, total fat 11 g, saturated fat 1.5 g, sodium 45 mg, carbohydrates 16 g, fiber 9 g, protein 6 g.

✓ Dairy-Free
✓ Vegetarian
✓ Gluten-Free

Southwestern Salad

8 ounces mixed greens
2 tablespoons guacamole
3 slices of Hass™ avocado
1 cup salsa
⅔ cup fresh cucumber, diced
1 cup grape or cherry tomatoes, halved
Juice of 1 lemon
4 to 5 flaxseed crackers, or Mary's Gone Raw Onion Crackers® crumbled on top

Optional: add chicken or ¼ cup of cooked black beans

Mix ingredients in a bowl and serve.

Makes 1 serving.

Nutrition per serving: calories 209, fat 10.95 g, cholesterol 0 mg, sodium 160 mg, carbohydrates 22 g, fiber 8.65 g, sugar 10.8 g, protein 5.55 g.

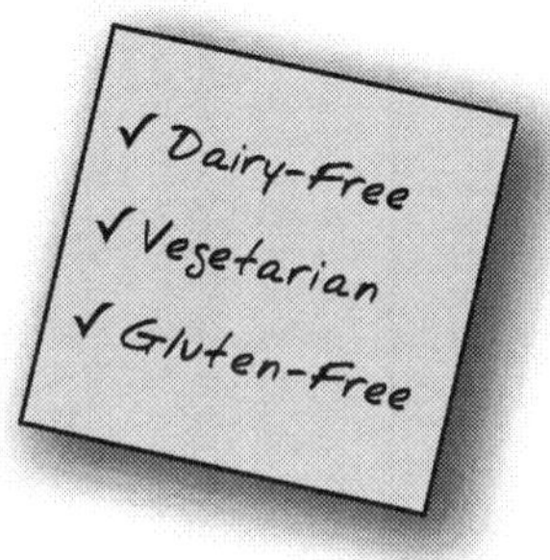

Spinach Salad with Strawberries and Pistachios

If strawberries aren't in season, substitute another fruit (such as blueberries, sliced apples or pears).

Vinaigrette:
3 tablespoons extra-virgin olive oil
2 tablespoons balsamic vinegar
1 tablespoon minced red onion
1 teaspoon Dijon-style mustard
1 teaspoon maple syrup

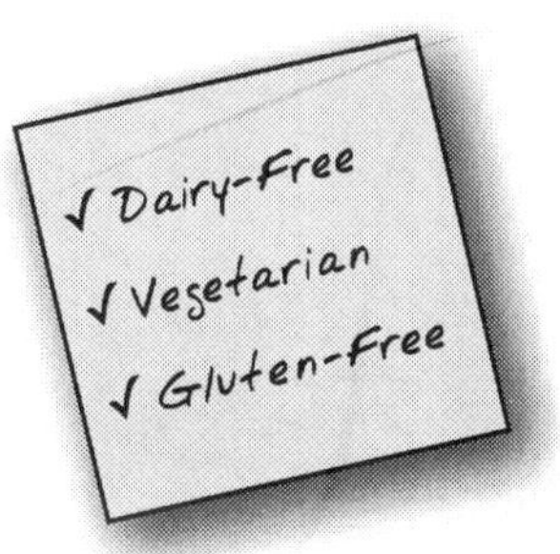

Salad:
1 bag (6 ounces) baby spinach
1 cup thinly sliced strawberries
¼ cup coarsely chopped pistachio nuts, toasted and cooled

To make the dressing, whisk together the olive oil, vinegar, red onion, mustard and maple syrup until well combined. Divide the spinach among four chilled bowls. Top each serving evenly with the strawberries and pistachio nuts. Drizzle with dressing and serve.

Makes 4 servings.

Nutrition per serving: calories 189, total fat 15 g, saturated fat 3 g, sodium 150 mg, carbohydrates 8 g, fiber 3 g, protein 5 g.

Spinach Strawberry Salad

1½ cup quartered strawberries
1 tablespoon finely chopped fresh mint
1 (6 ounce) package organic baby spinach
2 tablespoons sliced almonds, toasted
¼ teaspoon freshly ground black pepper

Combine the first 4 ingredients in a large bowl; toss gently to coat.

Makes 4 servings.

Nutrition per serving: calories 136, total fat 10.3 g, saturated fat 0.7 g, sodium 113 mg, carbohydrates 11 g, fiber 3.6 g, protein 2.1 g.

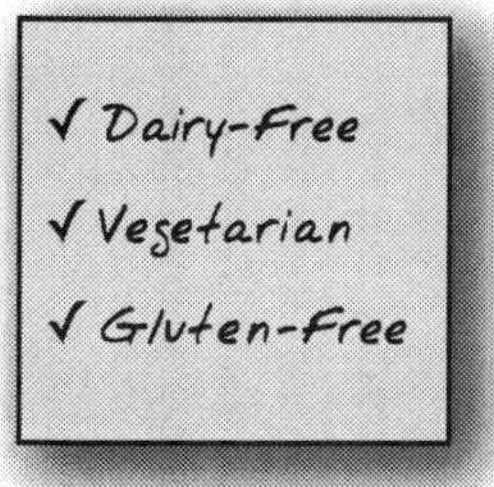

Spinach Walnut Salad[11]

2 tablespoons freshly squeezed lemon juice
⅓ cup olive oil
1 small garlic clove, minced
½ teaspoon Dijon-style mustard
½ teaspoon fine sea salt
⅛ teaspoon freshly ground black pepper
6 green onions, with tops, thinly sliced
1 pound spinach, well washed, stems removed and leaves torn in pieces
1 cup raw walnuts, toasted and finely chopped

Put the lemon juice, olive oil, garlic, mustard, salt and pepper in a small jar. Cover with the lid and shake until the ingredients are well mixed. In a salad bowl, toss together the green onions, spinach and walnuts. Shake the lemon garlic dressing and pour it over the salad. Toss until well coated.

Makes 4 servings.

Nutrition per serving: calories 421, total fat 37.1 g, saturated fat 4.2 g, sodium 300 mg, carbohydrates 13.8 g, fiber 5.2 g, protein 8 g.

√ Dairy-Free
√ Vegetarian
√ Gluten-Free

Stuffed Avocado Salad[12]

2 small ripe tomatoes
½ red onion, chopped
2 tablespoons olive oil
2 tablespoons chopped parsley
1 tablespoon red wine vinegar
1 teaspoon oregano
2 large avocados

Optional:
⅔ cup crumbled feta cheese
Chopped olives and balsamic vinegar to taste
Chopped chicken to taste

In a medium bowl, squeeze the juice from one half of the lemon over the crab and stir to combine—along with a large pinch of salt and a few grinds of black pepper. Season to taste with salt and pepper. Spoon mixture into each avocado half.

Makes 4 servings.

Nutrition per serving (not including optional ingredients): calories 334, fat 29 g, cholesterol 22 mg, sodium 290 mg, carbohydrates 14.6 g, fiber 8.9 g, sugar 3.6 g, protein 6.5 g.

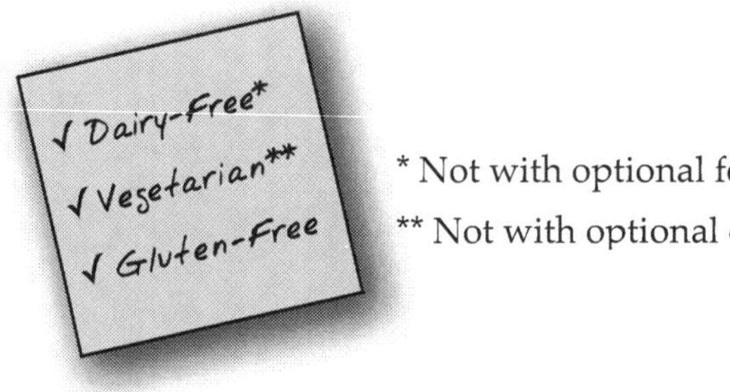

* Not with optional feta cheese.
** Not with optional chicken.

Summer Salad

6 to 8 unsulfured, sun-dried tomatoes (soaked in lukewarm water until soft, then chopped)
¼ pound fresh baby greens
3 to 4 slices cucumber
2 to 3 baby tomatoes
3 ounces Alta Dena raw cheddar style goat cheese
¼ cup fresh chopped basil
1 tablespoon chopped oregano
1 tablespoon fresh lemon juice
Dressing choice of: *Tahini Dressing* (page 428) or *Lemon Oregano Vinaigrette* (page 408)
Sea salt to taste
Pepper to taste

Mix all ingredients together in a bowl.

Makes 1 serving.

Nutrition per serving: calories 249, fat 9.09 g, cholesterol 30 mg, sodium 330 mg, carbohydrates 14 g, fiber 6 g, fiber 3 g, protein 17 g.

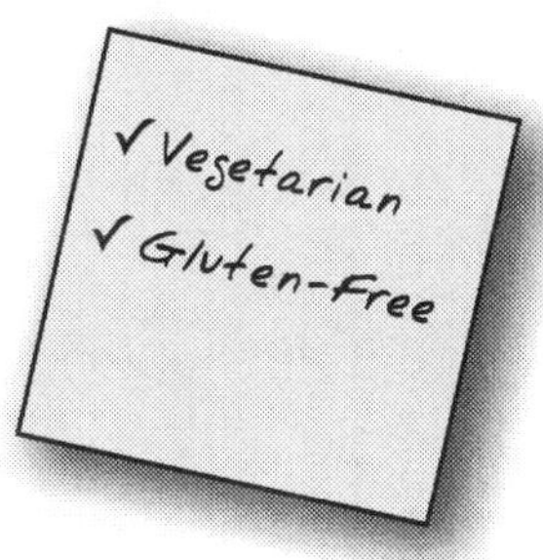

Tahini Dressing

½ cup raw tahini
¼ to ½ cup water
3 tablespoons fresh lemon juice or lime juice
¼ to ½ teaspoon cayenne pepper
¼ to ½ teaspoon crystal salt

Blend all ingredients until smooth.

Makes 3 to 4 servings.

Nutrition per serving: calories 100, fat 8 g, cholesterol 0 mg, sodium 420.8 mg, carbohydrates 5.88 g, fiber 6.6 g, sugar 0.26 g, protein 3.06 g.

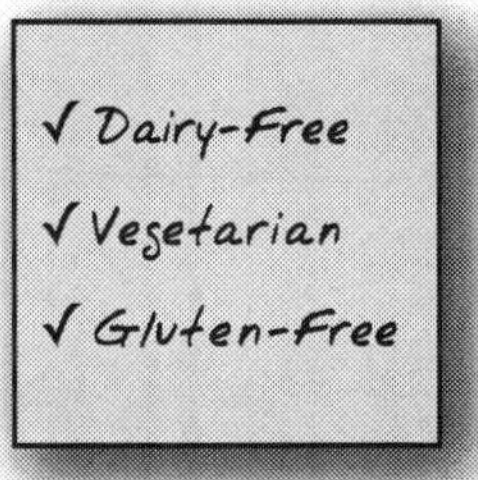

Tropical Fruit Salad with Arugula[13]

1 medium shallot, sliced into thin rings
2 tablespoons rice vinegar or champagne
3 tablespoons extra virgin olive oil
1 teaspoon red wine vinegar
2 cups baby arugula or watercress
¼ cup roasted, salted pistachios, coarsely chopped
1 tablespoon sliced fresh mint
1 tablespoon fresh basil
Ground pepper
Sea salt
3 avocados—medium, firm and ripe
2 kiwis, peeled, halved and sliced ¼-inch thick
1 mango, sliced ¼-inch thick
½ pineapple, cut into ½-inch diameter

✓ Dairy-Free
✓ Vegetarian
✓ Gluten-Free

In a medium bowl, toss the shallot with the champagne vinegar and add a pinch of salt and set aside for 10 minutes, stirring once. Drain the shallot into a small bowl and save the vinegar. Whisk olive oil and red wine vinegar into the shallot vinegar. In a medium bowl, tow 1 tablespoon of the vinaigrette with the pickled shallots, arugula (or watercress), pistachios, mint, basil, ¼ teaspoon salt and a few grinds of pepper. Arrange the avocado, kiwi, mango and pineapple on a platter. Drizzle with remaining vinaigrette and season to taste with salt and pepper. Top with arugula mixture and serve immediately. Add chicken or turkey for added protein.

Makes 5 to 6 servings.

Nutrition per serving: calories 215, fat 13.8 g, cholesterol 0 mg, sodium 12 mg, carbohydrates 28.8 g, fiber 7.65 g, sugar 9.95 g, protein 3.74 g.

Turkey Pilgrim Salad

6 ounces fresh cooked turkey breast, shredded or chopped
1 to 2 tablespoons dried cranberries
1 to 2 tablespoons pistachios
1 to 2 tablespoons olive oil
1 tablespoon goat cheese
2 to 3 slices of orange
¼ cup chopped tomato
2 handfuls of romaine
1 handful of spinach
1 onion
1 teaspoon butter
¼ cup citrus vinaigrette (mix ⅔ cup rice wine vinegar, ⅓ cup orange juice, 2 tablespoons olive oil, 2 tablespoons fresh cilantro, 1 tablespoon Dijon-style mustard, 2 teaspoons minced garlic and 1 teaspoon honey)

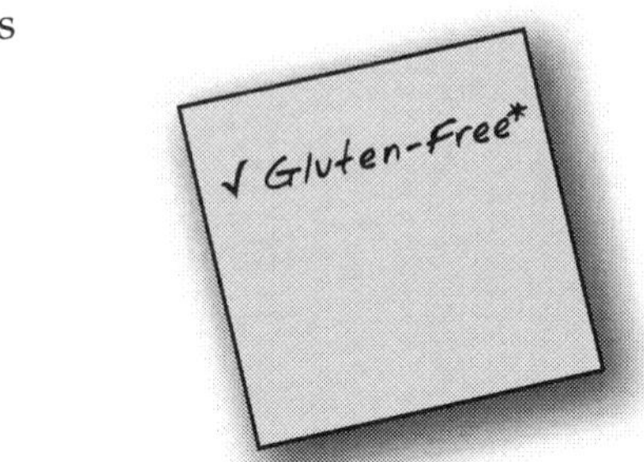

* Basting solutions injected in turkey during processing may contain gluten. Be sure to read label.

Cut onions in half, then slice onions lengthwise. Coat pan with olive oil and 1 teaspoon butter. Heat pan until oil is shimmering. Add onions and stir to coat onions with oil. Cook for 10 minutes, then sprinkle with a pinch of salt. Let cook for 30 more minutes on low heat to brown, while stirring to avoid burning. Mix remaining ingredients (except for goat cheese) with onions and toss with ¼ cup citrus vinaigrette. Top with goat cheese.

Makes 1 to 2 servings.

Nutrition per serving: calories 250, fat 12.6 g, cholesterol 22 mg, sodium 199 mg, carbohydrates 34.3 g, fiber 5.25 g, sugar 17.2 g, protein 8.33 g.

Turkey Salad

½ cup low-fat plain yogurt
1 teaspoon curry
½ teaspoon ground ginger
½ teaspoon dried thyme
2 portions cooked turkey breast (about ½ pound), chopped
1 stalk celery, sliced
2 cups mixed salad greens
4 tablespoons sliced almonds

In a large mixing bowl, combine yogurt, curry, ginger and thyme. Stir in raisins, then cover and refrigerate for 15 minutes. Combine pre-cooked, chopped turkey and celery with yogurt mixture. Line 2 plates with mixed salad greens. Top each with a portion of turkey mixture and sprinkle with sliced almonds.

Makes 4 servings.

Nutrition per serving: calories 170, total fat 7.7 g, saturated fat 1.3 g, sodium 88 mg, carbohydrates 14 g, fiber 6.1 g, protein 9.6 g.

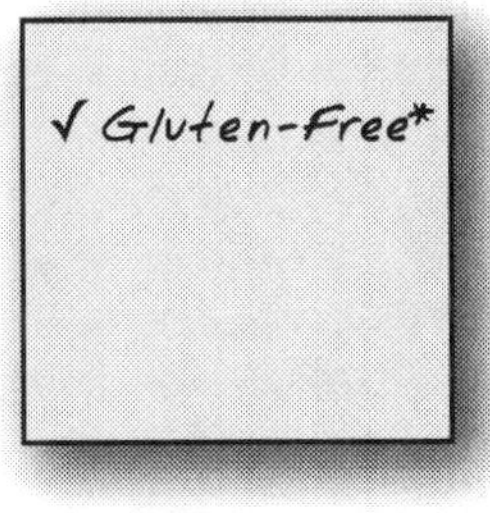

* Basting solutions injected in turkey during processing may contain gluten. Be sure to read label.

Recipes: Soups

"An old-fashioned vegetable soup, without any enhancement, is a more powerful anticarcinogen than any known medicine."
— James "Red" Duke M.D.

Avocado Coconut Soup

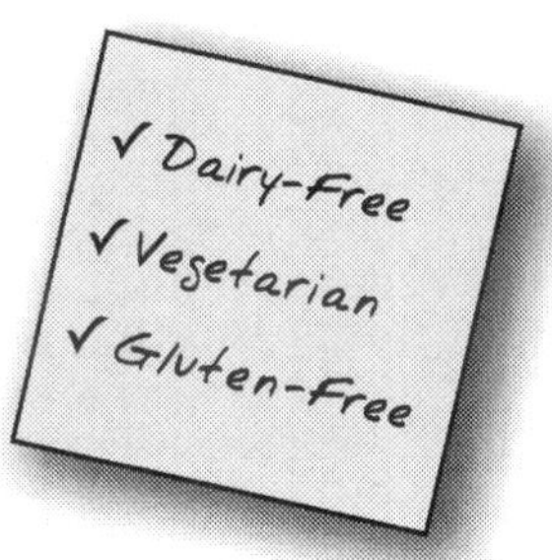

1 avocado
2 young coconuts
1¼ cup coconut water
Sea salt to taste
Stevia to taste

Blend ingredients in blender. Serve cold.

Makes 2 servings.

Nutrition per serving: calories 260, fat 10.5 g, cholesterol 0 mg, sodium 303 mg, carbohydrates 39.6 g, fiber 9 g, sugar 15 g, protein 4.6 g.

Blended Creamy Tomato Soup[1]

5 ripe Holland tomatoes halved
¼ cup fresh cilantro
½ avocado
Sea salt to taste
Fresh ground pepper to taste
1 tablespoon agave nectar or 2 dates

Blend until smooth. Add chopped apple for more flavor.

Makes 2 servings.

Nutrition per serving: calories 129, fat 4 g, cholesterol 0 mg, sodium 1.75 mg, carbohydrates 12.35 g, fiber 4 g, sugar 7.75 g, protein 1.05 g.

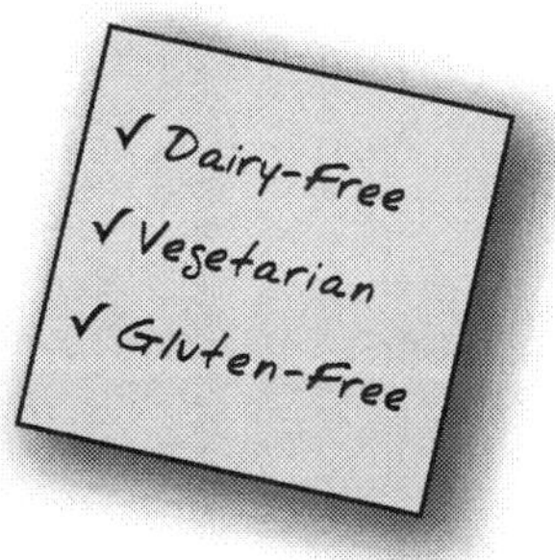

Butternut Squash Soup with Toasted Pecans

1 large leek
2 tablespoons olive oil
1 medium sweet onion, chopped
1 medium butternut squash, peeled, seeded and cut into 1-inch pieces
5 cups vegetable stock
Sea salt to taste
Fresh ground black pepper to taste
⅓ cup toasted pecans, chopped

Halve the leek lengthwise, rinse thoroughly and chop the white and light green parts only. Discard the tough dark green parts. Heat oil in a large saucepan over medium heat. Add onion and leek and sauté until they start to turn golden—8 to 10 minutes. Add squash, then stir to coat with oil and continue cooking 10 minutes longer. Add stock and bring to a boil. Reduce heat to a simmer and cook until squash is tender—about 20 minutes. Let soup cool slightly. In a food processor, purée half of the soup until smooth. Take extreme care when puréeing a hot liquid. Mix purée back into soup and season to taste with salt and pepper. Top with toasted pecans and serve.

Makes 4 servings.

Nutrition per serving: calories 220, fat 15 g, cholesterol 0 mg, sodium 350 mg, carbohydrates 22 g, fiber 3 g, sugar 6 g, protein 4 g.

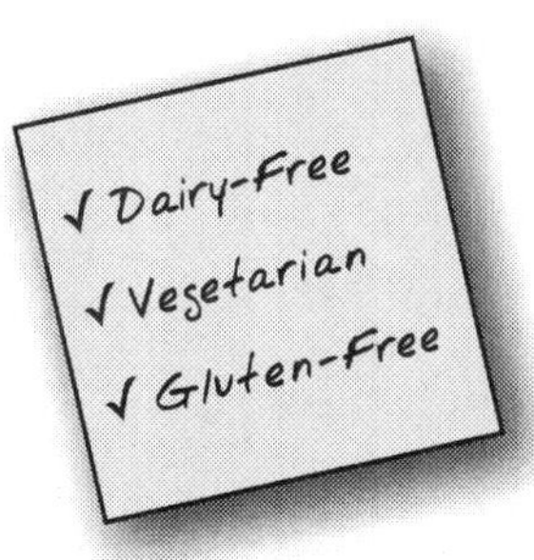

Creamy Curried Cauliflower Soup

¼ cup raw sunflower kernels
3½ cups unsweetened almond milk or hemp milk
3 teaspoons curry powder, divided, more to taste
1 cup chopped yellow onion
3 cloves of garlic, chopped
5 cups cauliflower florets

Preheat oven to 350°F. In a medium bowl, toss sunflower kernels with 1 teaspoon almond milk and 1 teaspoon curry powder. Spread out on a small parchment paper-lined baking sheet and bake, tossing once or twice—about 6-8 minutes—and then set aside. Heat ½ cup almond milk in large pot over medium heat. Add onion and garlic, then cook while stirring occasionally, until soft—about 10 minutes. Add cauliflower, remaining 2 teaspoons curry powder and almond milk, then cover and simmer until cauliflower is tender—about 40 minutes. Taste and adjust seasoning with more curry powder if you like. Working in batches, puree in blender until smooth. Garnish with sunflower seeds.

Makes 4 servings.

Nutrition per serving: calories 140, fat 7 g, cholesterol 0 mg, sodium 200 mg, carbohydrates 16 g, fiber 6 g, sugar 5 g, protein 6 g.

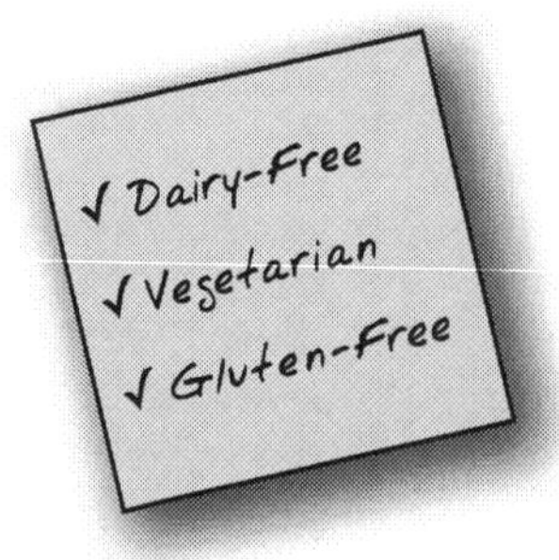

Creamy Roasted Butternut Squash Soup with Cardamom[2]

5 pounds butternut squash, peeled and cut into ¾-inch pieces
2 medium yellow onions, chopped
1 tablespoon chopped thyme
3 tablespoons extra virgin olive oil
6 cups chicken and vegetable broth
½ cup dry white wine
1 teaspoon ground cardamom
Salt and pepper to taste

Optional: add shredded, roasted chicken

Preheat oven to 425. Toss squash, onions and thyme in oil. Spread mixture onto 1 or 2 large baking sheets. Season with salt and pepper. Roast 20 to 30 minutes until tender, stirring once or twice. Remove from oven and transfer to a large pot. Add broth, wine and cardamom. Simmer 10 minutes. Working in batches, puree the soup in a blender or food processor until smooth. Transfer to a clean pot and check seasoning. When ready to serve, bring soup back to a simmer, then remove from heat.

Makes 8 to 10 servings.

Nutrition per serving: calories 260, fat 11 g, cholesterol 25 mg, sodium 340 mg, carbohydrates 35 g, fiber 5 g, protein 6 g.

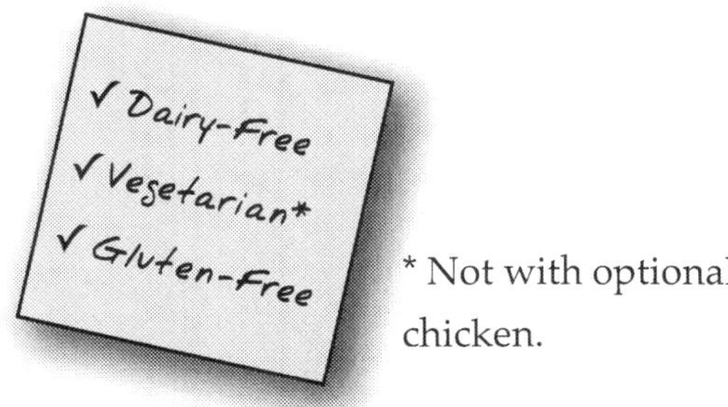

* Not with optional chicken.

Easy Minestrone Soup[3]

1 pound extra-lean, grass-fed ground beef
4 cups organic chicken broth
8 ounces kidney beans
2 cups canned or fresh tomatoes
1 clove garlic minced
¼ teaspoon black pepper
¼ cup dry white wine

Brown ground beef in a large stockpot or deep skillet. Add chicken broth, kidney beans, tomatoes, garlic, pepper and white wine. Simmer 1 hour to blend flavors.

Makes 8 servings (serving size of 1 cup).

Nutrition per serving: calories 205, protein 17 g, carbohydrates 10 g, fat 8 g.

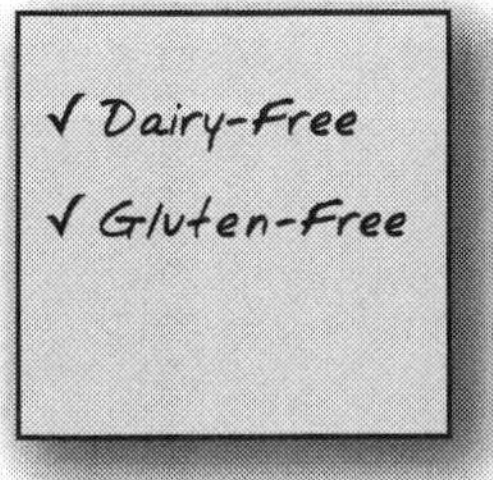

Fifteen-Minute Vegetarian Chili[4]

1 onion, chopped
1 teaspoon olive oil
2 cloves garlic, minced
1 can (16 ounces) organic red kidney beans
1 can (16 ounces) organic stewed tomatoes
½ teaspoon garlic powder
⅛ teaspoon dried oregano
⅛ teaspoon dried basil
1 tablespoon chili powder

Heat olive oil in a large pot. Lightly brown onion and garlic. Add kidney beans, tomatoes and spices. Simmer uncovered over medium heat for 15 minutes, stirring frequently.

Makes 4 servings.

Nutrition per serving: calories 105, carbohydrate 23 g, protein 7 g.

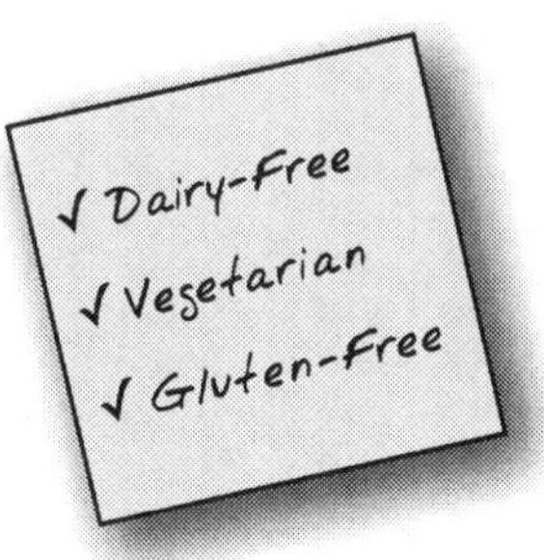

Indian-Spiced Chickpea and Fire-Roasted Tomato Soup

¼ cup olive oil
2 garlic cloves, chopped
1 can (15 ounces) chick peas, rinsed and drained (use dried beans to further reduce sodium)
½ small onion, coarsely chopped
1 teaspoon ground cumin
½ teaspoon ground cardamom
½ teaspoon ground turmeric
Black pepper
1 cup organic chicken stock
1 can (28 ounces) organic fire-roasted tomatoes

Heat the olive oil in a medium pot over medium heat. Add the garlic and cook for 2 to 3 minutes. Combine the chickpeas and onions in a food processor and process until finely chopped. Add them to the pot and cook for 5 minutes to sweeten the onions. Season the chickpeas with the cumin, cardamom, turmeric and pepper. Stir in the stock, then the tomatoes, and simmer the soup for 5 to 10 minutes to combine the flavors.

Makes 4 servings (serving size of 1¾ cups).

Nutrition per serving: calories 246, total fat 8.4 g, saturated fat 1.1 g, sodium 400 mg, carbohydrates 36.5 g, fiber 7.2 g, protein 7.6 g.

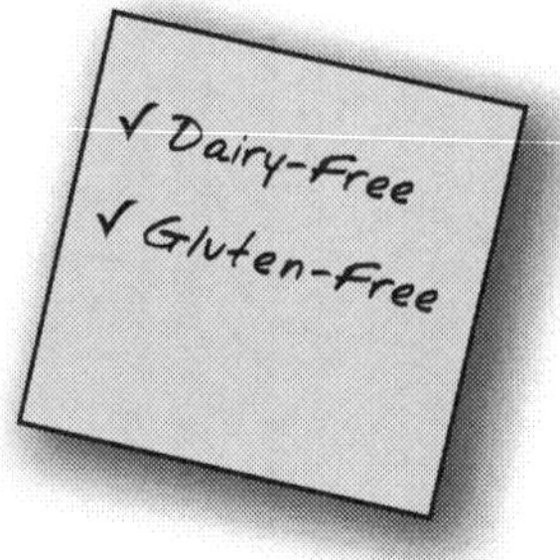

Italian Vegetable Soup[5]

1 large bunch kale
1 tablespoon olive oil
1 medium onion
1 large carrot, peeled and chopped
1 stalk celery, chopped
2 cloves garlic, minced
1 cup tomato puree
2 tablespoons tomato paste
6 cups water
1 piece Parmesan cheese (2 inches)
¼ teaspoon cayenne pepper

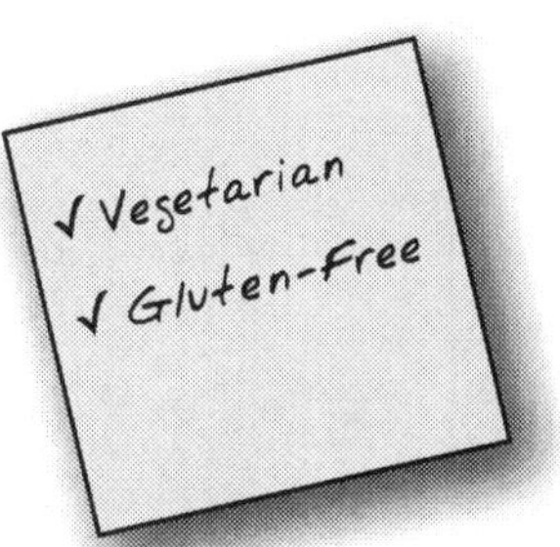

Wash the kale well. Remove the leaves from the stems and tear the leaves into medium-size pieces. Set aside. Place a large nonstick pan over medium-high heat and add the olive oil. Add the onion and cook for about 5 minutes, or until softened. Add the carrot, celery and garlic, then cook for 5 minutes longer, stirring often. Stir in the tomato puree, tomato paste and the water, then bring to a boil. Add the Parmesan and kale. Reduce the heat and simmer for 30 minutes. Add the cayenne pepper.

Makes 4 servings.

Nutrition per serving: calories: 127, total fat 6 g, saturated fat 2 g, carbohydrates 16 g, fiber 3 g, protein 6 g.

Lentil Soup

1 medium onion, chopped (about 1 cup)
2 garlic cloves, minced
1 tablespoon olive oil
3 carrots, chopped
2 stalks celery, chopped
1 cup dried lentils, picked over and rinsed
5 cups vegetable, chicken broth or water
1 cup peeled and chopped tomato (fresh or canned)
1 teaspoon ground cumin

Optional: ½ teaspoon crushed red pepper

In a large saucepan, cook the onion and the garlic in the oil over moderately low heat for 5 minutes, or until they are softened. Add the carrots, celery, lentils, broth and cumin. Bring the soup to a boil and simmer for 30 minutes. Add the tomatoes and red pepper flakes, if using, and simmer for 10 minutes or until the lentils are tender.

Hint: To reduce sodium content use water instead of chicken broth.

Makes 6 to 7 servings (serving size of 1 cup).

Nutrition per serving: calories 174, total fat 2.8 g, saturated fat 0.3 g, sodium 581 mg, carbohydrates 26 g, fiber 11.5 g, protein 10.9 g.

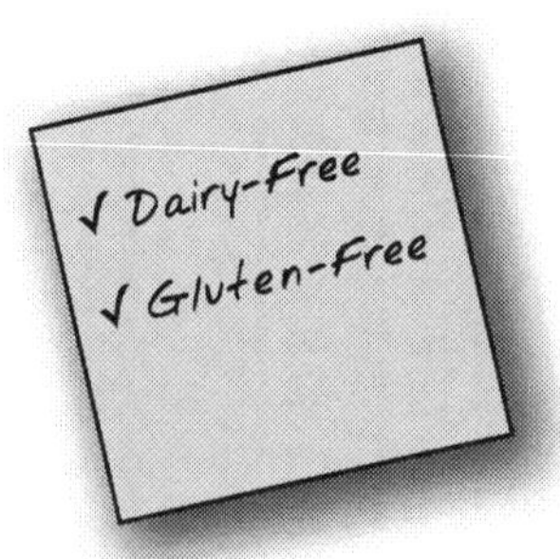

Mexican Chicken Soup with Ancho Chilies[6]

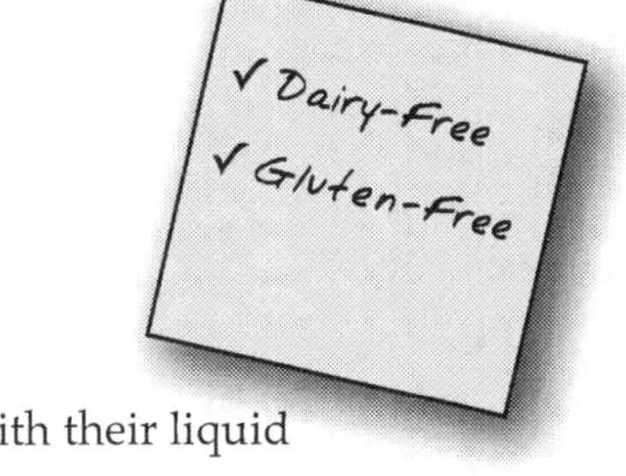

2 to 3 dried ancho chilies, stemmed
1 quart low-sodium chicken broth
2 carrots, chopped
Chopped cilantro
1 clove garlic, mashed into a paste
1 (15-ounce) can chopped tomatoes, with their liquid
½ pound skinless, boneless chicken breasts, cut into small strips
Salt and pepper to taste

Tortilla chips (during Phase 2, not during Phase 1)
Diced avocados
Lime wedges

Optional: crumbled feta or grated Monterey Jack cheese

Put chilies into a medium size heatproof bowl with water and bring to boil, then cover and set aside to let soak until softened—about 10 minutes. Transfer chilies and about ½ cup of their soaking liquid to a blender and purée, adding more of the chilies' soaking liquid (if needed) to make a smooth, thin paste. Set aside. Put broth into a large pot and bring just to a boil. Add carrots, garlic, tomatoes and 2 to 3 tablespoons of the reserved chili purée, then simmer until carrots are almost tender—15 to 20 minutes. (Save leftover chili purée for another use. It keeps well in the refrigerator for up to a week, or the freezer for up to 2 months.) Add chicken and simmer over low heat just until cooked through. Remove soup from heat, season with salt and pepper, then serve garnished with cilantro, cheese, tortilla chips, avocados and lime wedges.

Makes 4 to 6 servings. Nutrition per serving: 170 calories, fat 4 g, sodium 710 mg, carbohydrates 16 g, fiber 5 g, sugar 4 g, protein 19 g.

Refresh Soup

2 cups fresh pineapple
5 ounces fresh, organic baby spinach
1 cup organic alfalfa sprouts
2 to 3 dried, Turkish figs
½ medium Hass avocado
5 frozen strawberries
1 to 2 cups of water
Stevia to taste

Blend in a high-speed blender until smooth.

Makes 4 to 5 servings.

Nutrition per serving: 121 calories, fat 3.02 g, sodium 18.75 mg, carbohydrates 24.5 g, fiber 4.075 g, sugar 15.7 g, protein 2.68 g.

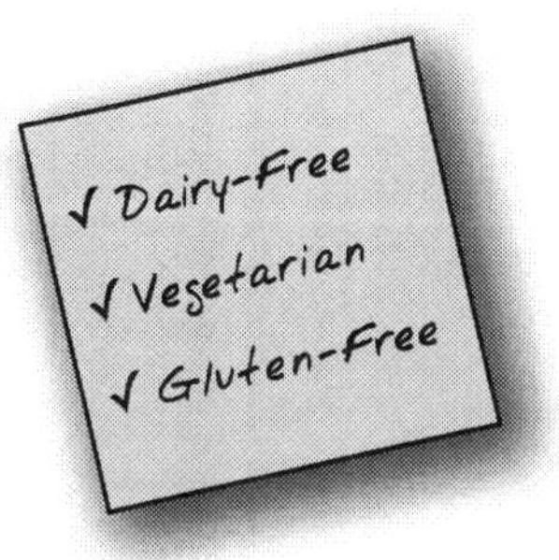

Sweet Potato Soup[7]—Option A

2 teaspoons olive oil
1 small onion, finely chopped
1 teaspoon ground cumin
1 sweet potato, peeled and cubed
2 cups organic low-sodium chicken or vegetable broth

In a large stockpot over medium heat, warm the olive oil. Add the onion and cumin and sauté for 10 minutes, stirring frequently. Add the sweet potato and the chicken broth, then raise the flame to high and bring the mixture to a boil. Reduce the heat and simmer the soup until the potato is tender—25 to 30 minutes. Remove the pot from the heat and allow the soup to cool slightly—about 10 minutes. Transfer the soup to a food processor or blender. If using a blender, work in batches, and do not fill the blender more than half way. Puree the soup at a low speed until smooth. Return the soup to the pot, and reheat it.

Makes 4 servings.

Nutrition per serving: calories 80, total fat 2 g, saturated fat 0 g, sodium 94 mg, carbohydrates 11 g, fiber 1 g, protein 3 g.

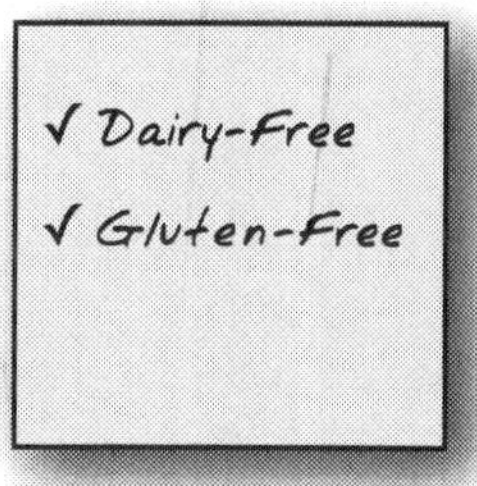

Sweet Potato Soup[8]*—Option B*

1 medium sweet potato (cubed, peeled) can use cooked or raw
2 cups of carrot juice (add more if too thick)
1 avocado (scooped out)
Several dashes of pumpkin pie spice

Optional: 4 dates, pitted

Blend until smooth.

Makes 4 to 5 servings (serving size of 1 cup).

Nutrition per serving: calories 169, fat 3.75 g, cholesterol 0 mg, sodium 61.5 mg, carbohydrates 36.28 g, fiber 6.3 g, sugar 22.83 g, protein 2 g.

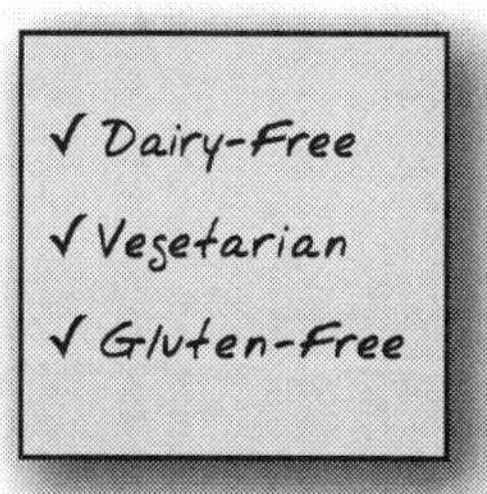

Thick & Chunky Tomato Soup

4 tomatoes
2 avocados
2 stalks celery
½ head cauliflower
2 zucchini
¼ cup olive oil
1 tablespoon basil
1 tablespoon oregano
½ tablespoon rosemary
1½ teaspoons Celtic Sea Salt®

Chop and marinate the cauliflower, zucchini and celery in olive oil and rosemary. Puree tomato and avocado, then stir in softened veggies and herbs. Salt to taste._Heat in pot to warm. Garnish with basil.

Makes 4 servings.

Nutrition per serving: calories 208, fat 17.42 g, cholesterol 0 mg, sodium 44.25 mg, carbohydrates 8.5 g, fiber 4.52 g, sugar 3.55 g, protein 2.97 g.

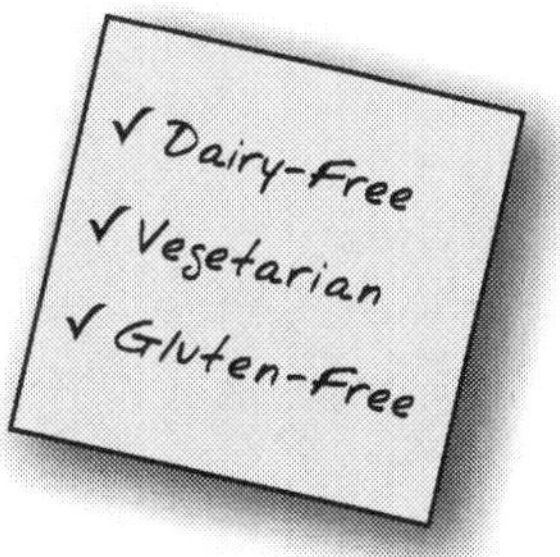

Tomato Minestrone

2 cups low sodium vegetable broth
¼ cup peeled and chopped Vidalia onion
½ cup chopped celery
½ cup peeled and diced sweet potatoes (for Phase 2)
1 cup drained and chopped canned plum tomatoes
2 tablespoons chopped basil
1 tablespoon parsley and chives
1 cup of chopped steamed kale
1 cup of steamed spinach

In a saucepan, combine ¼ cup of stock with onions, celery and sweet potatoes. Sweat vegetables for about 8 minutes over medium heat, stirring. Add tomatoes and rest of stock, simmering until vegetables are all soft. Add basil, parsley, chives, spinach and kale, then simmer for another 5 minutes.

Makes 1 to 2 servings.

Nutrition per serving: calories 197, fat 0.5 g, cholesterol 0 mg, sodium 1130.5 mg, carbohydrates 37.45 g, fiber 11.35 g, sugar 20.75 g, protein 7.97 g.

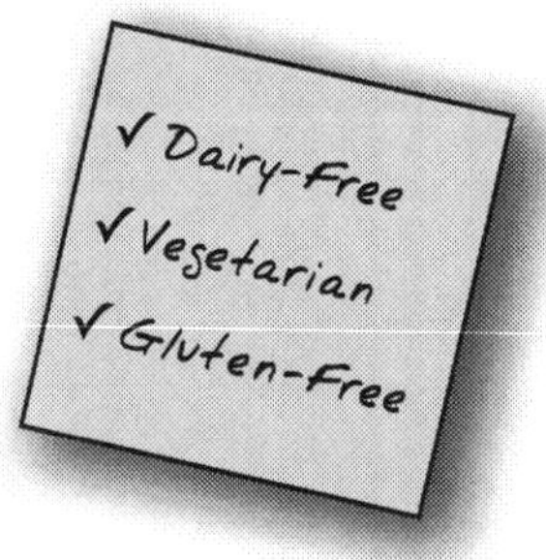

Turkey Soup

1 yellow onion, quartered
10 cloves garlic, minced
2 leeks
1 bunch asparagus tips
3 stalks celery
1 parsnip, chopped
1 handful of thyme
2 sprigs of rosemary
2 low-sodium vegetable bullion cubes
12 cups of water
1 bunch parsley, minced
2 pounds boneless, skinless turkey breast
1 tablespoon soy sauce
1 to 2 pounds kale

√ Dairy-Free
√ Gluten-Free*

* Basting solutions injected in turkey during processing may contain gluten. Be sure to read label.

Rub the turkey with half the garlic, half the rosemary, half the thyme, soy sauce and half the parsley. In a soup pot, add remaining ingredients except for the kale, then sauté on medium heat about 10 minutes so the vegetables start to brown. Cover with water and add bullion, then simmer about 3 hours so the vegetables are cooked. Strain broth. Place turkey with seasonings in a covered roasting pan into a 370°F oven. Roast about 1½ hours or until cooked. Take out of the oven, uncover and let cool about an hour. Shred the turkey and add it to the strained broth. Take the stems out of the kale, chop the kale and add to the broth, then cook another hour. Serve garnished with fresh parsley and a splash of soy sauce to taste.

Makes 5 to 6 servings. Nutrition per serving: calories 141, fat 0.58 g, cholesterol 50.8 mg, sodium 276.4 mg, carbohydrates 11.2 g, fiber 3.6 g, sugar 4.6 g, protein 20.2 g.

Tuscan Minestrone Soup[9]

2 tablespoons olive oil
1 medium zucchini, cut into ½-inch slices, about 2 cups
1 medium summer squash, cut into ½-inch slices, about 2 cups
1 large carrot, finely diced, about ¾ cup
1 small onion, finely diced, about ¾ cup
2 cloves garlic minced
1 teaspoon Italian seasoning
4 cups reduced-sodium chicken or vegetable broth
1 can (15 ounces) cannelli beans, drained and rinsed
1 can (15 ounces) diced tomatoes or 2 cups fresh tomatoes diced

Heat the oil in a Dutch oven over medium-high heat. Add the zucchini, summer squash, carrot, onion, garlic,and Italian seasoning to the Dutch oven and cook while stirring frequently, until the vegetables start to soften—about 10 minutes. Stir in the broth and diced tomatoes, cover the mixture then bring it to a boil. Add the beans and cook uncovered at a low boil for about 10 minutes.

Makes 6 servings.

Nutrition per serving: calories 176, total fat 5.3 g, saturated fat 0.7 g, sodium 456 mg, carbohydrates 24.7 g, fiber 6.3 g, protein 7.7 g.

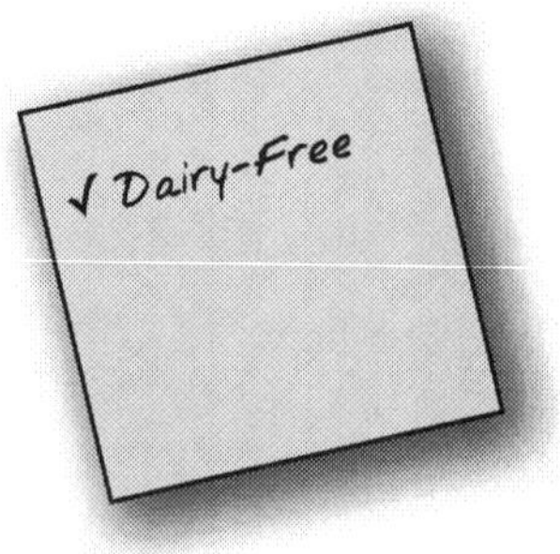

Vegetable Soup

1 zucchini, chopped
1 yellow onion, chopped
10 stalks of celery, chopped
1 bunch of kale
1 bunch collard greens
4 cups of vegetable broth
Salt and pepper to taste

Place chopped vegetables and vegetable broth into a soup pot. Add salt and pepper to taste, or add herbs for flavoring, such as basil, parsley, Italian seasoning. Cook until vegetables are soft. Serve

Makes 2 to 3 servings.

Nutrition per serving: calories 143, fat 0.2 g, cholesterol 0 mg, sodium 555.75 mg, carbohydrates 30.3 g, fiber 10.6 g, sugar 19.2 g, protein 2.7 g.

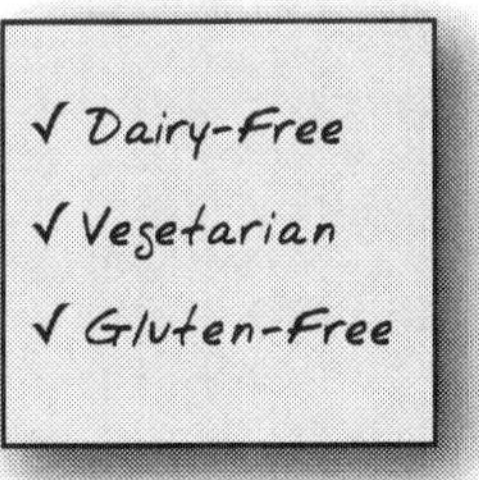

Vitamix® Tomato Onion Cheese Soup

1 large tomato, quartered
¼ cup onion
1 tablespoon tomato paste
1 cup organic chicken, vegetable or beef broth

Optional: ¼ cup sharp cheddar or Swiss cheese

Place all ingredients in container in order listed. Secure 2-part lid and select low speed. Turn machine on and then switch to high speed. Process for 5 to 6 minutes, or until steam escapes through the lid plug opening.

Makes 2½ servings (serving size of 1 cup).

Nutrition per serving: calories 85, total fat 5 g, saturated fat 3 g, cholesterol 14 mg, sodium 360 mg, carbohydrates 6 g, fiber 1 g, protein 6 g.

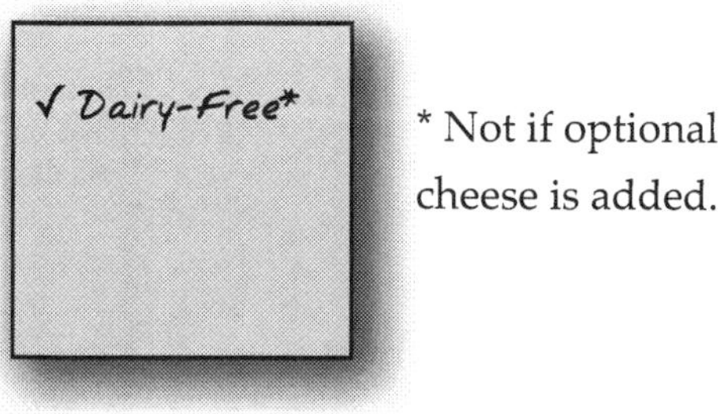

* Not if optional cheese is added.

Vitamix® Vegetable Soup

¼ cup peas, fresh or frozen (thawed)
¼ cup lima beans, canned or frozen (thawed)
1 cup canned tomatoes or 1 large tomato
¼ cup celery
¼ cup fresh carrots
1-inch thick, sweet green or red pepper slice
1 cup organic vegetable, chicken or beef broth
Dash onion powder
Pepper to taste

Optional: 1 teaspoon coriander

Place all ingredients in container in order listed. Secure 2-part lid and select low speed. Turn machine on and then switch to high speed. Process for 4 to 5 minutes or until steam escapes through the lid plug opening.

Makes 2 servings (serving size of 1 cup).

Nutrition per serving: calories 81, total fat 1 g, saturated fat 0 g, sodium 350 mg, carbohydrates 14 g, fiber 4 g, protein 6 g.

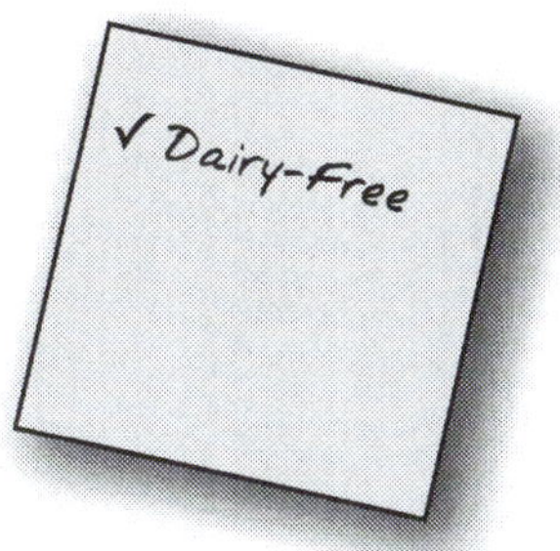

White Bean Soup with Kale and Sausage

2 ounces turkey sausage
1 cup chopped onion
3 garlic cloves, minced
3 cups organic chicken broth
2 (15 ounce) cans organic cannellini beans, rinsed and drained
4 cups chopped kale
½ teaspoon freshly ground black pepper

Heat a large saucepan over medium-high heat. Add turkey sausage to pan, then sauté 1 minute. Add onion and garlic to pan, then sauté another 5 minutes, or until tender. Add broth and beans to pan and bring to a boil. Partially mash beans with potato masher. Stir in kale and ½ teaspoon pepper, then cook over medium heat for 6 minutes.

Makes 4 servings (serving size of 1¼ cups).

Nutrition per serving: calories 235, total fat 7.3 g, saturated fat 2.1 g, sodium 586 mg, carbohydrates 30.7 g, fiber 7.6 g, protein 13.4 g.

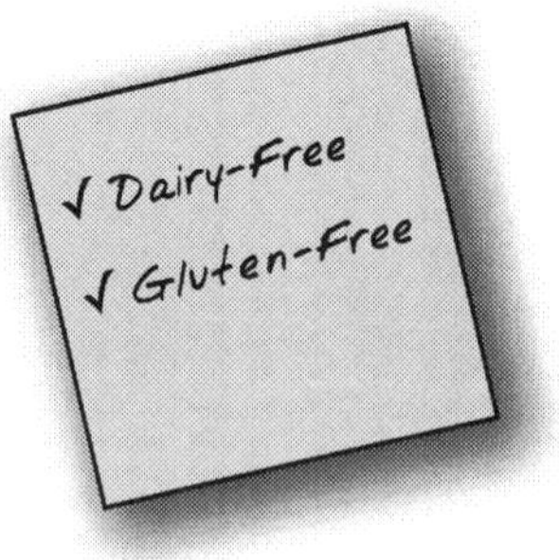

Recipes: Desserts and Snacks

"All I really need is love,
but a little chocolate now and then doesn't hurt!"
— *Charles Schulz*

Chocolate Banana Soft Serve

✓ Vegetarian
✓ Gluten-Free

1 frozen banana
1 tablespoon cocoa powder
1 tablespoon maple syrup, agave, or honey
¼ teaspoon vanilla extract
1 splash of almond milk for desired consistency

Optional:
   Add almond butter or natural peanut butter
   Add mint leaves for chocolate mint

Place ingredients in blender and blend until creamy.

Makes 2 servings.

Nutrition per serving: calories 110, fat 1.13 g, cholesterol 0 mg, sodium 26.13 mg, carbohydrates 26.45 g, fiber 3.01 g, sugar 17.12 g, protein 1.615 g.

Chocolate Dipped Raw Cookie Balls

5 Medjool dates, soaked
1 cup of nuts (choose from almonds, cashews, walnuts)
4 tablespoons dried coconut
1 to 2 tablespoons agave, raw honey or maple syrup
1 cup chocolate chips

Soak dates in water for 2 hours. Remove pit and coarsely chop. Place nuts in food processor and process until small, but do not over process because it will turn into nut butter. Add coconut and maple syrup into food processor and process until mixed. Remove from food processor and mix in chocolate chips. Form into 1-inch balls and place in refrigerator to set. Melt chocolate chips and dip balls into chocolate and place on wax paper to set.

Optional: add 1 teaspoon of cinnamon or cocoa—or dried pineapple—to mixture.

Makes 6 to 7 servings.

Nutrition per serving: calories 143, fat 5.76 g, cholesterol 0 mg, sodium 11 mg, carbohydrates 22.6 g, fiber 2.5 g, sugar 15.8 g, protein 2 g.

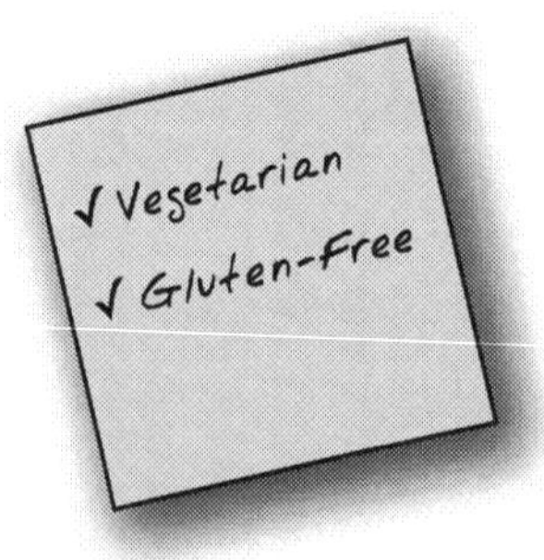

Chocolate Peanut Butter Cups

½ cup Earth Balance Butter
¼ cup peanut butter, almond butter or walnut butter
¾ cup graham cracker crumbs (or gluten free graham cracker crumbs)
¼ cup maple sugar or other granulated sweetener
1 cup dark chocolate
¼ cup rice milk or nut milk
¼ cup chopped pecans, almonds or peanuts

Line a 12 cup muffin tin with paper liners. Melt the butter in a small saucepan over medium heat. Stir in the peanut butter, graham cracker crumbs and maple sugar, then mix well. Remove the mixture from the heat. Evenly divide the mixture—approximately 2 tablespoons per cup—among the muffin cups. Let that cool and harden. Into another pan, combine the chocolate and milk. Stir over medium heat until chocolate has melted. Evenly spoon the chocolate mixture over the peanut butter mixture. Top with chopped nuts, then place in the refrigerator to set for at least 2 hours before serving.

Makes 15 servings.

Nutrition per serving: calories 145, fat 13.24 g, cholesterol 0 mg, sodium 67 mg, carbohydrates 4.63 g, fiber 3.8 g, sugar 2.81 g, protein 2.616 g.

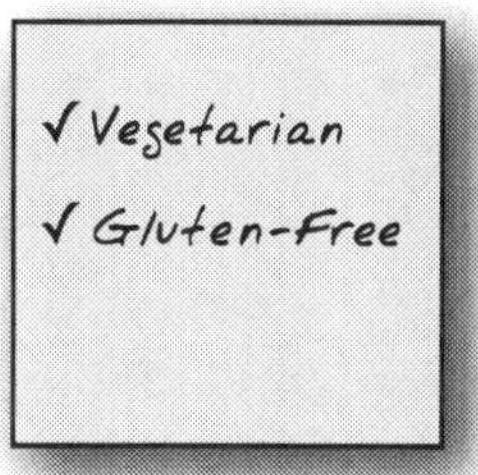

Dark Chocolate Clementines

4 clementines
16 ounces dark chocolate
2 tablespoons shredded coconut
2 tablespoons almonds, toasted and finely chopped

Peel and segment the clementines. Melt chocolate in a double boiler. Dip clementine segments into melted chocolate and sprinkle with toasted, chopped almonds or shredded coconut.

Can also use for dipping berries, bananas, pineapple, etc.

Makes 4 servings.

Nutrition per serving: calories 100, fat 4.84 g, cholesterol 0 mg, sodium 9.45 mg, carbohydrates 14.9 g, fiber 2.55 g, sugar 9.3 g, protein 1.6 g.

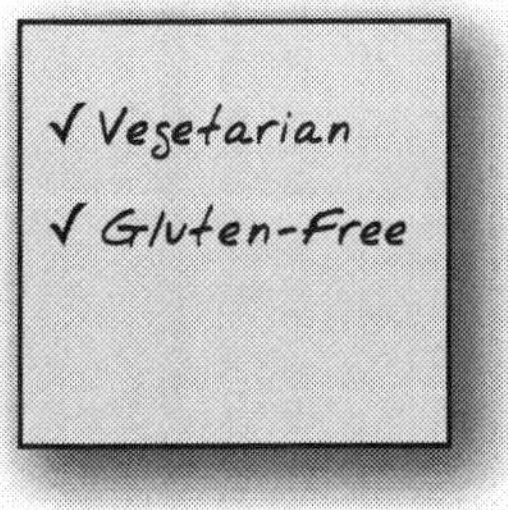

Dark Chocolate Pecan Butter

1 cups raw pecans
½ cup dark chocolate chips
1 to 2 tablespoons agave
1 teaspoon coconut oil
¼ teaspoon salt

Toast raw pecans for 10 minutes at 325°F. Watch so they don't burn. Place pecans in food processor and process for 10 minutes—until it forms nut butter. Add ½ cup chocolate chips and 1 teaspoon coconut oil to small pot, then melt on low heat. Avoid burning chocolate. Add melted chocolate to pecan butter in food processor and process until mixed. Add salt and process. Store in refrigerator. Use Dark Chocolate Pecan Butter to top raw vanilla ice cream, banana, toast, etc.

Makes 10 servings (serving size of 1 tablespoon).

Nutrition per serving: calories 108, fat 10.06 g, cholesterol 0 mg, sodium 0 mg, carbohydrates 4.73 g, fiber 1.76 g, sugar 3.08 g, protein 1.57 g.

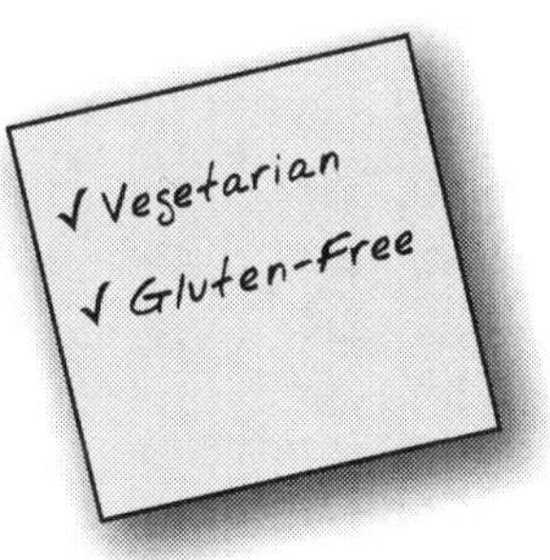

Doughnut Holes

⅔ cup raw cashews

⅓ cup oats (not instant)

3 tablespoons agave

1 teaspoon vanilla extract

¼ cup chocolate chips (bittersweet, milk, or white chocolate chips)

Optional:

For high omega-3 doughnut holes, add cocoa powder, carob powder, shredded coconut, hemp seeds or flaxseeds and 2 tablespoons coconut oil.

For cinnamon raisin doughnut holes, add 1 to 2 teaspoons cinnamon and 2 tablespoons raisins.

Blend oats and cashews into a flour-like consistency (use food processor—don't blend too much or will turn into butter). Place flour mix into blender. Add agave and vanilla extract, then blend until dough-like texture. Add chocolate chips, then stir by hand. Refrigerate for 30 minutes to an hour. Remove from blender and roll into tablespoon size cookie balls. Refrigerate.

Makes 16 to 18 servings.

Nutrition per serving: calories 50, fat 2.3 g, cholesterol 0 mg, sodium 0.45 mg, carbohydrates 6.26 g, fiber 0.6 g, sugar 3.75 g, protein 1 g.

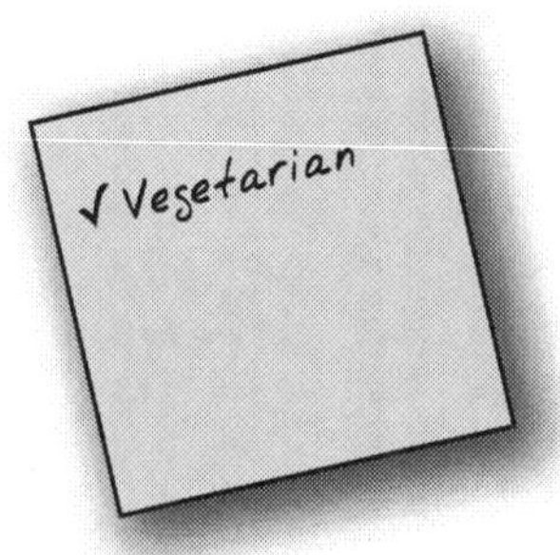

Frozen Fudge

¾ cup coconut oil, liquefied
½ cup honey or maple syrup
1 cup (crunchy or smooth) sunflower seed butter, almond butter or macadamia butter
10 drops of vanilla liquid stevia
½ teaspoon Celtic Sea Salt®

Optional:

For a crunch, add favorite cereal or quinoa flakes.
Add 2 tablespoons cocoa for chocolate fudge (adjust sweetener to taste).
Add peppermint extract for peppermint chocolate fudge.

Blend ingredients. Pour into a large glass dish, lined with parchment paper. Top with dark chocolate or dairy free chocolate chips. Freeze for 2 hours, then slice and store in the freezer.

Makes 10 to 12 servings.

Nutrition per serving: calories 180, fat 16.6 g, cholesterol 0 mg, sodium 13.3 mg, carbohydrates 10 g, fiber 0 g, sugar 4.6 g, protein 1 g.

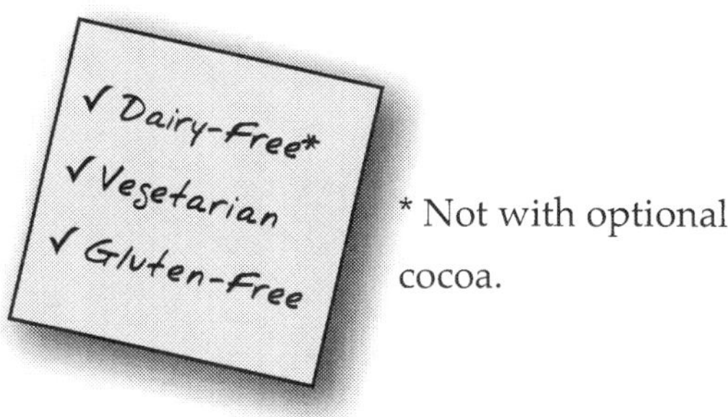

* Not with optional cocoa.

Oatmeal Cookies

½ cup oil
¾ cup honey
1 egg
¼ cup water
1 teaspoon vanilla
1 cup whole wheat flour
½ cup dry milk powder
½ teaspoon baking soda
1 teaspoon cinnamon
2 cup rolled oats
1 cup wheat germ
½ cup goji berries
½ cup chia seeds

Blend oil, honey, egg, water and vanilla with electric mixer. Add flour, dry milk powder, soda and cinnamon. Beat well. Mix in oats, wheat germ, goji berries and chia seeds. Drop by teaspoonfuls onto greased cookie sheets. Bake at 350°F for 10 to 12 minutes, or until lightly browned.

Makes approximately 40 servings (serving size of 1 cookie).

Nutrition per serving: calories 123, total fat 4.3 g, saturated fat 0.5 g, carbohydrates 17.1 g, fiber 2.3 g, protein 3.6 g.

Raw Chocolate Pudding

1 avocado, pitted
2 tablespoons cocoa powder
3 tablespoons vanilla almond milk
2 to 3 tablespoons maple syrup or honey
1 splash of vanilla extract or 1 vanilla bean
1 pinch of sea salt

Optional:
¾ cup frozen cherries, strawberries, blueberries
1 splash of almond extract

Throw all ingredients in a food process and blend. Add more milk for desired consistency. For variety, add any type of frozen fruit—such as cherries, strawberries, blueberries.

Makes 2 servings.

Nutrition per serving: calories 120, fat 18 g, cholesterol 0 mg, sodium 4 mg, carbohydrates 19.45 g, fiber 6.75 g, sugar 8.25 g, protein 2.25 g.

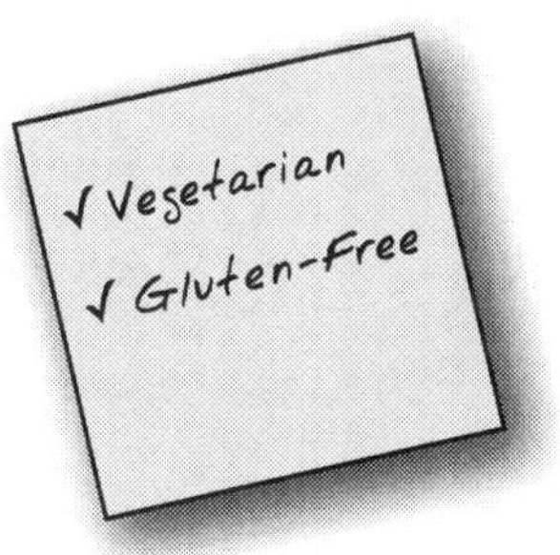

Raw Strawberry Ice Cream

Meat of 2 young coconuts and 1 cup coconut water
5 cups organic strawberries
3 organic dates, pitted
4 cups ice cubes (14 cubes)

Optional:
1 teaspoon organic strawberry extract
Fresh basil leaves

Place coconut meat, strawberries, stevia, dates, strawberry extract and 1 cup of ice in a blender. Blend at highest speed and add remaining ice as long as mixture is flowing and blending well. You may not need to use all the ice, just enough to make the mixture thick. Add a little coconut water to facilitate blending. For other flavors, add 3 tablespoons cocoa powder and mint extract for mint chocolate—or add freshly scraped vanilla beans for French vanilla.

Makes 4 servings.

Nutrition per serving: calories 180, fat 1.75 g, cholesterol 0 g, sodium 151.25 mg, carbohydrates 45 g, fiber 7.75 g, sugar 28 g, protein 3.25 g.

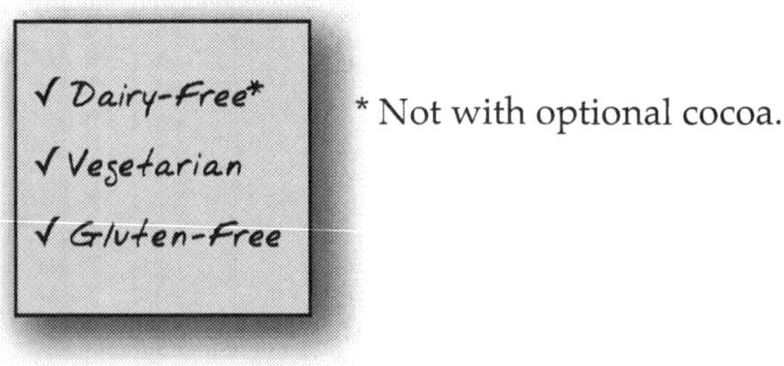

* Not with optional cocoa.

Raw Pie Crust

4 Medjool dates (or ⅓ cup honey or agave nectar)

2 cups of nuts (use one type—or for a good mixture, use cashews and macadamia nuts)

Soak Medjool dates in water for 1 to 2 hours. Place nuts in food processor and process until ground, but not too long or else it will turn into nut butter. Add dates (or agave) until mixed in. Press into pie dish. Top with seasonal fruit, *Raw Chocolate Pudding* (page 463) or a scoop of ice cream.

Makes 10 servings.

Nutrition per serving: calories 154, fat 10.3 g, cholesterol 0 mg, sodium 4 mg, carbohydrates 14.4 g, fiber 4 g, sugar 7.11 g, protein 3.2 g.

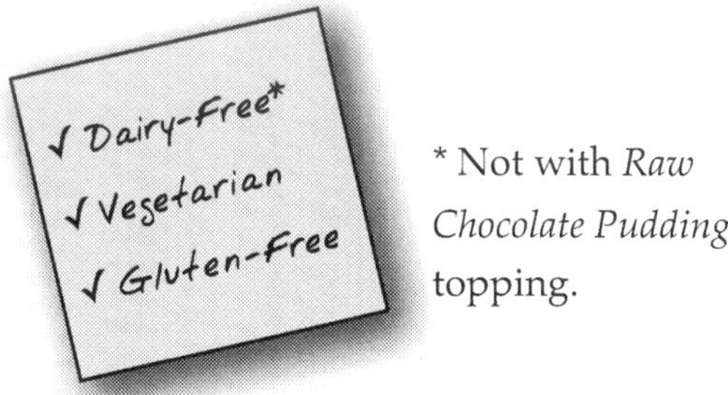

* Not with *Raw Chocolate Pudding* topping.

Trail Mix

1 cup raw almonds
½ cup raw sunflower seeds
½ raw pumpkins seeds
½ cup goji berries
4 tablespoons honey or maple syrup
1 teaspoon cinnamon

Toss the almonds and sunflower seeds with the honey and cinnamon. Spread on a baking sheet sprayed with cooking spray, or lined with parchment paper. Bake in a 300°F oven for 20 minutes. Stir in goji berries after cooked. (they will burn if cooked with other ingredients)

Makes 8 servings (serving size of ¼ cup).

Nutrition per serving: calories 281, total fat 15.5 g, saturated fat 1.6 g, sodium 69 mg, carbohydrates 26.5 g, fiber 4.5 g, protein 8.9 g.

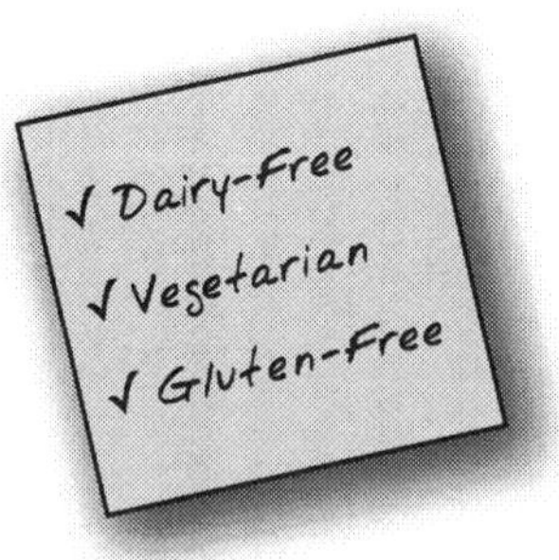

Vanilla Bean Cake[1]

2 cups cooked white beans, room temperature
6 eggs
¾ teaspoon vanilla liquid stevia
1 teaspoon vanilla extract
⅓ cup honey or maple syrup
¼ cup coconut oil, liquefied
⅓ cup coconut flour, sifted
1 teaspoon baking soda
⅕ teaspoon baking powder
¾ cup chocolate chips
½ cup coconut milk
2 tablespoons honey
2 to 4 tablespoons coconut flour

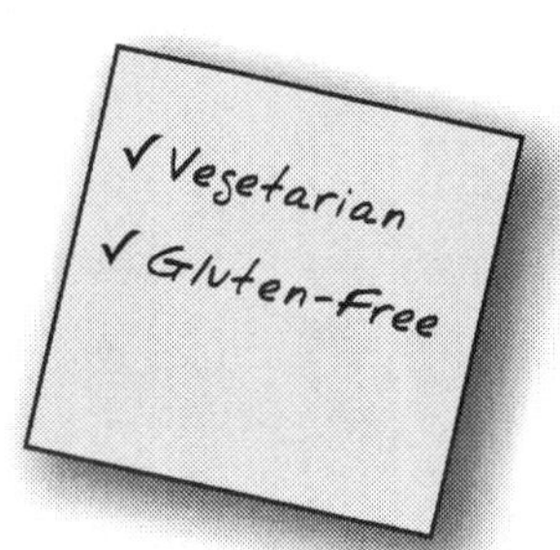

Add white beans, eggs, stevia, vanilla extract and honey to food processor. Puree for 2 minutes—until well blended. Add coconut oil, coconut flour, salt, baking soda and baking powder, then puree. Pour into spring-form pan, lined with parchment paper and greased with coconut oil spray or organic butter. Bake at 325°F for 30 minutes. For cupcakes, bake for 22 minutes. For frosting, melt ¾ cup chocolate chips and ½ cup coconut milk over double boiler. After it's melted, remove from heat and add 2 tablespoons honey and 2 to 4 tablespoons coconut flour, then refrigerate for 15 minutes.

Makes 15 servings.

Nutrition per serving: calories 152, fat 9.6 g, cholesterol 76 mg, sodium 44 mg, carbohydrates 13.6 g, fiber 3 g, sugar 4.2 g, protein 5 g.

Vanilla Pudding

½ cup cashews, soaked in water for 3 hours and drained
½ cup coconut oil, liquefied
¼ cup maple syrup, honey, or 2 to 3 dates
1 tablespoon vanilla extract
½ to ¾ cup coconut milk
1 pinch of salt

Add cashews and coconut oil into food processor. Add remaining ingredients and process for 2 minutes—until smooth. Put more coconut milk for thinner consistency, or only ½ cup for thicker consistency. Pour into dish and refrigerate. Top with bananas, raisins, granola or strawberries.

Makes 8 servings.

Nutrition per serving: calories 138, fat 11 g, cholesterol 0 mg, sodium 3.75 mg, carbohydrates 10.25 g, fiber 0.25 g, sugar 6.63 g, protein 1.375 g.

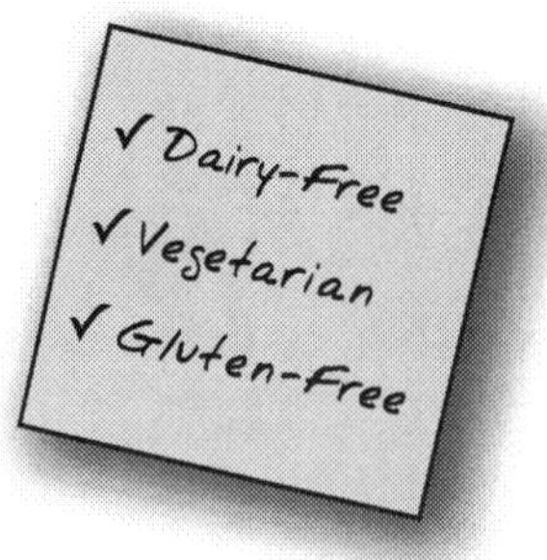

White Chocolate Mango Cookie Dough Balls

⅔ cup raw cashews
⅓ cup oats
3 tablespoons maple syrup
¼ cup chopped, unsweetened dried mango
¼ cup of white chocolate chips (or chopped bar)

Place cashews and oats in food processor or high speed blender and process until fine. Add maple syrup. Add chopped mango and white chocolate chunks and mix in by hand—or for 2 pulses in food processor. Form into 16 to 18 dough balls and place in freezer for 30 minutes to set. For variety: replace mango with dried apples and use dark chocolate instead of white chocolate, then add ½ teaspoon cinnamon.

Makes 16 servings.

Nutrition per serving: calories 62, fat 2.96 g, cholesterol 1.25 mg, sodium 6.5 mg, carbohydrates 7.5 g, fiber 0.34 g, protein 1.18 g, sugar 5.46 g.

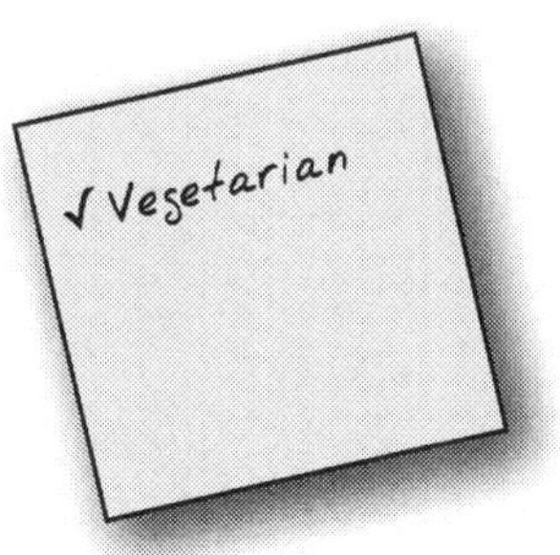

Zucchini Chocolate Chip Cookies

1 egg
⅓ cup warm water
⅓ cup applesauce
⅓ cup brown sugar, coconut sugar, or date sugar
¼ cup honey or agave
1 tablespoon vanilla extract
2 cups whole wheat flour or spelt flour
½ teaspoon baking soda
¼ teaspoon baking powder
¼ teaspoon salt
¼ teaspoon cinnamon
¼ teaspoon nutmeg
1 cup finely shredded zucchini
1 pinch of salt
12 ounces chocolate chips

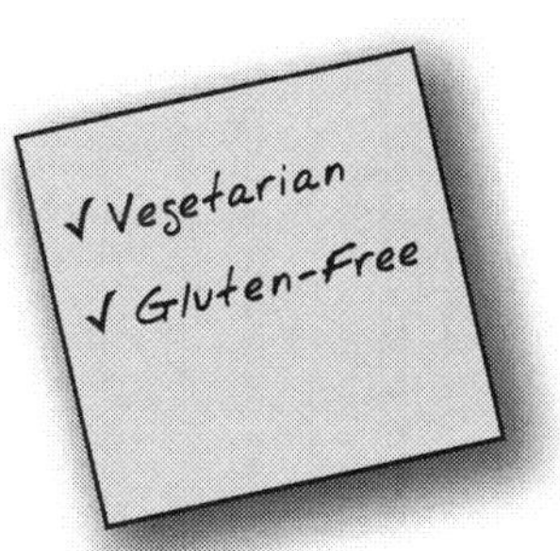

Optional: add 1 teaspoon melted coconut oil for more moisture

Preheat oven to 350°F. Line cookie sheet with parchment paper. In a large bowl, whisk together egg and water until frothy. Stir in applesauce, brown sugar, honey and vanilla extract. In a small bowl, stir together flour, baking soda, baking powder, salt, cinnamon and nutmeg. Stir dry ingredients into wet ingredients until combined. The dough may seem a little dry, but the zucchini will give moisture. Add grated zucchini and chocolate chips, stirring until incorporated. Spoon dough onto cookie sheets and bake at 350°F for 12 to 15 minutes.

Makes 12 to 15 servings (serving size of 1 cookie).

Nutrition per serving: calories 150, fat 6.9 g, cholesterol 5 mg, carbohydrates 20.9 g, fiber 0.8 g, sugar 13.7 g, protein 1.4 g.

Appendix A: Diagnosing Insulin Resistance

My criteria for diagnosing insulin resistance is somewhat modified and is based on a fasting insulin and fasting glucose blood test. As for my particular criteria (not the criteria of the American Diabetes Association), if the fasting insulin level is above five microIU/mL and the glucose is above 81, then you have pre-diabetes or insulin resistance. A recent study published in an endocrinology journal noted a fasting insulin level above nine microIU/mL has an 80 percent chance in diagnosing pre-diabetes with the definition of fasting glucose of 100 to 125.[1]

However, if your doctor waits for a fasting glucose above 100 to inform you that you have pre-diabetes, then your doctor is not aware that pre-diabetes actually starts *before* a fasting glucose above 100. A beautiful study published in the New England Journal of Medicine looked at 13,163 healthy men in the Israel armed forces and followed them for close to six years. It was determined that if a fasting blood glucose is between 91 and 99 mg/dL, that person has an eight times higher risk of developing diabetes when compared to someone with a fasting glucose of 86 mg/dL. So, if you are overweight with a fasting glucose of 99 mg/dL, then you are technically "normal" in the conventional medicine criteria. Normal blood glucose is less than 100 mg/dL. However; you really have an eight times higher risk of developing diabetes if you continue the same lifestyle—because you already have insulin resistance. Also, in the study if someone had a fasting glucose of less than 81 mg /dL, than their risk for developing diabetes was the lowest. Because of that study, I use the criteria of a fasting glucose of less than 81 mg/dL to be optimal.[2]

The optimal fasting insulin level of less than five microIU/ml is my criteria. By the way, most laboratories list their normal fasting insulin levels up to 24.9 microIU/ml. There are no medical studies to answer the question, "What are the optimal insulin levels?" Some of my physician friends that practice Age Management Medicine or Functional Medicine use the criteria of fasting insulin level less than 2 microIU/ml. I have not seen any data on less than 2 microIU/ml.

There are some medical studies and data suggesting the optimal fasting insulin level is less than five microIU/ml. In a classic study on insulin resistance by Dr. Wallace and Dr. Matthews, they looked at a group of 290 healthy patients and the most common fasting insulin level for this group was five microIU/ml, although some of the healthy group had higher levels. However, the diabetic group had fasting levels of an average of twelve microIU/ml, and some had levels in the 40 microIU/ml.[3]

In a recent study on the Paleolithic diet (high intake of vegetables, fruits and meat; moderate intake of nuts, berries and honey; low intake of grains and no intake of milk or dairy products, legumes, salt, alcohol or refined carbohydrates), it was shown that healthy medical student volunteers from Sweden improved on their insulin resistance (according to the HOMA test) on the Paleolithic diet.

Their fasting insulin was measured in pmol/l, and to convert to microIU/ml you need to divide by seven. The fasting insulin levels started at 4.37 and after 21 days on the Paleolithic diet, the fasting insulin levels dropped to 3.5 microIU/ml. Also, the insulin resistance improved with the Paleolithic diet.[4]

Regarding these studies, I consider the optimal fasting insulin level to be less than five microIU/ml.

The American Diabetes Association has been lowering their criteria for the definition of diabetes and pre-diabetes. Currently, they do not recommend a fasting insulin level or 2-hour insulin levels after a glucose challenge test. Hopefully, over time, the American Diabetes Association will change their criteria for the definition of pre-diabetes and thereby become more aggressive in picking up insulin resistance sooner, rather than later.

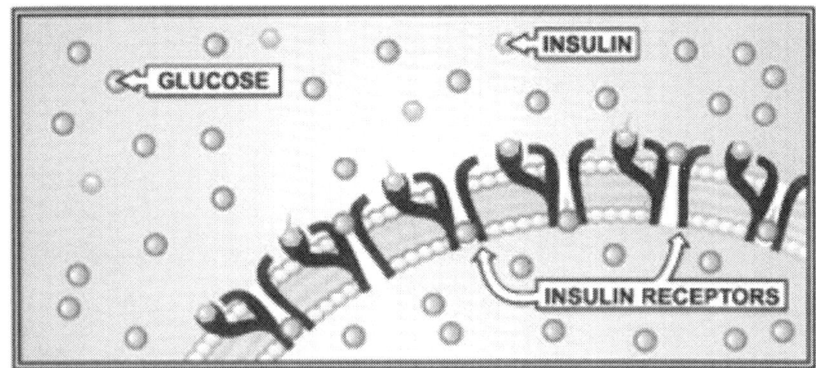

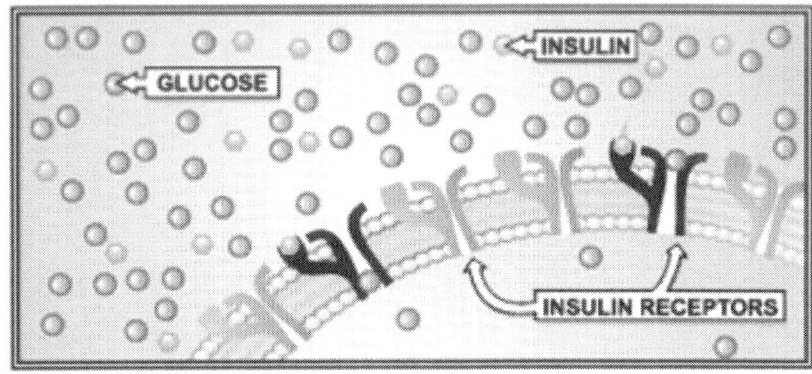

Insulin resistance reduces the insulin sensitivity of cells, which means that it impairs the processing of glucose through the cell wall for conversion to energy. As a result, instead of glucose passing from the blood into the cells, glucose remains in the blood stream - causing elevated levels of blood sugar, which are sent to the liver. Once there, the sugar is converted into fat and stored by the blood stream throughout the body - leading to weight gain and obesity.

The current gold standard test for diagnosing insulin resistance is the Glucose Clamp Study. It requires an infusion of insulin and glucose for two hours. The blood sugars are monitored frequently and maintained at a certain level by adjusting the insulin infusion. The last 30 minutes determine insulin sensitivity. The more insulin required for the Glucose Clamp Study, then more insulin resistance. On the other hand, the less insulin required means that one has insulin sensitivity, or no insulin resistance. However, this test is rarely performed in the community and is usually done in University centers or research centers. I believe that the fasting insulin and glucose is an inexpensive way to diagnosis insulin resistance.

Another way to measure insulin resistance is the HOMA (Homeostatic Model Assessment). It's a special mathematical test measuring insulin resistance by using a fasting insulin and glucose level. Dr. Matthews first described it in 1985. Later, a newer model called the HOMA2 was developed to better measure insulin resistance.[5]

Another mathematical test that has been developed is the QUICKI (Quantitative Insulin Sensitivity Check Index). This test does correlate well with the glucose clamp studies. The lower numbers reflect a higher insulin resistance.[6]

Appendix B: Dirty Dozen™ and Clean 15™

Dirty Dozen™

(These non-organics are highest in pesticides—buy organic instead)

1. Apples
2. Celery
3. Strawberries
4. Peaches
5. Spinach
6. Nectarines (imported)
7. Grapes (imported)
8. Sweet bell peppers
9. Potatoes
10. Blueberries (domestic)
11. Lettuce
12. Kale / collard greens

Clean 15™

(These non-organics are lowest in pesticides)

1. Onions
2. Corn
3. Pineapples
4. Avocado
5. Asparagus
6. Sweet peas
7. Mangoes
8. Eggplant
9. Cantaloupe (domestic)
10. Kiwi
11. Cabbage
12. Watermelon
13. Sweet potatoes
14. Grapefruit
15. Mushrooms

With this helpful guide, you'll know which fruits and vegetables have the most pesticide residues and are therefore the most important to buy organic. You can lower your pesticide intake substantially just by avoiding the twelve most contaminated non-organic fruits and vegetables (Dirty Dozen™). For this and other helpful information from the Environmental Working Group, please visit www.foodnews.org.

Appendix C: Your New Grocery List

Whether you're in Phase One or Phase Two, Option A or Option B, your grocery shopping routine is going to change. In some cases, you may even have to find a more appropriate grocery store or farmers market. Just remember that as you improve upon the ingredients of your nutrition, your best investment improves as well.

While you probably won't be buying everything on this list all at once, these are the typical items for which you'll be shopping. Also, remember to buy what is currently in season and, whenever possible, from local sources.

Produce (best to buy what is in season)

Romaine or red leaf lettuce
Dark leafy greens: collard greens, Swiss chard, mustard greens, kale
Spinach and arugula
Zucchini
Bell peppers
Cucumbers
Celery
Cabbage

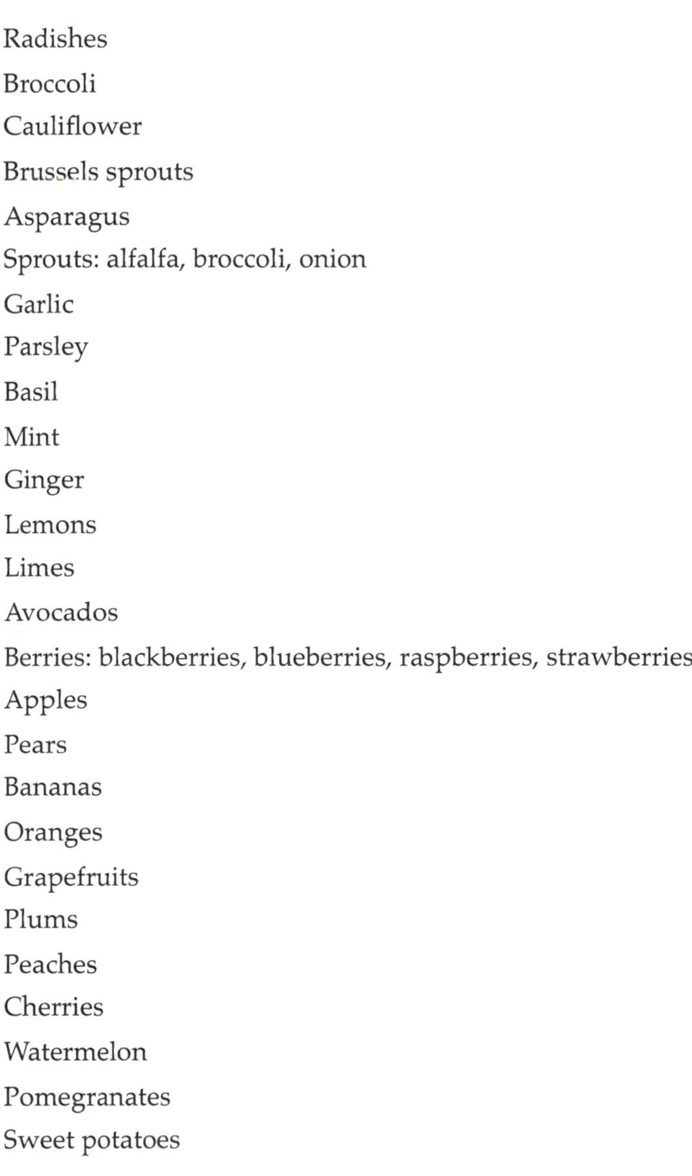

Radishes

Broccoli

Cauliflower

Brussels sprouts

Asparagus

Sprouts: alfalfa, broccoli, onion

Garlic

Parsley

Basil

Mint

Ginger

Lemons

Limes

Avocados

Berries: blackberries, blueberries, raspberries, strawberries

Apples

Pears

Bananas

Oranges

Grapefruits

Plums

Peaches

Cherries

Watermelon

Pomegranates

Sweet potatoes

Starch

Miracle Noodle®

Brown rice pasta

Brown rice

100 percent buckwheat soba noodles

Quinoa

Black beans—dried or canned (if canned, low sodium organic beans)

Nuts/seeds/dried fruit

Walnuts

Almonds and almond flour

Raw cashews

Raw sunflower seeds

Raw pumpkin seeds

Raw pistachios

Dried cranberries or golden raisins

Protein

Organic frozen chicken

Eggs

Alternative Dairy

Hemp milk or almond milk (Pacific Foods, Almond Breeze®)

Light coconut milk

Soup

Pacific Foods organic vegetable broth

Desserts

70 percent dark chocolate (such as Dagoba® or Green & Black's®)

Purely decadent or coconut bliss coconut milk ice cream

Rice milk ice cream

Laloo's® Goat's Milk Ice Cream (Vanilla Snowflake is delicious!)

Dark chocolate chips or dairy free chocolate chips

Sweeteners

NuNaturals stevia

Raw agave, raw honey, or coconut nectar

Spices/powder

Cayenne pepper

Ground cinnamon

Curry or garam masala

Turmeric or curcumin

Ginseng powder

Oils/Butters

Coconut oil (for cooking)

Almond butter or cashew butter

Extra virgin olive oil (cold pressed)

Appendix D: Miracle Noodle®

A slower digestion process allows your body to absorb more nutrients from the foods you eat. Soluble fiber acts to slow digestion overall, while prolonging the sensation of fullness—essential elements of a successful weight management program.

In addition, a slower digestive process equals a slower absorption of glucose, which in turn requires a slower release of insulin, which aids in the normalization of blood glucose after eating a meal.

For more than two-thousand years in Asia, there has been a noodle recipe capable of all that and more. Miracle Noodle® is based on that recipe. It's made from water-soluble fiber, contains no fat, sugar, starch or gluten, and is a great tasting way to slow you digestion process.

As if that wasn't enough, soluble fiber helps control cholesterol by binding with bile acids that are secreted from the gall bladder. These bile acids have cholesterol in them, but when bound with the soluble fiber in Miracle Noodle®, they are harmlessly excreted.

Miracle Noodle® makes a perfect addition to most of the recipes in Phase One and Phase Two, or as a substitute for rice. The many varieties of Miracle Noodle® (such as angel hair and fettucini) are easy to prepare, and readily absorb the flavors of any soup, dish or sauce.

Visit miraclenoodle.com for more information on this truly amazing, multitasking source of plant-based fiber.

Glossary

A

acidic—The pH scale (which measures the acidity or alkalinity of a fluid) ranges from 0 to 14. A pH of 7 is considered neutral, a pH of less than 7 is considered acidic, whereas a pH greater than 7 is considered alkaline.

adrenal cortex—Outer portion of the adrenal gland which produces cortisol, which regulate carbohydrate and fat metabolism, and aldosterone (salt) hormones, which regulate salt and water balance in the body. The deepest layer of the adrenal cortex makes the sex hormone DHEA.

adrenal fatigue—Condition where the adrenal glands do not make enough cortisol and/or DHEA and/or aldosterone (adrenal hormones).

adrenal glands—Triangle-shaped glands that sit on top of the kidneys and regulate stress response through the synthesis of hormones which include cortisol, DHEA, aldosterone (salt hormone) and adrenaline.

adrenal hormone—The four major hormones made by the adrenal gland: cortisol, aldosterone, DHEA and adrenaline.

adrenal insufficiency—See adrenal fatigue.

ALA (alpha-linolenic acid)—Type of omega-3 fatty acid found in plants. Similar to the omega-3 fatty acids that are in fish oil (eicosapentaenoic acid, or EPA, and docosahexaenoic acid, or DHA) and can be converted into EPA and DHA in the body. Is highly concentrated in flaxseed oil and, to a lesser extent, in canola, soy, perilla, and walnut oils. (Not to be confused with alpha-lipoic acid, which may sometimes be called ALA as well.)

ALCAT (Antigen Leukocyte Cellular Antibody Test)—Food allergies and sensitivities testing procedures developed Cell Science Systems.

alkaline—The pH scale (which measures the acidity or alkalinity of a fluid) ranges from 0 to 14. A pH of 7 is considered neutral, a pH of less than 7 is considered acidic, whereas a pH greater than 7 is considered alkaline.

alkaline water—Water with a pH greater than 7. Alkaline water is not found in bottled water, vitamin water or sport drinks. Drinking alkaline water helps lower the devastating effects of acidity in our bodies. (See Kangen Water®.)

alpha-linolenic acid—See ALA. (Not to be confused with alpha-lipoic acid, which may sometimes be called ALA as well.)

alpha-lipoic acid—Universal antioxidant for energy production, blood sugar regulation and the maintenance of a healthy neural system. Helps reduce the complications associated with diabetes, such as pain and numbness. Has the ability to neutralize many different types of free-radicals, and provides a broad spectrum of support to the body's antioxidant network. (Not to be confused with alpha-linolenic acid, which may sometimes be called ALA as well.)

Antigen Leukocyte Cellular Antibody Test—See ALCAT.

B

bioidentical hormones—Compounds that have exactly the same chemical and molecular structure as hormones that are produced in the human body.

BMI (body mass index)—Derived from the weight and height of a person, a BMI above 30 will usually reveal obesity; although, weight lifters with more muscle and lower amounts of body fat may also have a BMI over 30.

body mass index—See BMI.

C

C-reactive protein (CRP)—Protein found in the blood that is elevated in response to inflammation. It is made in the liver and is a marker for inflammation. (CRP is not to be confused with C-peptide.)

celiac disease (gluten sensitive enteropathy)—Digestive disease that damages the small intestine because of a sensitivity to gluten, which is found in wheat, rye, barley, and oats. This hereditary disorder interferes with the absorption of nutrients from food.

cholesterol—White crystalline substance found in animal tissues and various foods that is normally synthesized by the liver, and is an important constituent of cell membranes as well as a precursor to steroid hormones.

chronic inflammation—Leads to a progressive shift in the type of cells which are present at the site of inflammation and is characterized by the simultaneous destruction and healing of the tissue from the inflammatory process. Without inflammation, wounds and infections would never heal and progressive destruction of the tissue would compromise survival; however, chronic inflammation can also lead to a host of diseases.

cortisol—Hormone produced by the adrenal gland which is involved in the stress response, reduces inflammation, opposes insulin so it increases glucose, and aids in fat and protein metabolism.

Cushing's syndrome (hypercortisolism)—Hormonal disorder caused by prolonged exposure of the body's tissues to high levels of the hormone cortisol.

cytokines—Any of various protein molecules secreted by cells of the immune system that serve to regulate the immune system.

D

dehydroepiandrosterone (DHEA)—Steroid hormone produced by the adrenal glands that helps build up muscle, improves memory and helps with vitality.

delayed food sensitivity (food intolerance)—Adverse responses to specific food(s) or food ingredient(s). Delayed allergic reactions, which are mediated by IgG, are different from a true food allergy that is mediated by IgE. Symptoms from delayed food sensitivity include chronic stuffy nose, chronic sinusitis, bad breath, tiredness, cough and headaches.

DHA (docosahexaenoic acid)—As part of omega-3, DHA is a major fatty acid in sperm and the retina. Low levels of DHA have been associated with Alzheimer's disease.

DHEA—See dehydroepiandrosterone.

diabetes—Disease in which blood glucose levels are above normal. The body of a person with diabetes either doesn't make enough insulin or can't use its own insulin as well as it should.

Docosahexaenoic acid—See DHA.

E

eicosapentaenoic acid (EPA)—Found in fish oils, especially from salmon and other cold-water fish, and acts to lower inflammation in the blood. EPA and docosahexaenoic acid (DHA) are the two principal omega-3 fatty acids. The body has a limited ability to manufacture EPA and DHA by converting alpha-linolenic acid, which is found in flaxseed oil, canola oil or walnuts.

endocrine disruptor—Natural and man-made chemicals that can either mimic or disrupt the action of hormones.

endocrinologist—Medical doctor that has done extra training in the field of hormones. Endocrinologists are specialists in diabetes, thyroid disease, thyroid nodules, thyroid cancer, calcium disorders, sodium disorders, short stature, growth hormone disorders, adrenal diseases, osteoporosis, and pituitary problems.

enlarged prostate—See benign prostatic hyperplasia.

EPA—See eicosapentaenoic acid.

estrogen—Group of steroid compounds that are the primary female sex hormones. They promote the development of female secondary sex characteristics and control aspects of regulating the menstrual cycle.

estrone—Type of estrogen that is mainly produced during menopause. High levels of estrone has been associated with breast cancer. Premarin® has estrone in it.

F

food allergy—Reaction to the ingestion of a food that causes adverse effects when the immune system does not recognize as safe a protein component (the allergen) of the food to which the individual is sensitive (such as some proteins in peanuts). The immune system then typically produces immunoglobulin E (IgE) antibodies to the allergen, which trigger other cells to release substances that cause inflammation. Allergic reactions are usually localized to a particular part of the body, and symptoms may include asthma, eczema, flushing, and swelling of tissues (such as the lips) or difficulty in breathing. A severe reaction may result in anaphylaxis (as with severe peanut allergy), in which there is a rapid fall in blood pressure and severe shock. Allergic reactions to foods vary in severity and can be potentially fatal.

food intolerance—See delayed food sensitivity.

free radicals—Molecule produced in the body that is necessary for life, such as destroying bacteria. Too much free radical production has been shown to cause DNA damage, which is not desirable. Vitamin A, vitamin E and vitamin C are antioxidants that can reduce free radicals.

free testosterone—Testosterone in the body that is biologically active and unbound to other molecules in the body, such as sex hormone binding globulin.

G

genetic testing—Tests on blood and other tissue to find genetic disorders.

gland—Organ that synthesizes a substance for release, such as hormones, often into the bloodstream (endocrine gland). An example of an endocrine gland is the thyroid gland that is found in the front of the neck and produces thyroxine (T4), triiodothyronine (T3) and calcitonin hormones.

glucagon—Hormone involved in carbohydrate metabolism or producing more glucose. Produced by the pancreas, it is released when the glucose level in the blood is low (hypoglycemia), causing the liver to convert stored glycogen into glucose and release it into the bloodstream. Glucagon levels are very high in diabetes.

gluten—Consisting of two proteins, gliadin and glutenin, gluten is found in wheat, rye and barley. Gluten is used in the food industry to help make baked food products chewier. Gluten is also used as a food stabilizing agent, and may be found in ketchup and ice cream.

gluten sensitive enteropathy—See celiac disease.

GnRH (gonadotropin releasing hormone)—Also known as luteinizing-hormone releasing hormone (LHRH), this peptide hormone is responsible for the release of gonadotropin (LH and FSH) from the anterior pituitary. GnRH is synthesized and released by the hypothalamus (an upper part of the brain).

gonads—Organ that makes gametes (sperm and egg cells). The gonads in males are the testes and the gonads in females are the ovaries.

gonadotropin—Hormone that stimulate the growth and activity of the gonads, especially any of several pituitary hormones that stimulate the function of the ovaries and testes.

gonadotropin releasing hormone—See GnRH.

glycemia—The concentration of glucose in the blood.

growth hormone—Secreted by the pituitary gland, it stimulates growth of bone and, essentially, all tissues of the body by building protein and breaking down fat to provide energy.

H

Hashimoto's thyroiditis—The most common cause of underactive thyroid disease, it is an autoimmune condition in which the immune system destroys the thyroid.

heavy metal toxicity—Condition where one has been exposed to a metal either by breathing, swallowing or skin exposure. Common heavy metal toxicity includes mercury, lead, cadmium and arsenic. Heavy metal toxicity is damaging to the body and needs to be removed from the body by chelation.

HGH (human growth hormone)—growth hormone that is mainly used to help children of short stature and also for adults with adult growth hormone deficiency. HGH is an injection that needs to be taken daily.

hormone—Made by endocrine glands, hormones are chemical messengers that travel in the bloodstream to tissues or organs. They affect many processes, including growth, metabolism, sexual function, reproduction and mood.

hormone therapy—The use of hormones in medical treatment, such as thyroid hormone replacement for thyroid deficiency.

hot flashes—Sudden wave of mild or intense body heat caused by dilation of capillaries in the skin resulting from decreased levels of estrogen.

human growth hormone—See HGH.

hypercortisolism— See Cushing's syndrome.

hypoglycemia (low blood sugar)—Occurs when the blood glucose level drops too low to provide enough energy for the body's activities.

hypothyroidism—Condition where the thyroid does not produce adequate thyroid hormone. A very common complaint of patients with hypothyroidism is that they are tired and also cold.

I — K

IgE—Certain class of antibody that has an important role against allergies and parasite infections.

IGF-1 (insulin-like growth factor-1)—Protein hormone similar in molecular structure to insulin. Secreted from the liver, it plays an important role in childhood growth and continues to have anabolic effects in adults. Also, it is used to screen for growth hormone deficiency.

IgG—Certain class of antibody that is involved in the secondary immune response. The initial response is IgM (another class of antibody). IgG is involved in delayed food sensitivity.

inflammation—Biological response for the body to heal. Without inflammation wounds and infections would never heal or get rid of infection. Inflammation is a complex reaction which involves many different cytokines.

insulin—A protein pancreatic hormone secreted by the beta cells of the islets of Langerhans that is especially essential for the metabolism of carbohydrates and the regulation of glucose levels in the blood; and, when insufficiently produced, results in diabetes mellitus.

insulin sensitizers—These make cells more responsive to insulin and are commonly used in patients with type 2 diabetes.

insulin-like growth factor-1—See IGF-1.

interleukin—A protein or cytokine that is involved in the immune system and with inflammation. While there are many different interleukins, interleukin-1 and interleukin-6 are also involved with regulating the immune system.

intestinal hyperpermeability (leaky gut)—An opening of the intestinal cell walls, or an opening up of the gut's mucosal barrier, which leads to chronic inflammation and thus to chronic disease. The breakdown of the gut barrier lets bacteria and toxins into the body's circulation, causing the immune system to work overtime.

L

leaky gut—See intestinal hyperpermeability.

LH (luteinizing hormone)—Necessary for proper reproductive function. In women it triggers ovulation, while in men it is involved in testosterone production.

longevity gene (Sirtuin 1 gene)—Activation of the Sirtuin 1 gene is believed to increase longevity. Resveratrol (supplement) has been shown to activate the Sirtuin 1 gene, which is the same gene that is activated with a very low calorie diet—but without the hunger.

low blood sugar—See hypoglycemia.

luteinizing hormone—See LH.

M

melatonin—Hormone that is produced in the pineal gland (in the brain) and helps with the sleep cycle. Melatonin is also an important antioxidant, and is involved with the immune system.

menopause—When the ovaries stop making estrogen and the monthly (menstrual) periods stop. Surgical menopause happens when the ovaries are surgically removed while a woman is still having menstrual cycles. Menopause is the dramatic decline in estrogen that impacts many organs including brain, skin, bone and heart.

metabolism—The complete set of chemical reactions inside a cell. The metabolism of an organism determines what it find nutritious, the pace at which it converts nutrients to energy, and how it stores excess nutrients.

Miracle Noodle®—A water-soluble fiber that contains no fat, sugar, starch or gluten.

N

necrosis—Death of a cell either from infection, toxin or trauma.

nuclear factor kappa beta (NFKB)—A protein complex that plays a key role in stress. NFKB controls the reading of the DNA, and are considered first responders to a toxic event like an infection. Once activated it can turn on the DNA to make other chemicals to respond to the toxic event. Incorrect regulation of NFKB has been linked to cancer, a weak immune system and autoimmune diseases.

O

obesity—Typically defined with a body mass Index (BMI) above 30. A BMI is derived from the weight and height of a person. Obesity increases mortality and the likelihood in developing heart disease, diabetes, cancer and sleep apnea. A BMI of 30 or more will usually reveal obesity; although, weight lifters with more muscle and lower amounts of body fat may also have a BMI over 30. Therefore, the best test is to measure the amount of body fat that a person has. Generally, a body fat of 30 percent or more is considered obese.

omega-3—Fatty acids that have been shown to reduce inflammation and may help prevent chronic diseases, such as heart disease and arthritis. In the body, these essential fatty acids are highly concentrated in the brain and may be particularly important for cognitive and behavioral health as well as normal growth and development. Important omega-3 fatty acids include alpha-linolenic acid, EPA (eicosapentaenoic acid) and DHA (docosahexaenoic acid).

osteoporosis—The diminishing of bone density, typically related to aging, low vitamin D levels and menopause in women. Also, osteoporosis happens in men with low testosterone and low vitamin D levels. Other causes are steroid induced bone loss, overactive thyroid and also hyperparathyroidism (high levels of parathyroid hormones that cause calcium to be lost from the bones).

ovaries—The egg producing organs found in females, they produce the hormones estrogen and progesterone

P — Q

pancreas—Organ that helps with digestion and also secretes several hormones including amylin, somatostatin, glucagon and insulin. Insulin is a hormone that helps glucose move from the blood into the cells where it is used for energy. The pancreas also secretes glucagon when the blood sugar is low to raise the glucose levels. Amylin is a hormone that is co-secreted with insulin to help lower glucose differently from insulin. Somatostatin regulates the secretion of insulin and glucagon.

PMS (premenstrual syndrome)—The appearance of physical and emotional symptoms during the second half of the menstrual cycle. Usual symptoms happens about 1 to 2 weeks before the period with issues of emotional instability, shorter fuse, water retention, insomnia, headaches and constipation.

polycystic ovary syndrome (PCOS)—An endocrine disorder with a host of symptoms related to small painful cysts on the ovaries. It is marked by the overproduction of male hormones in females. PCOS presents itself with irregular periods, is a leading cause of infertility and is related with metabolic syndrome or with insulin resistance.

premenstrual syndrome—See PMS.

progesterone—Female hormone that acts on the uterus (womb) to prepare it for receiving an egg following fertilization. When progesterone levels go down each month, this causes the bleeding associated with menstrual (monthly) periods. Progesterone is a hormone that can help prevent breast cancer and prostate cancer, helps with insomnia, improves bones and helps with reducing anxiety. Progesterone is also produced in men but in much smaller quantities.

progestin—Synthetic form of progesterone, this class of drugs was developed in the 1950s to allow absorption by mouth for use in birth control pills. Medroxyprogesterone is also considered progestin, or synthetic progesterone, and not bioidentical progesterone. Provera® has medroxyprogesterone acetate.

R

resveratrol—Chemical that is found in the skin of red grapes and in red wine that may have an effect of improving longevity. In animal studies, resveratrol has been shown to be anti-inflammatory and have anti-cancer effects. Resveratrol has also been shown to activate the Sirtuin 1 gene that is believed to be involved with longevity. Drinking one glass of red wine has about one milligram of resveratrol, whereas I recommend a dose over 200 mg. Resveratrol comes in a pill form.

S

Sirtuin 1 gene—See longevity gene.

sleep apnea—Condition where one stops breathing while sleeping. Significant levels are when one stops breathing more than five times per hour. An overnight sleep study is needed to make a proper diagnosis.

steroid—Any of various molecules, including hormones, that contain a particular arrangement of carbon rings. Some common steroids include sex steroids, corticosteroids, anabolic steroids and cholesterol.

T

T cells—A certain type of white blood cells that are involved with the immune system. Certain T cells assist other white blood cells and are called T helper cells. Another class of T cells, cytotoxic T cells, destroy virally infected cells and tumor cells.

testosterone—As a steroid, an androgen hormone and the primary male sex hormone, testosterone is produced by the testes in men and ovaries in women. It plays key roles in libido, energy and the immune function in both men and women. Testosterone also helps with muscle and bone formation, and also with hair growth.

thyroid—Gland located inside the neck, it regulates metabolism, which is the body's ability to break down food and convert it to energy. The thyroid gland secretes the hormones thyroxine (T4), triiodothyronine (T3), and calcitonin. The thyroid also is involved in growth. Thyroid disorders result from too little or too much thyroid hormone. Symptoms of hypothyroidism (too little hormone) include decreased energy, slow heart rate, dry skin, constipation, irritability, increased serum cholesterol, irregular menstrual cycles and feeling cold.

thyroid-stimulating hormone (TSH or thyrotropin)—Stimulates the thyroid to secrete the hormones thyroxine (T4) and triiodothyronine (T3). TSH is made in the anterior pituitary gland and regulates the thyroid to make more or less of the thyroid hormones, T4 and T3.

TNF (tumor necrosis factor)—A class of chemical substances involved with inflammation, that is used to measure inflammation. TNF is considered a cytokine (chemical substance) that is involved with cell death. Too much production of TNF has been linked to cancer and chronic health disease (e.g., rheumatoid arthritis).

tumor necrosis factor—See TNF.

U — Z

vitamin D—A fat soluble vitamin that can be found in some foods, but is mostly made by the skin when exposed to ultraviolet rays from the sun. Active vitamin D functions as a hormone because it sends messages to the intestines to increase the absorption of calcium and phosphorus. Vitamin D deficiency is known to cause several bone diseases, including rickets and osteoporosis. Improving on vitamin D levels can reduce the risk of certain cancers and improve the immune system.

zonulin—A protein that is produced in the gut that is consider the "gatekeeper" of the gut. Zonulin is what opens those billions of gateway spaces between those billions of cells, allowing some substances to pass through, while keeping harmful bacteria and toxins out. Zonulin is produced in the gut, and if it is elevated, then the tight junctures of your gut will open up even more—allowing harmful bacteria and toxins to pass through. Those opened junctures will not close until your zonulin level goes back down. For testing purposes, zonulin can be measured in your blood.

References

Chapter 1: America's Secret Recipe for Obesity

1 Mahmood, M., et al. Health effects of soda drinking in adolescent girls in the United Arab Emirates. J Crit Care, 2008 Sep;23(3):434-40.

2 Swithers, S.E., et al. Fat substitutes promote weight gain in rats consuming high-fat diets. Behav Neurosci, 2011 Jun 20. Epub ahead of print.

3 Remig, V., et al. Trans fats in America: a review of their use, consumption, health implications and regulation. J Am Diet Assoc, 2010 Apr;110(4):585-92.

4 Shearn, C.T., et al. Carbonyl reductase inactivation may contribute to mouse lung tumor promotion by electrophilic metabolites of butylated hydroxytoluene: protein alkylation in vivo and in vitro. Chem Res Toxicol, 2008 Aug;21(8):1631-41. Epub 2008 Jul 3.

5 Environmental Working Group. EWG's Shopper's Guide to Pesticides in Produce. www.foodnews.org

6 Campbell, T. C. The China Study: The Most Comprehensive Study of Nutrition Ever Conducted and the Startling Implications for Diet, Weight Loss and Long-term Health (pages 151–152). BenBella Books, 2006, ISBN 1-932100-38-5.

7 Harvard School of Public Health. Food Pyramids and Plates: What Should You Really Eat? www.hsph.harvard.edu/nutritionsource/what-should-you-eat/pyramid-full-story/index.html#dga2005

8 Harvard School of Public Health. Food Pyramids and Plates: What Should You Really Eat? www.hsph.harvard.edu/nutritionsource/what-should-you-eat/pyramid-full-story/index.html#dga2005

9 Centers for Disease Control and Prevention. Obesity and Overweight. www.cdc.gov/nchs/fastats/overwt.htm

10 Willett, W.C. and Stampfer, M.J. Rebuilding the food pyramid. Sci Am, 2003 Jan;288(1):64-71.

Chapter 2: The Consequences of Insulin Resistance

1 Wahrenberg, H., et al. Use of waist circumference to predict insulin resistance: retrospective study. BMJ, 2005 Jun 11;330(7504):1363-4.

2 Proceedings of the American College of Endocrinology Insulin Resistance Syndrome Conference. Washington, DC, USA, August 25-26, 2002. Endocr Pract, 2003 Sep-Oct;9 Suppl 2:22-112.

3 Bingham, E.M., et al. The role of insulin in human brain glucose metabolism: a fluoro-deoxyglucose positron emission tomography study. Diabetes, 2002;51(12):3384-3390.

4 Benedict, C., et al. Intranasal insulin enhances postprandial thermogenesis and lowers postprandial serum insulin levels in healthy men. Diabetes, 2011 Jan;60(1):114-8. Epub 2010 Sep 28.

5 Thambisetty, M., et al. Association of plasma clusterin concentration with severity, pathology, and progression in Alzheimer disease. Arch Gen Psychiatry, 2010 Jul;67(7):739-48.

[6] McGuinness, B., et al. Apolipoprotein epsilon4 and neuropsychological performance in Alzheimer's disease and vascular dementia. Neurosci Lett, 2010 Oct 8;483(1):62-6. Epub 2010 Aug 1.

[7] Weller, R.O., et al. Microvasculature changes and cerebral amyloid angiopathy in Alzheimer's disease and their potential impact on therapy. Acta Neuropathol, 2009 Jul;118(1):87-102. Epub 2009 Feb 22.

[8] Baker, L.D., et al. Insulin resistance and Alzheimer-like reductions in regional cerebral glucose metabolism for cognitively normal adults with pre-diabetes or early type 2 diabetes. Arch Neurol, 2011 Jan;68(1):51-7. Epub 2010 Sep 13.

[9] Schrijvers, E.M., et al. Insulin metabolism and the risk of Alzheimer disease: the Rotterdam Study. Neurology, 2010 Nov 30;75(22):1982-7.

[10] Schrijvers, E.M., et al. Insulin metabolism and the risk of Alzheimer disease: the Rotterdam Study. Neurology, 2010 Nov 30;75(22):1982-7.

[11] McGeer, E.G. and McGeer, P.L. Neuroinflammation in Alzheimer's disease and mild cognitive impairment: a field in its infancy. J Alzheimers Dis. 2010;19(1):355-61.

[12] McGeer, E.G. and McGeer, P.L. Neuroinflammation in Alzheimer's disease and mild cognitive impairment: a field in its infancy. J Alzheimers Dis. 2010;19(1):355-61.

[13] Matsuzaki, T., et al. Insulin resistance is associated with the pathology of Alzheimer disease: the Hisayama study. Neurology, 2010 Aug 31;75(9):764-70. Epub 2010 Aug 25.

[14] de la Monte, S.M. and Wands, J.R. Alzheimer's disease is type 3 diabetes - evidence reviewed. J Diabetes Sci Technol, 2008 Nov;2(6):1101-13.

[15] American Health Assistance Foundation. Plaques and Tangles. http://www.ahaf.org/alzheimers/about/understanding/plaques-and-tangles.html

16 Qingguang, J., et al. ApoE promotes the proteolytic degradation of Aβ. Neuron, 2008 June 12;58(5):681-93.

17 Soczynska, J.K., et al. Mood disorders and obesity: understanding inflammation as a pathophysiological nexus. Neuromolecular Med, 2011 Jun;13(2):93-116. Epub 2010 Dec 17.

18 Morris, J.K., et al. Measures of striatal insulin resistance in a 6-hydroxydopamine model of Parkinson's disease. Brain Res, 2008 Nov 13;1240:185-95. Epub 2008 Sep 11.

19 Bazar, K.A., et al. Obesity and ADHD may represent different manifestations of a common environmental oversampling syndrome: a model for revealing mechanistic overlap among cognitive, metabolic, and inflammatory disorders. Med Hypotheses, 2006;66(2):263-9.

20 Ashwood, P., et al. Elevated plasma cytokines in autism spectrum disorders provide evidence of immune dysfunction and are associated with impaired behavioral outcome. Brain Behav Immun, 2011 Jan;25(1):40-5. Epub 2010 Aug 10.

21 Howard, G., et al. Insulin sensitivity and atherosclerosis. The Insulin Resistance Atherosclerosis Study (IRAS) Investigators. Circulation, 1996 May 15;93(10):1809-17.

22 Duvnjak, L. and Duvnjak, M. The metabolic syndrome - an ongoing story. J Physiol Pharmacol, 2009 Dec;60 Supplement 7:19-24.

23 Madjid, M., et al. Lipoprotein-associated phospholipase A2 as a novel risk marker for cardiovascular disease: a systematic review of the literature. Tex Heart Inst J, 2010;37(1):25-39.

24 Kloner, R.A. Erectile dysfunction as a predictor of cardiovascular disease. Int J Impot Res, 2008 Sep-Oct;20(5):460-5. Epub 2008 May 15.

25 Endemann, D.H. and Schiffrin, E.L. Endothelial dysfunction. J Am Soc Nephrol, 2004 Aug;15(8):1983-92.

[26] Shin, D., et al. Erectile dysfunction: a disease marker for cardiovascular disease. Cardiol Rev, 2011 Jan-Feb;19(1):5-11.

[27] Hsing, A.W., et al. Insulin resistance and prostate cancer risk. J Natl Cancer Inst, 2003 Jan 1;95(1):67-71.

[28] Jonasson, J.M., et al. Insulin glargine use and short-term incidence of malignancies-a population-based follow-up study in Sweden. Diabetologia, 2009 Sep;52(9):1745-54. Epub 2009 Jul 9.

[29] Hemkens, L.G., et al. Risk of malignancies in patients with diabetes treated with human insulin or insulin analogues: a cohort study. Diabetologia, 2009 Sep;52(9):1732-44. Epub 2009 Jun 30.

[30] Colhoun, H.M., et al. Use of insulin glargine and cancer incidence in Scotland: a study from the Scottish Diabetes Research Network Epidemiology Group. Diabetologia, 2009 Sep;52(9):1755-65. Epub 2009 Jul 15.

[31] Currie, C.J., et al. The influence of glucose-lowering therapies on cancer risk in type 2 diabetes. Diabetologia, 2009 Sep;52(9):1766-7.

[32] O'Callaghan, T. President's panel analyzes environmental cancer impact. http://healthland.time.com/2010/05/06/presidents-panel-analyzes-environmental-cancer-impact

[33] Samy, N., et al. Clinical significance of inflammatory markers in polycystic ovary syndrome: their relationship to insulin resistance and body mass index. Dis Markers, 2009;26(4):163-70.

[34] González, F., et al. Evidence of proatherogenic inflammation in polycystic ovary syndrome. Metabolism, 2009 Jul;58(7):954-62.

[35] Schauer, I.E., et al. CREB downregulation in vascular disease: a common response to cardiovascular risk. Arterioscler Thromb Vasc Biol, 2010 Apr;30(4):733-41. Epub 2010 Feb 11.

[36] Bleckmann, S.C., et al. Activating transcription factor 1 and CREB are important for cell survival during early mouse development. Mol Cell Biol, 2002 Mar;22(6):1919-25.

[37] Roth, G.S., et al. Biomarkers of caloric restriction may predict longevity in humans. Science, 2002 Aug 2;297(5582):811.

[38] Vaarala, O., et al. The "perfect storm" for type 1 diabetes: the complex interplay between intestinal microbiota, gut permeability, and mucosal immunity. Diabetes, 2008 Oct;57(10):2555-62.

[39] de Kort, S., et al. Leaky gut and diabetes mellitus: what is the link? Obes Rev, 2011 Jun;12(6):449-58. Epub 2011 Mar 8.

[40] Fasano, A., et al. Mechanisms of disease: the role of intestinal barrier function in the pathogenesis of gastrointestinal autoimmune diseases. Nat Clin Pract Gastroenterol Hepatol, 2005 Sep;2(9):416-22.

[41] Liu, Z., et al. Tight junctions, leaky intestines, and pediatric diseases. Acta Paediatr, 2005 Apr;94(4):386-93.

[42] Sidiropoulos, P.I., et al. Metabolic syndrome in rheumatic diseases: epidemiology, pathophysiology, and clinical implications. Arthritis Res Ther, 2008;10(3):207. Epub 2008 May 8.

[43] Sabio, J.M., et al. Effects of low or medium-dose of prednisone on insulin resistance in patients with systemic lupus erythematosus. Clin Exp Rheumatol, 2010 Jul-Aug;28(4):483-9. Epub 2010 Aug 30.

[44] Dessein, P.H., et al. Effects of disease modifying agents and dietary intervention on insulin resistance and dyslipidemia in inflammatory arthritis: a pilot study. Arthritis Res, 2002;4(6):R12. Epub 2002 Sep 16.

[45] Pérez-López, F.R., et al. Effects of the Mediterranean diet on longevity and age-related morbid conditions. Maturitas, 2009 Oct 20;64(2):67-79. Epub 2009 Aug 31.

Chapter 3: Fighting an Epidemic Battle of the Bulge

1 Mattson, M.P. Perspective: Does brown fat protect against diseases of aging? Ageing Res Rev, 2010 Jan;9(1):69-76. Epub 2009 Dec 5.

2 Indulekha, K., et al. Association of visceral and subcutaneous fat with glucose intolerance, insulin resistance, adipocytokines and inflammatory markers in Asian Indians (CURES-113). Clin Biochem, 2011 Mar;44(4):281-7. Epub 2011 Jan 8.

3 Després, J.P., et al. Abdominal obesity and the metabolic syndrome: contribution to global cardiometabolic risk. Arterioscler Thromb Vasc Biol, 2008 Jun;28(6):1039-49. Epub 2008 Mar 20.

4 Greenberg, A.S. and Obin, M.S. Obesity and the role of adipose tissue in inflammation and metabolism. Am J Clin Nutr, 2006 Feb;83(2):461S-465S.

5 Fabbrini, E., et al. Surgical removal of omental fat does not improve insulin sensitivity and cardiovascular risk factors in obese adults. Gastroenterology, 2010 Aug;139(2):448-55. Epub 2010 May 7.

6 World Health Organization. Obesity and Overweight. www.who.int/mediacentre/factsheets/fs311/en/index.html

7 Pereira, M.A., et al. Fast-food habits, weight gain, and insulin resistance (the CARDIA study): 15-year prospective analysis. Lancet, 2005 Jan 1-7;365(9453):36-42.

8 Warner, J. and Chang, L. Corn Oil Used Most Often for French Fries: Most Fast Food Restaurants Using Corn Oil Rather Than Healthier Oils. www.webmd.com/diet/news/20100119/corn-oil-used-most-often-french-fries

9 Egan, K. FDA's Total Diet Study: Monitoring U.S. Food Supply Safety. www.fda.gov/Food/FoodSafety/FoodContaminantsAdulteration/TotalDietStudy/ucm186140.htm

[10] Kandaraki, E., et al. Endocrine disruptors and polycystic ovary syndrome (PCOS): elevated serum levels of bisphenol A in women with PCOS. J Clin Endocrinol Metab, 2011 Mar;96(3):E480-4. Epub 2010 Dec 30.

[11] Ropero, A.B., et al. Bisphenol A disruption of the endocrine pancreas and blood glucose homeostasis. Int J Androl, 2008 Apr;31(2):194-200. Epub 2007 Oct 31.

Chapter 4: You Cannot Not Choose Your Lifestyle

[1] Roth, S.M., et al. Strength training for the prevention and treatment of sarcopenia. J Nutr Health Aging, 2000;4(3):143-55.

[2] Jones, T.H., et al. Testosterone replacement in hypogonadal men with type 2 diabetes and/or metabolic syndrome (the TIMES2 study). Diabetes Care, 2011 Apr;34(4):828-37. Epub 2011 Mar 8.

[3] Villareal, D.T. and Holloszy, J.O. Effect of DHEA on abdominal fat and insulin action in elderly women and men: a randomized controlled trial. JAMA, 2004 Nov 10;292(18):2243-8.

Chapter 5: Don't Give Up… There Are Other Options

[1] Ayoub, W.A., et al. Exenatide-induced acute pancreatitis. Endocr Pract, 2010 Jan-Feb;16(1):80-3

[2] Ahmad, S.R. and Swann, J. Exenatide and rare adverse events. N Engl J Med, 2008 May 1;358(18):1970-1; discussion 1971-2.

[3] Garg, R., et al. Acute pancreatitis in type 2 diabetes treated with exenatide or sitagliptin: a retrospective observational pharmacy claims analysis. Diabetes Care, 2010 Nov;33(11):2349-54. Epub 2010 Aug 3.

[4] Badman, M.K. and Flier, J.S. The gut and energy balance: visceral allies in the obesity wars. Science, 2005 Mar 25;307(5717):1909-14.

[5] Smith, S.R., et al. Sustained weight loss following 12-month pramlintide treatment as an adjunct to lifestyle intervention in obesity. Diabetes Care, 2008 Sep;31(9):1816-23. Epub 2008 Jun 20.

[6] Aronne, L., et al. Progressive reduction in body weight after treatment with the amylin analog pramlintide in obese subjects: a phase 2, randomized, placebo-controlled, dose-escalation study. J Clin Endocrinol Metab, 2007 Aug;92(8):2977-83. Epub 2007 May 15.

[7] Pournaras, D.J., et al. Remission of type 2 diabetes after gastric bypass and banding: mechanisms and 2 year outcomes. Ann Surg, 2010 Dec;252(6):966-71.

[8] Christou, N.V., et al. Weight gain after short- and long-limb gastric bypass in patients followed for longer than 10 years. Ann Surg, 2006 Nov;244(5):734-40.

[9] Robb-Nicholson, C. By the way, doctor. I've been trying to lose weight for a long time and nothing seems to work. What do you know about the HCG diet? Harv Womens Health Watch, 2010 May;17(9):8.

[10] Bosch, B., et al. Human chorionic gonadotrophin and weight loss. A double-blind, placebo-controlled trial. S Afr Med J, 1990 Feb 17;77(4):185-9.

[11] Lijesen, G.K., et al. The effect of human chorionic gonadotropin (HCG) in the treatment of obesity by means of the Simeons therapy: a criteria-based meta-analysis. Br J Clin Pharmacol, 1995 Sep;40(3):237-43.

[12] Drucker, D.J., et al. Exenatide once weekly versus twice daily for the treatment of type 2 diabetes: a randomised, open-label, non-inferiority study. Lancet, 2008 Oct 4;372(9645):1240-50. Epub 2008 Sep 7.

Chapter 6: Your Weight Loss Secret Weapon is ALCAT

1 Fasano, A. Zonulin and its regulation of intestinal barrier function: the biological door to inflammation, autoimmunity, and cancer. Physiol Rev, 2011 Jan;91(1):151-75.

2 Drago, S., et al. Gliadin, zonulin and gut permeability: Effects on celiac and non-celiac intestinal mucosa and intestinal cell lines. Scand J Gastroenterol, 2006 Apr;41(4):408-19.

3 Kaats, G.R., et al. The Short Term Efficacy of the ALCAT Test of Food Sensitivities to Facilitate Changes in Body Composition and Self-Reported Disease Symptoms: A Randomized Controlled Study. The Bariatrician, 1996 spring;18-23.

4 Berardi, L., et al. ALCAT Test results in the treatment of gastrointestinal symptoms. Findings presented on June 13, 2011 at the European Academy of Allergy and Clinical Immunology 30th Annual Congress in Istanbul, Turkey.

5 De Amici, M., et al. Evaluation of ALCAT Test results in the non IgE-mediated pathology of the skin. Findings presented on June 13, 2011 at the European Academy of Allergy and Clinical Immunology 30th Annual Congress in Istanbul, Turkey.

6 Akmal, M., et al. The Effect of The ALCAT Test Diet Therapy for Food Sensitivity in Patient's With Obesity. Middle East Journal of Family Medicine, 2009, April;7(3).

7 Lecke, S.B., et al. Leptin and adiponectin in the female life course. Braz J Med Biol Res, 2011 May;44(5):381-7. Epub 2011 Mar 29.

8 Hajri, T., et al. Regulation of adiponectin production by insulin: interactions with tumor necrosis factor-α and interleukin-6. Am J Physiol Endocrinol Metab, 2011 Feb;300(2):E350-60. Epub 2010 Nov 9.

Chapter 7: Nutraceuticals, Minerals and Botanicals

1 Knowler, W.C., et al. Reduction in the incidence of type 2 diabetes with lifestyle intervention or metformin. N Engl J Med, 2002 Feb 7;346(6):393-403.

2 Moreno-Aliaga, M.J., et al. Regulation of adipokine secretion by n-3 fatty acids. Proc Nutr Soc, 2010 Aug;69(3):324-32.

3 Tsitouras, P.D., et al. High omega-3 fat intake improves insulin sensitivity and reduces CRP and IL-6, but does not affect other endocrine axes in healthy older adults. Horm Metab Res, 2008 Mar;40(3):199-205.

4 Figueras, M., et al. Effects of eicosapentaenoic acid (EPA) treatment on insulin sensitivity in an animal model of diabetes: improvement of the inflammatory status. Obesity (Silver Spring), 2011 Feb;19(2):362-9.

5 Balasubramanian, R., et al. Combination peroxisome proliferator-activated receptor gamma and alpha agonist treatment in Type 2 diabetes prevents the beneficial pioglitazone effect on liver fat content. Diabet Med, 2010 Feb;27(2):150-6.

6 Svegliati-Baroni, G., et al. A model of insulin resistance and nonalcoholic steatohepatitis in rats: role of peroxisome proliferator-activated receptor-alpha and n-3 polyunsaturated fatty acid treatment on liver injury. Am J Pathol, 2006 Sep;169(3):846-60.

7 Anderson, B.M. and Ma, D.W. Are all n-3 polyunsaturated fatty acids created equal? Lipids Health Dis, 2009 Aug 10;8:33.

8 Pauwels, E.K. and Kostkiewicz, M. Fatty acid facts, Part III: Cardiovascular disease, or, a fish diet is not fishy. Drug News Perspect, 2008 Dec;21(10):552-61.

9 Marik, P.E. and Varon, J. Omega-3 dietary supplements and the risk of cardiovascular events: a systematic review. Clin Cardiol, 2009 Jul;32(7):365-72.

10 Gonzales, A.M. and Orlando, R.A. Curcumin and resveratrol inhibit nuclear factor-kappaB-mediated cytokine expression in adipocytes. Nutr Metab (Lond), 2008 Jun 12;5:17.

11 Baur, J.A., et al. Resveratrol improves health and survival of mice on a high-calorie diet. Nature, 2006 Nov 16;444(7117):337-42.

12 Sun, C., et al. SIRT1 improves insulin sensitivity under insulin-resistant conditions by repressing PTP1B. Cell Metab, 2007 Oct;6(4):307-19.

13 Prasain, J.K., et al. Flavonoids and age-related disease: risk, benefits and critical windows. Maturitas, 2010 Jun;66(2):163-71.

14 Walle, T., et al. High absorption but very low bioavailability of oral resveratrol in humans. Drug Metab Dispos, 2004 Dec;32(12):1377-82.

15 Knekt, P., et al. Flavonoid intake and risk of chronic diseases. Am J Clin Nutr, 2002 Sep;76(3):560-8.

16 Mink, P.J., et al. Flavonoid intake and cardiovascular disease mortality: a prospective study in postmenopausal women. Am J Clin Nutr, 2007 Mar;85(3):895-909.

17 Brasnyó, P., et al. Resveratrol improves insulin sensitivity, reduces oxidative stress and activates the Akt pathway in type 2 diabetic patients. Br J Nutr, 2011 Aug;106(3):383-389. Epub 2011 Mar 9.

18 Reed, L.J., et al. Cristalline alpha-lipoic acid: a catalytic agent associated with pyruvate dehydrogenase. Science, 1951;114(2952):93-94.

19 Berkson, B.M., et al. Revisiting the ALA/N (alpha-lipoic acid/low-dose naltrexone) protocol for people with metastatic and nonmetastatic pancreatic cancer: a report of 3 new cases. Integr Cancer Ther, 2009 Dec;8(4):416-22.

20 Melhem, A., et al. Treatment of chronic hepatitis C virus infection via antioxidants: results of a phase I clinical trial. J Clin Gastroenterol, 2005 Sep;39(8):737-42.

21 Guais, A. Adding a combination of hydroxycitrate and lipoic acid (METABLOC™) to chemotherapy improves effectiveness against tumor development: experimental results and case report. Invest New Drugs, 2010 Oct 8. Epub ahead of print.

22 Jacob, S., et al. Enhancement of glucose disposal in patients with type 2 diabetes by alpha-lipoic acid. Arzneimittelforschung, 1995 Aug;45(8):872-4.

23 Sugimoto, K., et al. Role of advanced glycation end products in diabetic neuropathy. Curr Pharm Des, 2008;14(10):953-61.

24 Ziegler, D., et al. Treatment of symptomatic diabetic polyneuropathy with the antioxidant alpha-lipoic acid: a meta-analysis. Diabet Med, 2004 Feb;21(2):114-21.

25 Vallianou, N., et al. Alpha-lipoic Acid and diabetic neuropathy. Rev Diabet Stud, 2009 Winter;6(4):230-6. Epub 2009 Dec 30.

26 Sola, S., et al. Irbesartan and lipoic acid improve endothelial function and reduce markers of inflammation in the metabolic syndrome: results of the Irbesartan and Lipoic Acid in Endothelial Dysfunction (ISLAND) study. Circulation, 2005 Jan 25;111(3):343-8. Epub 2005 Jan 17.

27 Gupte, A.A., et al. Lipoic acid increases heat shock protein expression and inhibits stress kinase activation to improve insulin signaling in skeletal muscle from high-fat-fed rats. J Appl Physiol. 2009 Apr;106(4):1425-34. Epub 2009 Jan 29.

28 Konrad, D., et al. The antihyperglycemic drug alpha-lipoic acid stimulates glucose uptake via both GLUT4 translocation and GLUT4 activation: potential role of p38 mitogen-activated protein kinase in GLUT4 activation. Diabetes, 2001 Jun;50(6):1464-71.

29 Pravst, I., et al. Coenzyme Q10 contents in foods and fortification strategies. Crit Rev Food Sci Nutr, 2010 Apr;50(4):269-80.

30 Soja, A.M. and,Mortensen, S.A. Treatment of chronic cardiac insufficiency with coenzyme Q10, results of meta-analysis in controlled

clinical trials. Ugeskr Laeger, 1997 Dec 1;159(49):7302-8. Article in Danish.

31 Sander, S., et al. The impact of coenzyme Q10 on systolic function in patients with chronic heart failure. J Card Fail, 2006 Aug;12(6):464-72.

32 Molyneux, S.L., et al. Coenzyme Q10: an independent predictor of mortality in chronic heart failure. J Am Coll Cardiol, 2008 Oct 28;52(18):1435-41.

33 Marcoff, L. and Thompson, P.D. The role of coenzyme Q10 in statin-associated myopathy: a systematic review. J Am Coll Cardiol, 2007 Jun 12;49(23):2231-7.

34 Hamilton, S.J., et al. Coenzyme Q10 improves endothelial dysfunction in statin-treated type 2 diabetic patients. Diabetes Care, 2009 May;32(5):810-2. Epub 2009 Feb 19.

35 Hodgson, J.M., et al. Coenzyme Q10 improves blood pressure and glycaemic control: a controlled trial in subjects with type 2 diabetes. Eur J Clin Nutr, 2002 Nov;56(11):1137-42.

36 Rosenfeldt, F.L. Coenzyme Q10 in the treatment of hypertension: a meta-analysis of the clinical trials. J Hum Hypertens, 2007 Apr;21(4):297-306. Epub 2007 Feb 8.

37 Singh, R.B., et al. Effect of hydrosoluble coenzyme Q10 on blood pressures and insulin resistance in hypertensive patients with coronary artery disease. J Hum Hypertens, 1999 Mar;13(3):203-8.

38 Shargorodsky, M., et al. Effect of long-term treatment with antioxidants (vitamin C, vitamin E, coenzyme Q10 and selenium) on arterial compliance, humoral factors and inflammatory markers in patients with multiple cardiovascular risk factors. Nutr Metab (Lond), 2010 Jul 6;7:55.

39 Schmelzer, C., et al. Effects of Coenzyme Q10 on TNF-alpha secretion in human and murine monocytic cell lines. Biofactors, 2007;31(1):35-41.

40 Shalansky, S. Risk of warfarin-related bleeding events and supratherapeutic international normalized ratios associated with complementary and alternative medicine: a longitudinal analysis. Pharmacotherapy, 2007 Sep;27(9):1237-47.

41 King, D.E., et al. Dietary magnesium and C-reactive protein levels. J Am Coll Nutr, 2005 Jun;24(3):166-71.

42 Chaudhary, D.P., et al. Implications of magnesium deficiency in type 2 diabetes: a review. Biol Trace Elem Res, 2010 May;134(2):119-29. Epub 2009 Jul 24.

43 Reinhart, R.A. Magnesium metabolism: a review with special reference to the relationship between intracellular content and serum levels. Arch Intern Med, 1988 Nov;148(11):2415-20.

44 Ulger, Z., et al. Intra-erythrocyte magnesium levels and their clinical implications in geriatric outpatients. J Nutr Health Aging, 2010 Oct;14(10):810-4.

45 Chaudhary, D.P., et al. Implications of magnesium deficiency in type 2 diabetes: a review. Biol Trace Elem Res, 2010 May;134(2):119-29. Epub 2009 Jul 24.

46 Lima, M.L., et al. Serum and intracellular magnesium deficiency in patients with metabolic syndrome - evidences for its relation to insulin resistance. Diabetes Res Clin Pract, 2009 Feb;83(2):257-62. Epub 2009 Jan 4.

47 Mooren, F.C., et al. Oral magnesium supplementation reduces insulin resistance in non-diabetic subjects: a double-blind, placebo-controlled, randomized trial. Diabetes Obes Metab, 2011 Mar;13(3):281-4.

48 Nadler, J.L., et al. Magnesium deficiency produces insulin resistance and increased thromboxane synthesis. Hypertension, 1993 Jun;21(6 Pt 2):1024-9.

[49] de Lordes, L.M., et al. The effect of magnesium supplementation in increasing doses on the control of type 2 diabetes. Diabetes Care, 1998 May;21(5):682-6.

[50] King, D.E., et al. Dietary magnesium and C-reactive protein levels. J Am Coll Nutr, 2005 Jun;24(3):166-71.

[51] Song, Y., et al. A prospective study of red meat consumption and type 2 diabetes in middle-aged and elderly women: the women's health study. Diabetes Care, 2004 Sep;27(9):2108-15.

[52] Lopez-Ridaura, R., et al. Magnesium intake and risk of type 2 diabetes in men and women. Diabetes Care, 2004 Jan;27(1):134-40.

[53] Meyer, K.A., et al. Carbohydrates, dietary fiber, and incident type 2 diabetes in older women. Am J Clin Nutr, 2000 Apr;71(4):921-30.

[54] de Lordes, L.M., et al. The effect of magnesium supplementation in increasing doses on the control of type 2 diabetes. Diabetes Care, 1998 May;21(5):682-6.

[55] Cefalu, W.T., et al. Characterization of the metabolic and physiologic response to chromium supplementation in subjects with type 2 diabetes mellitus. Metabolism, 2010 May;59(5):755-62.

[56] Martin, J., et al. Chromium picolinate supplementation attenuates body weight gain and increases insulin sensitivity in subjects with type 2 diabetes. Diabetes Care, 2006 Aug;29(8):1826-32.

[57] Lai, M.H. Antioxidant effects and insulin resistance improvement of chromium combined with vitamin C and e supplementation for type 2 diabetes mellitus. J Clin Biochem Nutr, 2008 Nov;43(3):191-8.

[58] Qiao, W., et al. Chromium improves glucose uptake and metabolism through upregulating the mRNA levels of IR, GLUT4, GS, and UCP3 in skeletal muscle cells. Biol Trace Elem Res, 2009 Nov;131(2):133-42.

[59] Jain, S.K., et al. Effect of chromium niacinate and chromium picolinate supplementation on lipid peroxidation, TNF-alpha, IL-6, CRP,

glycated hemoglobin, triglycerides, and cholesterol levels in blood of streptozotocin-treated diabetic rats. Free Radic Biol Med, 2007 Oct 15;43(8):1124-31.

60 Wiernsperger, N. and Rapin, J. Trace elements in glucometabolic disorders: an update. Diabetol Metab Syndr, 2010 Dec 19;2:70.

61 Ried, K., et al. Aged garlic extract lowers blood pressure in patients with treated but uncontrolled hypertension: a randomised controlled trial. Maturitas, 2010 Oct;67(2):144-50.

62 Sobenin, I.A., et al. Metabolic effects of time-released garlic powder tablets in type 2 diabetes mellitus: the results of double-blinded placebo-controlled study. Acta Diabetol, 2008 Mar;45(1):1-6.

63 Weisberg, S.P., et al. Dietary curcumin significantly improves obesity-associated inflammation and diabetes in mouse models of diabesity. Endocrinology, 2008 Jul;149(7):3549-58.

64 Srinivasan, M. Effect of curcumin on blood sugar as seen in a diabetic subject. Indian J Med Sci, 1972 Apr;26(4):269-70.

65 Park, J. and Conteas, C.N. Anti-carcinogenic properties of curcumin on colorectal cancer. World J Gastrointest Oncol, 2010 Apr 15;2(4):169-76.

66 Vuksan, V., et al. Similar postprandial glycemic reductions with escalation of dose and administration time of American ginseng in type 2 diabetes. Diabetes Care, 2000 Sep;23(9):1221-6.

67 Ma, S.W., et al. Effect of Panax ginseng supplementation on biomarkers of glucose tolerance, antioxidant status and oxidative stress in type 2 diabetic subjects: results of a placebo-controlled human intervention trial. Diabetes Obes Metab, 2008 Nov;10(11):1125-7.

68 Vuksan, V., et al. Korean red ginseng (Panax ginseng) improves glucose and insulin regulation in well-controlled, type 2 diabetes: results of a randomized, double-blind, placebo-controlled study of efficacy and safety. Nutr Metab Cardiovasc Dis, 2008 Jan;18(1):46-56.

69 Jang, D.J., et al. Red ginseng for treating erectile dysfunction: a systematic review. Br J Clin Pharmacol, 2008 Oct;66(4):444-50.

70 Oh, K.J., et al. Effects of Korean red ginseng on sexual arousal in menopausal women: placebo-controlled, double-blind crossover clinical study. J Sex Med, 2010 Apr;7(4 Pt 1):1469-77.

71 Bettuzzi, S., et al. Chemoprevention of human prostate cancer by oral administration of green tea catechins in volunteers with high-grade prostate intraepithelial neoplasia: a preliminary report from a one-year proof-of-principle study. Cancer Res, 2006 Jan 15;66(2):1234-40.

72 Hakim, I.A., et al. Effect of increased tea consumption on oxidative DNA damage among smokers: a randomized controlled study. J Nutr, 2003 Oct;133(10):3303S-3309S.

73 Luo, H., et al. Phase IIa chemoprevention trial of green tea polyphenols in high-risk individuals of liver cancer: modulation of urinary excretion of green tea polyphenols and 8-hydroxydeoxyguanosine. Carcinogenesis, 2006 Feb;27(2):262-8.

74 Fu, Z., et al. Epigallocatechin gallate delays the onset of type 1 diabetes in spontaneous non-obese diabetic mice. Br J Nutr, 2010 Dec 9:1-8.

75 Yun, J.M., et al. Effects of epigallocatechin gallate on regulatory T cell number and function in obese v. lean volunteers. Br J Nutr, 2010 Jun;103(12):1771-7.

76 Iso, H., et al. The relationship between green tea and total caffeine intake and risk for self-reported type 2 diabetes among Japanese adults. Ann Intern Med, 2006 Apr 18;144(8):554-62.

77 Nagao, T., et al. A catechin-rich beverage improves obesity and blood glucose control in patients with type 2 diabetes. Obesity (Silver Spring), 2009 Feb;17(2):310-7.

78 Taher, M., et al. "A proanthocyanidin from Cinnamomum zeylanicum stimulates phosphorylation of insullin receptor in 3T3-L1 adipocyties. Jurnal Teknologi, 44(F) Jun 2006: 53–68.

79 Cao, H., et al. Cinnamon extract and polyphenols affect the expression of tristetraprolin, insulin receptor, and glucose transporter 4 in mouse 3T3-L1 adipocytes. Arch Biochem Biophys, 2007 Mar 15;459(2):214-22.

80 Crawford, P. Effectiveness of cinnamon for lowering hemoglobin A1C in patients with type 2 diabetes: a randomized, controlled trial. J Am Board Fam Med, 2009 Sep-Oct;22(5):507-12.

81 Khan, A.,et al. Cinnamon improves glucose and lipids of people with type 2 diabetes. Diabetes Care, 2003 Dec;26(12):3215-8.

82 Akilen, R., et al. Glycated haemoglobin and blood pressure-lowering effect of cinnamon in multi-ethnic Type 2 diabetic patients in the UK: a randomized, placebo-controlled, double-blind clinical trial. Diabet Med, 2010 Oct;27(10):1159-67.

83 Wang, J.G., et al. The effect of cinnamon extract on insulin resistance parameters in polycystic ovary syndrome: a pilot study. Fertil Steril, 2007 Jul;88(1):240-3.

84 Giovannucci, E., et al. "25-hydroxyvitamin D and risk of myocardial infarction in men: a prospective study." Arch Intern Med, 2008 Jun 9;168(11):1174-80.

85 Nagpal, S., et al. "Noncalcemic actions of vitamin D receptor ligands." Endocr Rev, 2005 Aug;26(5):662-87.

86 Freedman, D.M., et al. "Prospective study of serum vitamin D and cancer mortality in the United States." J Natl Cancer Inst, 2007 Nov 7;99(21):1594-602.

87 Lappe, J.M., et al. "Vitamin D and calcium supplementation reduces cancer risk: results of a randomized trial." Am J Clin Nutr, 2007 Jun;85(6):1586-91.

[88] Alvarez, J.A. and Ashraf, A. Role of vitamin d in insulin secretion and insulin sensitivity for glucose homeostasis. Int J Endocrinol, 2010;2010:351385.

[89] Chiu, K.C., et al. Hypovitaminosis D is associated with insulin resistance and beta cell dysfunction. Am J Clin Nutr, 2004 May;79(5):820-5.

[90] Schleithoff, S.S., et al. Vitamin D supplementation improves cytokine profiles in patients with congestive heart failure: a double-blind, randomized, placebo-controlled trial. Am J Clin Nutr, 2006 Apr;83(4):754-9.

[91] Judd, S. and Tangpricha, V. Vitamin D deficiency and risk for cardiovascular disease. Circulation, 2008 Jan 29;117(4):503-11.

[92] Mach, T. Clinical usefulness of probiotics in inflammatory bowel diseases. J Physiol Pharmacol, 2006 Nov;57 Suppl 9:23-33.

Recipes: Breakfast

[1] Adapted from www.greenlemonade.com.

[2] Adapted from The UltraMetabolism Cookbook.

[3] Adapted from The Thrive Diet.

[4] Adapted from www.centeredchef.com.

[5] Adapted from www.ohsheglows.com.

[6] Adapted from www.welloflifecenter.com.

[7] Adapted from www.ohsheglows.com.

[8] Adapted from Tracy Anderson's 30-day Method.

[9] Adapted from Women's Health Magazine.

[10] Adapted from www.wholefoodsmarket.com.

[11] Adapted from www.healthfulpursuit.com.

Recipes: Smoothies

[1] Adapted from www.ohsheglows.com.

[2] Adapted from Women's Health Magazine.

Recipes: Lunch and Dinner

[1] Adapted from From Belly Fat to Belly Flat.

[2] Adapted from From Belly Fat to Belly Flat.

[3] Adapted from www.self.com.

[4] Adapted from www.wholefoodsmarket.com.

[5] Adapted from From Belly Fat to Belly Flat.

[6] Adapted from www.simplyrecipes.com.

[7] Adapted from From Belly Fat to Belly Flat.

[8] Adapted from From Belly Fat to Belly Flat.

[9] Adapted from www.wholefoodsmarket.com.

[10] Adapted from From Belly Fat to Belly Flat.

[11] Adapted from From Belly Fat to Belly Flat.

[12] Adapted from Food for Life.

[13] Adapted from From Belly Fat to Belly Flat.

[14] Adapted from The Insulin-Resistance Diet.

[15] Adapted from The UltraMetabolism Cookbook.

[16] Adapted from www.tastebook.com.

[17] Adapted from www.wholefoodsmarket.com.

[18] Adapted from Cooking Light.

[19] Adapted from The UltraMetabolism Cookbook.

[20] Adapted from From Belly Fat to Belly Flat.

[21] Adapted from The 02 Diet.

[22] Adapted from www.wholefoodsmarket.com.

[23] Adapted from Better Homes and Gardens.

[24] Adapted from The UltraMetabolism Cookbook.

[25] Adapted from The UltraMetabolism Cookbook.

[26] Adapted from www.self.com.

[27] Adapted from www.pure2raw.com.

Recipes: Salads and Dressings

[1] Adapted from The UltraMetabolism Cookbook.

[2] Adapted from www.ohsheglows.com.

[3] Adapted from The UltraMetabolism Cookbook.

[4] Adapted from www.wholefoodsmarket.com.

[5] Adapted from www.choosingraw.com.

[6] Adapted from The UltraMetabolism Cookbook.

[7] Adapted from www.renegadehealth.com.

[8] Adapted from www.wholefoodsmarket.com.

[9] Adapted from The Kind Diet.

[10] Adapted from From Belly Fat to Belly Flat.

[11] Adapted from May All Be Fed.

[12] Adapted from www.food.com.

[13] Adapted from www.yumsugar.com.

Recipes: Soups

[1] Adapted from Detox 4 Women.

[2] Adapted from www.wholefoodsmarket.com.

[3] Adapted from The Insulin-Resistance Diet.

[4] Adapted from The Insulin-Resistance Diet.

[5] Adapted from www.bestliferecipes.com.

[6] Adapted from www.wholefoodsmarket.com.

[7] Adapted from www.bestliferecipes.com.

[8] Adapted from Detox 4 Women.

[9] Adapted from www.bestliferecipes.com.

Recipes: Desserts and Snacks

[1] Adapted from www.thespunkycoconut.com.

Appendix A: Diagnosing Insulin Resistance

[1] Johnson, J.L., et al. Identifying pre-diabetes using fasting insulin levels. Endocr Pract, 2010 Jan-Feb;16(1):47-52.

[2] Tirosh, A., et al. Normal fasting plasma glucose levels and type 2 diabetes in young men. N Engl J Med, 2005 Oct 6;353(14):1454-62.

[3] Wallace ,T.M. and Matthews, D.R. The assessment of insulin resistance in man. Diabet Med, 2002 Jul;19(7):527-34.

[4] Osterdahl, M., et al. Effects of a short-term intervention with a Paleolithic diet in healthy volunteers. Eur J Clin Nutr, 2008 May;62(5):682-5. Epub 2007 May 16.

[5] Rudenski, A.S., et al. Understanding insulin resistance: both glucose resistance and insulin resistance are required to model human diabetes. Metabolism, 1991 Sep;40(9):908-17.

[6] Katz, A., et al. Quantitative insulin sensitivity check index: a simple, accurate method for assessing insulin sensitivity in humans. J Clin Endocrinol Metab, 2000 Jul;85(7):2402-10.

INDEX

Charts and Illustrations

A

C

D

E

F

G

H

I

J

K

L

M

N

O

P

Q

R

S

T—U

V

W—Y

Z

Biographies and Additional Reading

Dr. Edwin Lee

Dr. Lee is an author and national spokesperson who—thanks in part to his groundbreaking insight in his field, and his many significant presentations at major medical conferences—is a respected proponent and authority on hormonal balance and wellness, and a leader in helping define the future of anti-aging medicine.

After graduating from Medical College of Pennsylvania, Dr. Edwin Lee completed three years of Internal Medicine residency and then completed two fellowships—in Critical Care Medicine and in Endocrinology and Metabolism—at the University of Pittsburgh.

Over the next ten years, Dr. Lee limited his practice to Endocrinology, Diabetes and Metabolism in central Florida. He also served as the Team Endocrinologist for the Cleveland Indians during their spring training in Florida.

Dr. Lee then went into private practice when he founded the Institute for Hormonal Balance in 2008. His driving purpose for opening the Institute was being able to focus on prevention of diseases, rather than just treating the impact of diseases—that in many cases could have been prevented.

Hormonal balance, with bioidentical or natural hormones, is the cornerstone for keeping the body and mind healthy. The Institute for Hormonal Balance has a holistic approach to integrating the best of western and eastern medicine, thereby improving the mind, body and soul so that one can heal naturally.

In addition to writing his books, *Feel Good Look Younger: Reversing Tiredness Through Hormonal Balance* and *Your Best Investment: Secrets to a Healthy Body and Mind,* Dr. Lee has published many articles in Internal Medicine and in Endocrinology.

He was also an author in the fourth edition of *Textbook of Critical Care* in the chapter entitled, *Neuroendocrine Immunology and the Role of Neuroendocrine Hormones in the Critically Ill Patient.*

Along with his achievements in academic medicine, he is currently board certified in Internal Medicine, Endocrinology, Diabetes, Metabolism and Anti-Aging. He is an active member of the American Diabetes Association, the American Academy of Anti-Aging and the American Association of Clinical Endocrinology. He also serves on volunteer staff at UCF College of Medicine.

He truly enjoys helping his patients achieve better health, and loves to practice what he preaches. Dr. Lee has completed many marathons, triathlons and finished the Great Floridian Triathlon (Ironman distance) in 2002. He has hiked the Grand Canyon south rim to north rim and back, and climbed to the summit of Mount Fuji. He also enjoys snowboarding, water skiing, fishing, golfing, mountaineering and surfing.

Alison Gordon

Alison Gordon grew up in a medical family where she was exposed to the traditional concepts of medication for health; however, it was her interest in food as medicine that led her to graduating Magna Cum Laude with a degree in Nutritional Sciences from San Diego State University.

Encouraged by her father (a nontraditional physician) to pursue higher credentials, Alison, realized that the greatest impact she could have on people was to become a physician specializing in Nutritional Medicine. In this capacity, she could bring to the table a new approach to medicine by using nutrition as a vital component to living a truly healthy lifestyle.

Through trial an error with such diets as juice feasting, veganism, raw foods and low carbohydrates, Alison has found the one thing that stayed true is that food should be edible and therefore, delicious. She has invested the past two years developing and compiling numerous recipes in which taste will not be sacrificed for health.

Alison is constantly self-educating and reads all the latest research articles, nutrition books and diet trends to ensure that she keeps pace with the evolving world of nutrition.

Laura Gavin

Nutrition, healthy cooking and fitness have always been passions for Laura Gavin, who decided to pursue nutrition as a career when her daughter was diagnosed with type 1 diabetes at age ten. Her personal experiences in dealing with the disease (her husband also has type 1 diabetes) have taught her how important a low carbohydrate diet is for controlling blood sugars.

Laura earned her Master of Science in Human Nutrition from the University of Alabama and is a Nutrition Educator for Women, Infants and Children (WIC) for the state of Florida. As a Nutrition Educator, she considers it a privilege to be improving people's lives through better nutrition.

Laura believes in the power of nutrition, and sees the effects—good and bad—at home and work every day. She encourages all her clients to develop an active lifestyle, which she says, "Keeps your weight down, while keeping your spirit up." Her goal in developing recipes for this book was to keep it simple, yet keep it tasty.

When Laura isn't reading and learning about developments in nutrition and healthy cooking, she enjoys walking, zumba dancing, yoga, pilates, aerobics and swimming.

Feel Good Look Younger

For more information, please be sure to read Dr. Lee's *Feel Good Look Younger: Reversing Tiredness Through Hormonal Balance*, available from Amazon.com and from InstituteOfHormonalBalance.com.

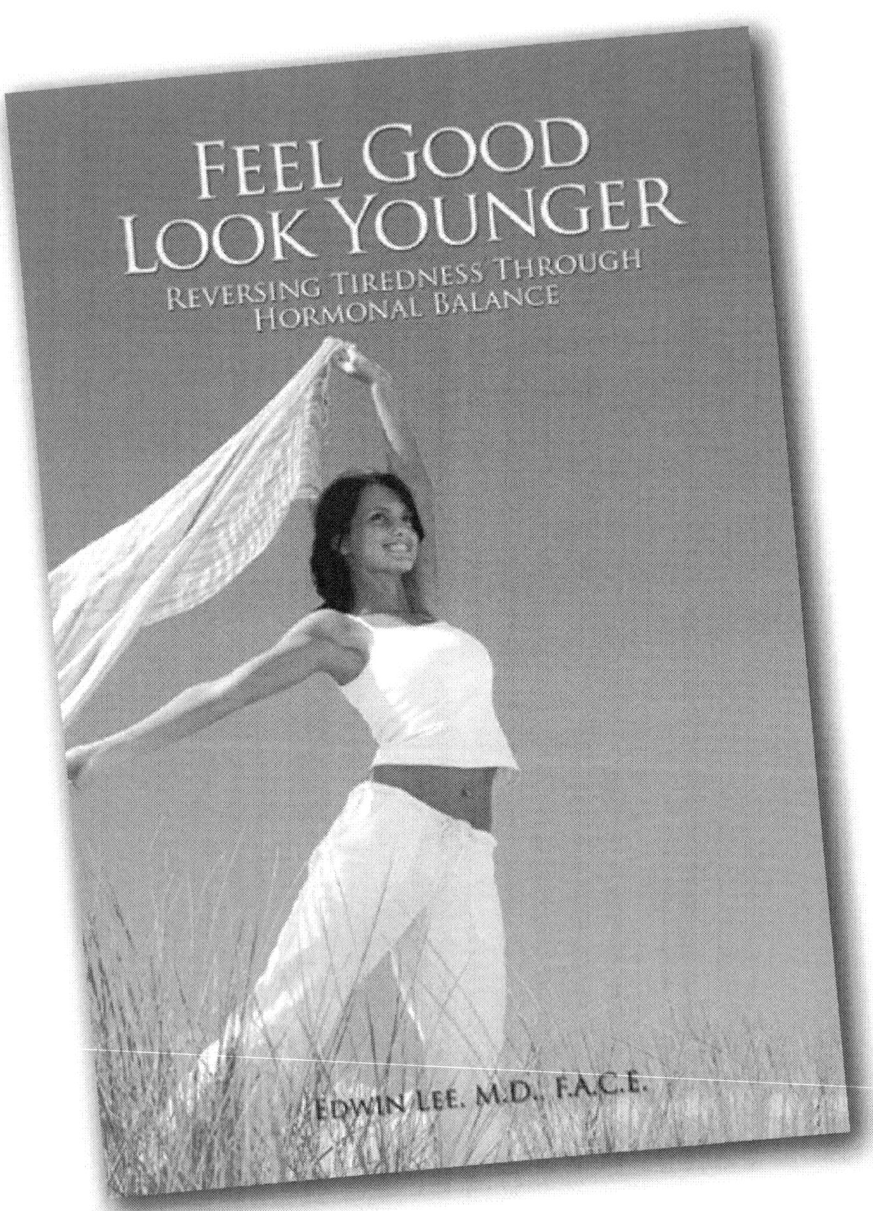

Written by Dr. Lee to address the root cause of tiredness—and to provide straightforward advice on how to overcome tiredness—*Feel Good Look Younger* has proven itself to be an easy-to-follow and valuable resource that physicians are now recommending to their patients for concise answers on the evolving subject of preventive medicine.

Dr. Edwin Lee has taken the elegant, simplex approach to hormone balance by making a complicated topic easy to understand. His book is a masterful, scientific and artful representation of how to effectively get back energy and vitality in tired, chaotic, stressful times.

— Deanna Minich, Ph.D., F.A.C.N., C.N.S.
author of Chakra Foods for Optimum Health
and The Complete Handbook to Quantum Healing

Dr. Lee's book is insightful and enlightening to those who wish to choose their own path in life regarding health, wellness and the means to achieve a balanced life. His knowledgeable ways of explaining issues to both patients and health care providers is welcomed. I hope to see more books from Dr. Lee.

— Sanjay Banerji, M.D.,
Clinical Professor UCLA Department of Neurology
Consultant Neurologist at Good Samaritan Hospital and
Saint Vincent's Medical Center
Los Angeles, California

Energetic and passionate are the words that describe Dr. Lee - and his book. His understanding of "where mainstream and alternate medicine meet" has delivered a must-read that is to-the-point.

— Mushtaq Syed, M.D.
Board Certified in Internal Medicine and Endocrinology
Indiana, Pennsylvania

This book is an excellent tool for physicians to give, or to recommend, to their patients as an educational enforcement of preventive medicine. It's written in such a way that the book is high science, yet easily readable. It's very real-life.

— Dr. Paul Hueseman
St. Louis, Missouri

With his book, Dr. Lee has given us a very insightful source for understanding what it takes to reverse tiredness. I highly recommend reading his book.

— Raul Santos, M.D.
Board Certified in Nephrology, Internal Medicine and Anti-Aging
Thomasville, Georgia

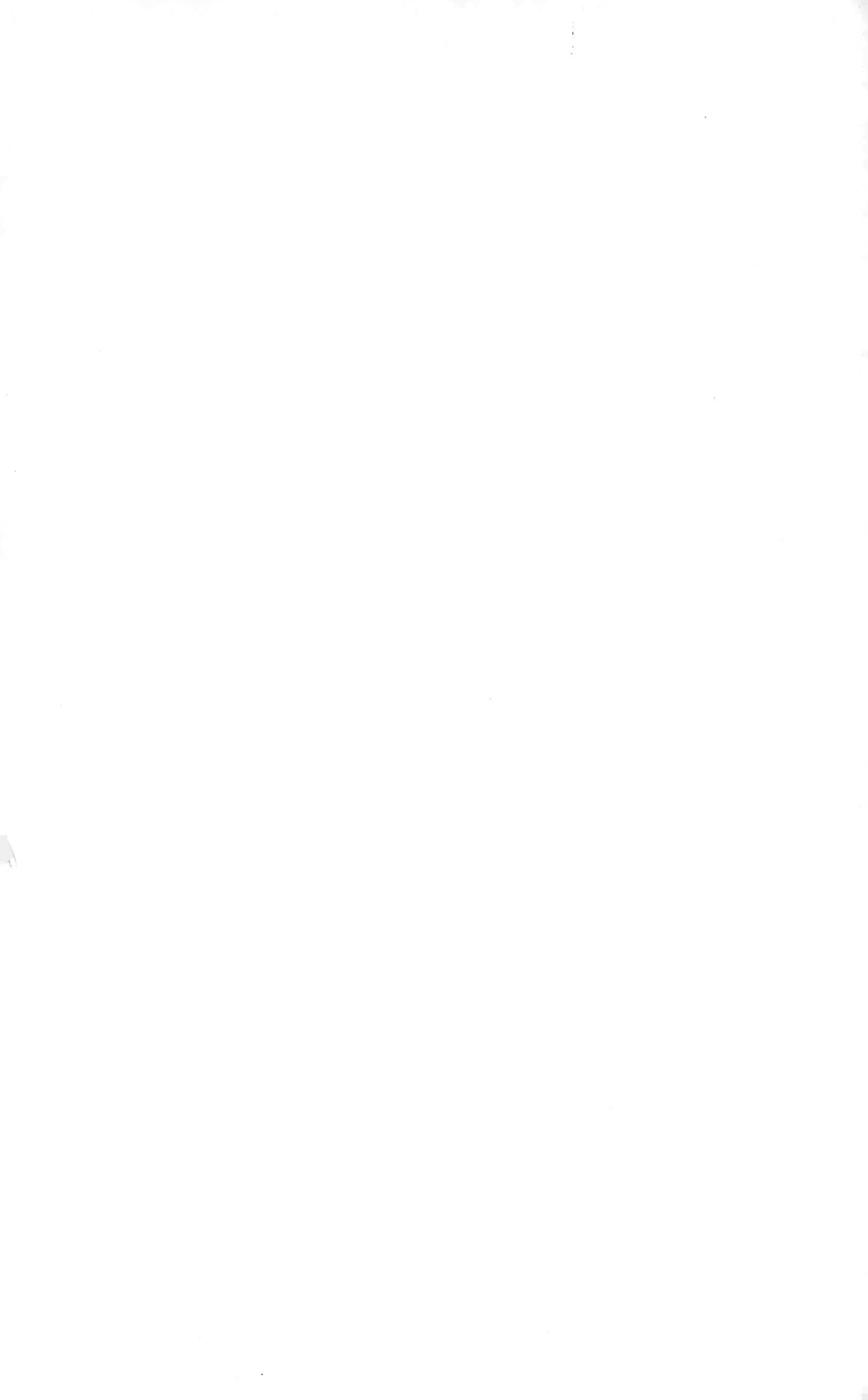

19100936R00296

Made in the USA
Lexington, KY
06 December 2012